Addiction

Guest Editors

ITAI DANOVITCH, MD
JOHN J. MARIANI, MD

PSYCHIATRIC CLINICS OF NORTH AMERICA

www.psych.theclinics.com

June 2012 • Volume 35 • Number 2

SAUNDERS an imprint of ELSEVIER, Inc.

W.B. SAUNDERS COMPANY
A Division of Elsevier Inc.

1600 John F. Kennedy Boulevard • Suite 1800 • Philadelphia, PA 19103-2899

http://www.theclinics.com

PSYCHIATRIC CLINICS OF NORTH AMERICA Volume 35, Number 2
June 2012 ISSN 0193-953X, ISBN-13: 978-1-4557-3926-4

Editor: Joanne Husovski
Developmental Editor: Donald Mumford

Psychiatric Clinics of North America (ISSN 0193-953X) is published quarterly by Elsevier Inc., 360 Park Avenue South, New York, NY 10010-1710. Months of issue are March, June, September, and December. Business and Editorial Offices: 1600 John F. Kennedy Blvd., Suite 1800, Philadelphia, PA 19103-2899. Periodicals postage paid at New York, NY and additional mailing offices. Subscription prices are $286.00 per year (US individuals), $504.00 per year (US institutions), $141.00 per year (US students/residents), $347.00 per year (Canadian individuals), $627.00 per year (Canadian Institutions), $431.00 per year (foreign individuals), and $627.00 per year (foreign institutions), and $210.00 per year (international & Canadian students/residents). Foreign air speed delivery is included in all *Clinics'* subscription prices. All prices are subject to change without notice. **POSTMASTER:** Send address changes to *Psychiatric Clinics of North America,* Elsevier Health Sciences Division, Subscription Customer Service, 3251 Riverport Lane, Maryland Heights, MO 63043. Customer Service: 1-800-654-2452 (US). From outside the United States, call 1-314-447-8871. Fax: 1-314-447-8029. E-mail: journalscustomerservice-usa@elsevier.com (for print support) and journalsonlinesupport-usa@elsevier.com (for online support).

Reprints. For copies of 100 or more, of articles in this publication, please contact the Commercial Reprints Department, Elsevier Inc., 360 Park Avenue South, New York, New York 10010-1710. Tel.: (212) 633-3813, Fax: (212) 462-1935, E-mail: reprints@elsevier.com.

Psychiatric Clinics of North America is covered in *MEDLINE/PubMed (Index Medicus), Current Contents/Social and Behavioral Sciences, Social Science Citation Index, Embase/Excerpta Medica,* and PsycINFO.

Printed and bound by CPI Group (UK) Ltd, Croydon, CR0 4YY
Transferred to Digital Print 2012

Contributors

GUEST EDITORS

ITAI DANOVITCH, MD
Chairman, Department of Psychiatry and Behavioral Neurosciences, Cedars-Sinai Medical Center, Los Angeles, California

JOHN J. MARIANI, MD
Assistant Professor of Clinical Psychiatry, Director, Substance Treatment and Research Service, Division of Substance Abuse, New York State Psychiatric Institute; Department of Psychiatry, College of Physicians and Surgeons of Columbia University, New York, New York

AUTHORS

WILSON M. COMPTON, MD, MPE
Director, Division of Epidemiology, Services, and Prevention Research, National Institute on Drug Abuse (NIDA), Bethesda, Maryland

JESSE DALLERY, PhD
Associate Professor, Department of Psychology, University of Florida, Gainesville, Florida

ITAI DANOVITCH, MD
Chairman, Department of Psychiatry and Behavioral Neurosciences, Cedars-Sinai Medical Center, Los Angeles, California

FRANCESCA DUCCI, MD, PhD
Institute of Psychiatry, Psychological Medicine, Kings College, London, United Kingdom

TIMOTHY W. FONG, MD
UCLA Gambling Studies Program; Department of Psychiatry and Biobehavioral Sciences, University of California, Los Angeles; UCLA Impulse Control Disorders Clinic, Semel Institute for Neuroscience and Biobehavioral Sciences, Los Angeles, California

DAVID GOLDMAN, MD
Laboratory of Neurogenetics, National Institute on Alcohol Abuse and Alcoholism, National Institutes of Health, Rockville, Maryland

ERIC GOPLERUD, PhD, MA
Senior Vice President, Substance Abuse, Mental Health, and Criminal Justice Studies, National Opinion Research Center (NORC) at the University of Chicago, Bethesda, Maryland

DAVID A. GORELICK, MD, PhD, DFAPA
Chemistry and Drug Metabolism Section, Intramural Research Program, National Institute on Drug Abuse, National Institutes of Health; Adjunct Professor, Department of Psychiatry, University of Maryland School of Medicine, Baltimore, Maryland

GRACE JUN
Department of Psychiatry and Biobehavioral Sciences, University of California, Los Angeles, Los Angeles, California

AARON KAUFMAN, MD
Department of Psychiatry and Biobehavioral Sciences, University of California, Los Angeles, Los Angeles, California

ALEXANDER KONG
Department of Psychiatry and Biobehavioral Sciences, University of California, Los Angeles, Los Angeles, California

FRANCES R. LEVIN, MD
Division of Substance Abuse, New York State Psychiatric Institute; Department of Psychiatry, College of Physicians and Surgeons of Columbia University, New York, New York

WALTER LING, MD
Professor, UCLA Department of Psychiatry and Biobehavioral Sciences, UCLA Integrated Substance Abuse Programs, Los Angeles, California

MARSHA F. LOPEZ, PhD, MHS
Branch Chief, Epidemiology Research Branch, Division of Epidemiology, Services, and Prevention Research, National Institute on Drug Abuse (NIDA), Bethesda, Maryland

JOHN J. MARIANI, MD
Assistant Professor of Clinical Psychiatry, Director, Substance Treatment and Research Service, Division of Substance Abuse, New York State Psychiatric Institute; Department of Psychiatry, College of Physicians and Surgeons of Columbia University, New York, New York

LISA A. MARSCH, PhD
Director, Center for Technology and Behavioral Health, Dartmouth Psychiatric Research Center; Associate Professor of Psychiatry, Department of Psychiatry, Dartmouth College, Lebanon, New Hampshire

JUDITH MARTIN, MD
Medical Director, BAART Turk Street Clinic, San Francisco, California

PETER R. MARTIN, MD
Professor of Psychiatry and Pharmacology, Director, Division of Addiction Psychiatry and Vanderbilt Addiction Center, Vanderbilt Psychiatric Hospital, Nashville, Tennessee

DIANA MARTINEZ, MD
Associate Professor of Psychiatry, Department of Psychiatry, Division of Substance Abuse, Columbia University; Department of Psychiatry, New York State Psychiatric Institute, New York, New York

MICHAEL M. MILLER, MD, FASAM, FAPA
Associate Clinical Professor, Department of Psychiatry, University of Wisconsin School of Medicine and Public Health; Medical Director, Herrington Recovery Center, Rogers Memorial Hospital, Oconomowoc, Wisconsin

KAREN MIOTTO, MD
Director of the Addiction Medicine Service, Clinical Professor, Department of Psychiatry and Biobehavioral Sciences, University of California, Los Angeles, Los Angeles, California

LARISSA MOONEY, MD
Assistant Professor, UCLA Department of Psychiatry and Biobehavioral Sciences, UCLA Integrated Substance Abuse Programs, University of California, Los Angeles, Los Angeles, California

BENJAMIN R. NORDSTROM, MD, PhD
Assistant Professor of Psychiatry, Dartmouth Medical School, Lebanon, New Hampshire

IMAN PARHAMI, MD, MPH
UCLA Gambling Studies Program; Department of Psychiatry and Biobehavioral Sciences, University of California, Los Angeles, Los Angeles, California

DAVID R. PATING, MD
Assistant Clinical Professor, Department of Psychiatry, University of California, San Francisco; Chief, Addiction Medicine, Kaiser Permanente San Francisco, San Francisco, California

ERNEST RASYIDI, MD
Addiction Psychiatry Fellow, Department of Psychiatry and Behavioral Neurosciences, Cedars-Sinai Medical Center, Los Angeles, California

RORY C. REID, PhD
UCLA Gambling Studies Program; Department of Psychiatry and Biobehavioral Sciences, University of California Los Angeles, Los Angeles, California

STEPHEN ROSS, MD
Assistant Professor of Psychiatry, Child and Adolescent Psychiatry, and Oral and Maxillofacial Pathology, Radiology and Medicine; Director, Division of Alcoholism and Drug Abuse, Bellevue Hospital; Director, Bellevue Opioid Overdose Prevention Program; Clinical Director, New York University (NYU) Langone Center of Excellence on Addiction; Director, Addiction Psychiatry, NYU Tisch Hospital; Director, NYU Addiction Psychiatry Fellowship, Department of Psychiatry, NYU School of Medicine, NYU College of Dentistry, New York, New York

JEFFREY D. SCHULDEN, MD
Medical Officer, Epidemiology Research Branch, Division of Epidemiology, Services, and Prevention Research, National Institute on Drug Abuse (NIDA), Bethesda, Maryland

JEFFREY SCHWARTZ, MD
Department of Psychiatry and Biobehavioral Sciences, University of California, Los Angeles, Los Angeles, California

NINA B.L. URBAN, MD, MSc
Assistant Professor of Clinical Psychiatry, Department of Psychiatry, Division of Substance Abuse, Columbia University; Department of Psychiatry, New York State Psychiatric Institute, New York, New York

JEFFERY N. WILKINS, MD
Department of Psychiatry and Behavioral Neurosciences, Cedars-Sinai Medical Center, Los Angeles, California

A.R. WILLIAMS, MD, MBE
Resident in Psychiatry, New York University, New York, New York

LI-TZY WU, ScD
Professor, Duke University School of Medicine, Duke University Medical Center, Durham, North Carolina

JESSICA L. YOUNG, MD
Assistant Professor of Obstetrics and Gynecology, Vanderbilt University Medical Center, Nashville, Tennessee

DOUGLAS M. ZIEDONIS, MD
Professor and Chair, Department of Psychiatry, University of Massachusetts Medical School and UMass Memorial Health Care, Worcester, Massachusetts

Contents

Recognizing the signs and symptoms of behavioral addictions can be confusing, at times, because the line between normative and pathological behaviors is not well defined. Behavioral addictions are conditions that create significant harm to individuals, families, and society. This article reviews the current and proposed diagnostic criteria of 3 prevalent behavioral addictions: (1) pathological gambling, (2) hypersexual disorders, and (3) compulsive shopping. Differential diagnoses are discussed and clinical characteristics are presented to facilitate clinicians in clarifying the difference between pathology and habit. Treatment options for these behavioral addictions are presented along with case studies.

Long-acting depot naltrexone, an opioid antagonist, inhibits the rewarding effects of exogenously introduced opioids, helping patients cease drug use. Although depot naltrexone formulations have demonstrated efficacy in reducing opioid use and improving abstinence rates in clinical studies, the utilization of depot naltrexone has not yet gained much traction since its approval for treatment of opioid addiction by the US Food and Drug Administration. This article provides a historical perspective of naltrexone, its practical use as a pharmacotherapy for opioid addiction, and issues regarding the current and future role of extended-release depot naltrexone for addiction treatment.

This article reviews treatment options for cannabis dependence. The evolving sociocultural context of cannabis use has contributed to decreased perceived risk and increased acceptability. The comparatively lower "severity" of cannabis-associated consequences makes it more difficult for users to recognize the impact of their use and establish an enduring commitment to change. As a result, many treatment seekers are reluctant to accept traditional abstinence-based goals. Psychotherapy studies are establishing a number of evidence-based models and techniques in the treatment resources for patients in need. Although no pharmacotherapy has been approved for cannabis dependence, a number of promising approaches are in development.

> We review the current systems of health care delivery for the treatment of substance use disorders and examine the expansion of addiction treatment to include new methods and settings, supported by changing technology, new financing/payment mechanisms, and expanded information management processes. We examine 3 subsets of patients who should be able to receive better, more frequent care through recent federally mandated health care reform. Finally, we provide recommendations for what we consider essential steps to facilitate the improvement of care for substance use disorders under health care reform.

> This article discusses the serotonergic hallucinogens (SHs) and includes classification systems, historical investigations, neurobiological mechanisms of action, addictive liability (from biological, behavioral, and epidemiologic perspectives), and potential therapeutic applications. The focus is on plausible neurobiologic mechanisms, though a small body of scholarship has also explored putative spiritual mechanisms of action. The article concludes with a discussion of an optimal study design to test SH treatment models for addictive disorders and review of the current state of the reemergence of research into these models at several major academic medical centers in the United States.

> Studies report that the direct effect of drug-related crime (ie, not including the cost of arrest, prosecution, and incarceration) is the largest single cost related to addiction. Addiction to illicit substances and its connection to people going through the criminal justice system are discussed in this review. Emphasis is on the efficacy of drug treatment in offender populations. Outcomes from large national studies and smaller studies are presented that deal with addiction treatment and criminal offenses; also discussed are operant conditioning in drug addiction, contingency management in a criminal justice context, coercion in the criminal justice setting, and drug courts.

> This discussion identifies risk factors for prescription use disorders and reviews key components of psychiatric screening for pain and addiction. The components of universal precautions for opioid treatment are discussed, including patient education, assessment, and monitoring as well as the use of drug testing. Additionally, this review identifies pharmacologic approaches that are useful in high-risk populations.

> Research on the epidemiology of illicit drug use disorders provides important insights into understanding these conditions and their impact on public health. Findings have indicated relatively high prevalence of illicit drug use and ongoing shifts in trends in use, for example highlighting elevated rates of prescription drug misuse. Building on an understanding of this research, it is important for clinicians in a range of settings to integrate strategies for prevention, screening, and linkage to substance abuse treatment programs. This paper focuses on highlights from research on the epidemiology of illicit drug use in the United States and its clinical implications.

> Substitution pharmacotherapy is an effective approach for treating opioid and nicotine dependence, and accumulating evidence indicates that stimulant pharmacotherapy for cocaine dependence is a promising strategy. To date, the available evidence is strongest for amphetamine analogs or dopaminergic agents combined with contingency management behavioral interventions as potential psychostimulant treatments for cocaine dependence. Most psychostimulants are controlled substances with inherent risks of misuse and diversion, and their use in patients with active substance use disorders is complex. As stimulant substitution treatment models for cocaine dependence are developed, particular attention to patient risk stratification is needed.

> Chronic use of opioids has short-term and long-term risks for the pregnant woman and the fetus. The treatment of opioid-dependent pregnant women presents a unique set of challenges for physicians. Standard of care for the pregnant woman with opioid dependence continues to be methadone maintenance. Buprenorphine has been shown to be safe in pregnancy, but further research is needed on

initiation during pregnancy. Collaboration between psychiatry, obstetrics, and social services in the form of a comprehensive treatment program can reduce risk and improve neonatal outcomes for the increasing problem of opioid dependence in pregnancy.

The current state of addiction training in medical schools, residencies including psychiatry, and addiction psychiatry and addiction medicine fellowships is presented. Deficits in addiction training are described as well as proposed models targeting training of relevant addiction clinical competencies. Specific recommendations address future roles for psychiatrists who specialize in addiction. Tables and boxes describe addiction training in medical school, residencies, and addiction fellowships, and outline a select history of physician contributions to the addiction field and physician education. Proposed competencies for primary care residents, principles of the patient-centered medical home, and recommended skillsets of tomorrow's psychiatry addiction specialists are outlined.

The authors present an overview of empirically supported psychosocial interventions for individuals with substance use disorders (SUDs), including recent advances in the field. They also identify barriers to the adoption of evidence-based psychosocial treatments in community-based systems of care, and the promise of leveraging technology (computers, web, mobile phone, and emerging technologies) to markedly enhance the reach of these treatments. Technology-based interventions may provide "on-demand," ubiquitous access to therapeutic support in diverse settings. A brief discussion of important next steps in developing, refining, and disseminating technology-delivered psychosocial interventions concludes the review.

The authors review genetic factors moderating vulnerability to addictions: heritability and mode of inheritance, developmental changes across the lifespan of genetic and environmental influences, shared and unshared inheritance, interplay between genetic and environmental factors, gene identification via candidate genes and genome-wide approaches, and the role of rare and common genetic variants in addiction.

Neuroimaging studies have been crucial in understanding changes in the various neurotransmitter systems implicated in addiction in the living human brain. The authors provide an overview of existing data from neuroimaging studies in addiction with a focus on psychostimulant, alcohol, and cannabis dependence. It addresses stimulant abuse and striatal dopamine transmission, neurocircuitry of reward in addiction, response to treatment, and clinical correlates of imaging dopamine transmission in addiction, including D2 receptors and dopamine transporters, as well as summarizing findings from imaging studies of other neurotransmitter systems such as the serotonergic system and opiate receptors, gamma-aminobutyric acid, and endogenous cannabinoid receptors.

PSYCHIATRIC CLINICS

Preface

Expanding Treatment Potential for Substance Use Disorders

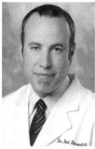 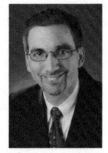

Itai Danovitch, MD   John J. Mariani, MD
Guest Editors

The treatment of substance use disorders is rapidly changing and the potential to identify and treat individuals suffering from addiction continues to increase. Advances in brain imaging technology and genetics have expanded our understanding of the neurobiology of addiction. New behavioral psychotherapies, as well as novel delivery mechanisms, are changing the nature of standard treatment approaches. Pharmacotherapy options continue to expand in terms of number of effective medications identified as well as treatment delivery models. Treatment methods for certain subpopulations of individuals with substance use disorders have been advanced greatly. This issue of the *Psychiatric Clinics of North America* provides an overview of cutting-edge developments in addiction science and treatment.

While the treatment expertise for managing patients with substance use disorders frequently is concentrated in subspecialists, it is of great importance for general psychiatry practitioners to be familiar with the developments in addiction science and treatment. Substance use disorders occupy a unique place in our system of care. Historically, much of the treatment of individuals with substance use disorders evolved outside of traditional medical and psychiatric care, with mutual assistance groups and other nonprofessionals playing a primary role. This model has changed in recent decades, with dramatic developments in the understanding of the neurobiological mechanisms underpinning the behavioral patterns of addiction. The treatment of substance use disorders has evolved into a scientifically based clinical model, with strong correlations between basic science knowledge and available effective treatments. General psychiatry practitioners in practically all treatment settings will inevitably encounter individuals with substance use disorders. Awareness of the state

Psychiatr Clin N Am 35 (2012) xiii–xiv
http://dx.doi.org/10.1016/j.psc.2012.04.003
0193-953X/12/$ – see front matter © 2012 Elsevier Inc. All rights reserved.

of development of addiction clinical science is necessary to achieve the best possible clinical outcomes.

This issue of the *Psychiatric Clinics of North America* provides a well-balanced sampling of cutting-edge developments in addiction science and clinical practice. We have been fortunate to have an impressive roster of prominent clinician-scientist contributors with a broad range of expertise. The review articles collected here represent an impressive sampling of the most important developments in addiction science. We hope you find this issue as interesting and valuable as we do.

Itai Danovitch, MD
Department of Psychiatry and Behavioral Neurosciences
Cedars-Sinai Medical Center
8730 Alden Drive, C-301
Los Angeles, CA 90048, USA

John J. Mariani, MD
Substance Treatment and Research Service
New York State Psychiatric Institute/Columbia University
1051 Riverside Drive, Unit 66
New York, NY 10010, USA

E-mail addresses:
itai.danovitch@cshs.org (I. Danovitch)
jm2330@columbia.edu (J.J. Mariani)

Behavioral Addictions
Where to Draw the Lines?

Timothy W. Fong, MD[a],*, Rory C. Reid, PhD[b,c],
Iman Parhami, MD, MPH[b,c]

KEYWORDS

- Behavioral addictions
- Hypersexual disorder
- Pathological gambling
- Compulsive shopping

KEY POINTS

- Providers need to accurately discern and be able to assess when excessive behavioral patterns require psychiatric intervention or whether presenting problems fall within the realm of normative behavior.
- Behavioral addictions involve compulsive behavior with inability to stop despite harmful consequences.
- Identifying when the line is crossed from recreation/habit to psychopathology relies on understanding current diagnostic criteria and consideration of cultural, ethnic, and local community standards.

Increased attention has been given to further understanding non–substance-related patterns of excessive behavior.[1] This attention has been accompanied by debate as to how these phenomena might best be conceptualized. Some categorize excessive behavioral patterns as addictive disorders, whereas others suggest they should be classified as obsessive compulsive spectrum disorders or as impulse control disorders.[2] Reliable classification is important in facilitating communication among

Financial Disclosures: Timothy W. Fong, MD, Speaker's Bureau: Reckitt Benckiser, Pfizer Pharmaceuticals; Grant Support: Psyadon Pharmaceuticals and National Institute on Drug Abuse (Grant #: K23DA 19522-2).
Rory C. Reid, PhD, and Iman Parhami, MD have nothing to disclose.
[a] UCLA Gambling Studies Program, Semel Institute for Neuroscience and Human Behavior, Department of Psychiatry and Biobehavioral Sciences, University of California Los Angeles, 760 Westwood Plaza, Los Angeles, CA 90024, USA; [b] UCLA Gambling Studies Program, 760 Westwood Plaza, Mailcode 175919, Los Angeles, CA 90064, USA [c] Department of Psychiatry and Biobehavioral Sciences, University of California Los Angeles, 760 Westwood Plaza, Los Angeles, CA 90064, USA
* Corresponding author.
E-mail address: tfong@mednet.ucla.edu

researchers, clinicians, and patients as well as providing a framework for developing therapeutic interventions.

Establishing validity is also crucial. In an era of limited psychiatric resources, it is particularly important to accurately differentiate psychiatric disease from mere aberrant behavior. Providers need to accurately discern and be able to assess when excessive behavioral patterns require psychiatric intervention or whether presenting problems fall within the realm of normative behavior. In an effort to help providers clarify these issues, this article highlights several important considerations with examples from pathological gambling, hypersexual behavior, and compulsive shopping. The focus of this article is on assessing common characteristics of these behaviors as well as considerations for therapeutic intervention. As with most disorders, classification of a diagnostic threshold is made by gathering as much information about the presenting problem from as many reliable sources as possible and then differentiating these symptoms from more parsimonious explanations of the chief complaint. In the case of behavioral addictions, it is important that patients be evaluated in the context of several other factors, including the extent to which their behavior (1) disrupts personal, family, social, or vocational pursuits; (2) causes significant personal distress to self or others; (3) has risk or potential for significant physical or emotional harm to self or others; (4) is uncontrollable or resistant to change (eg, patient feels out of control or unable to reduce or change the behavior), and (5) is not better accounted for by an alternate psychiatric diagnosis.

HYPERSEXUAL DISORDER

The proposed diagnostic criteria for hypersexual disorder (HD)—also known as sexual addiction, excessive sexuality, problem sexual behaviors, or compulsive sexual behavior—are currently under consideration for inclusion in the Diagnostic and Statistical Manual of Mental Disorders (DSM)-V (**Box 1**). The distinguishing characteristic of this phenomenon is the presence of repetitive and intense preoccupations with sexual fantasies, urges, and behaviors, leading to adverse consequences and clinically significant distress or impairment in social, occupational, or other important areas of functioning.[3-7] Patients seeking help for HD frequently experience multiple unsuccessful attempts to control or diminish the amount of time spent engaging in sexual fantasies, urges, and behaviors in response to dysphoric mood states or stressful life events.[6] HD has received increased attention among mental health professionals and researchers in an effort to understand more clearly the etiology, consequences, and associated features of HD, including possible health risks associated with sexually transmitted infections.[8-11]

Clinical Characteristics

Individuals seeking help for HD often seek treatment first for co-occurring psychopathology including mood, anxiety, attention-deficit, and substance-related disorders.[12-15] Personality characteristics, such as boredom proneness, impulsivity, interpersonal sensitivity, alexithymia, loneliness, low self-esteem, and shame have also been observed in association with hypersexual behavior.[16-19] When hypersexual disorder occurs among married individuals, relationships are often adversely impacted and divorce is common.[20]

Prevalence and Etiology

Estimates suggest that 3% to 6% of the general population in the United States may suffer from hypersexual disorder.[21,22] Studies indicate men (particularly those reporting

---

Box 1
DSM-V proposed criteria for hypersexual disorder

A. Over a period of at least 6 months, recurrent and intense sexual fantasies, sexual urges, and sexual behavior in association with 4 or more of the following 5 criteria:

　1. Excessive time is consumed by sexual fantasies and urges and by planning for and engaging in sexual behavior

　2. Repetitively engaging in these sexual fantasies, urges, and behavior in response to dysphoric mood states (eg, anxiety, depression, boredom, irritability)

　3. Repetitively engaging in sexual fantasies, urges, and behavior in response to stressful life events

　4. Repetitive but unsuccessful efforts to control or significantly reduce these sexual fantasies, urges, and behavior

　5. Repetitively engaging in sexual behavior while disregarding the risk for physical or emotional harm to self or others

B. There is clinically significant personal distress or impairment in social, occupational, or other important areas of functioning associated with the frequency and intensity of these sexual fantasies, urges, and behavior[20]

C. These sexual fantasies, urges, and behaviors are not due to direct physiologic effects of exogenous substances (eg, drugs of abuse or medications) or to manic episodes.

D. The person is at least 18 years of age

Specify if: Masturbation, pornography, sexual behavior with consenting adults, cybersex, telephone sex, strip clubs

---

homosexual preference) are more likely to have HD than women. In a study that loosely defined hypersexual behavior as "out of control" sexual fantasies and urges leading to sexual behavior that caused disturbances to activities in daily living, a prevalence rate of HD was 0.8% for men (n = 474) and 0.6% (n = 466) for women in a nonclinical sample from New Zealand.[23] One online study of men (n = 5834) and women (n = 7251) designed to help the researchers investigate differences between sexually dysregulated behavior and high levels of sexual desire, found that 1.83% of men and 0.95% of women had significantly elevated scores on the Sexual Compulsivity Scale and a history of having sought treatment for sexual compulsivity, addiction, or impulsivity.[24]

To date, research has focused largely on white samples of heterosexual and homosexual men, although the few comparisons studies of hypersexual men, many of whom are "straight" or bisexual, who have sex with other men reflect more similarities than differences across racial and ethnic groups.[9] It has been hypothesized that gay and bisexual men may be at a greater risk for HD development given reports of higher levels of lifetime sex partners compared with other social groups. Moreover, gay and bisexual hypersexual men tend to frequent a greater variety of sexual outlets such as bathhouses or sex clubs.[25] Among the dearth of studies about HD in adult women, some evidence suggests that childhood sex abuse is more common than among hypersexual men. Thus, childhood sexual abuse may be a predisposing risk factor in the development of HD in women. Although some have suggested that HD may emerge as a compensation strategy for developmental attachment ruptures or childhood trauma, no research has emerged to provide convincing support for this hypothesis. Finally, studies seeking to assess neurobiological mechanisms associated with HD have found mixed results with some findings supporting executive deficits[26,27] and others failing to find such support.[17]

Assessment and Diagnostic Considerations

A number of self-report measures have been developed in an attempt to capture the associated characteristics of hypersexual behavior.[22,28] Of particular interest is the Hypersexual Behavior Inventory, given its close alignment with the DSM-V criteria for HD and excellent psychometric properties.[17] The 19-item scale captures aspects of HD such as engaging in sex in response to stress (eg, "Doing something sexual helps me cope with stress") or dysphoric mood (eg, "I turn to sexual activities when I experience unpleasant feelings") or multiple unsuccessful attempts to diminish or control sexual thoughts, urges, and behaviors (eg, "Even though I promised myself I would not repeat a sexual behavior, I find myself returning to it over and over again"). Impairment in social, occupational, or other important areas of functioning is also captured by several items, which helps to identify pathological behaviors (eg, "My sexual activities interfere with aspects of my life such as work or school" and "My sexual thoughts and fantasies distract me from accomplishing important tasks").

If HD is suspected, clinicians should also take time to assess important domains such as human immunodeficiency virus risk behavior including the number of sex partners and presence of unprotected sexual transactions. Other risks for physical or emotional harm should also be considered. For example, risks reported from clinical populations recruited to the DSM-V field trial for hypersexual disorders, include masturbating to pornography while operating a motor vehicle, entering high-crime neighborhoods to engage with a commercial sex worker, and potential loss of employment because of sexual activities in the workplace. Relationships with romantic partners are often compromised when an individual engages in hypersexual behavior, and children may be at risk for premature exposure to sexual stimuli and situations. Inquiries should be made about levels of personal distress and perceived control related to sexual fantasies, urges, and behaviors. Additionally, Axis I comorbidity should be considered, as HD is not diagnosed if it occurs *exclusively* in the context of a substance-related disorder, a manic episode, or if the period of sexual activities has not persisted for a period of 6 months or longer. Collectively, these domains can help a clinician evaluate the degree to which a patient may struggle with hypersexual behavior and its associated features.

Interventions and Treatment Approaches

A number of self-help materials and workbooks containing anecdotal suggestions for change have been published to help hypersexual patients; however, there is a dearth of rigorous outcome studies assessing the efficacy or effectiveness of treatment interventions in this population.[3] Case studies and nonrandomized open clinical trials have reported successful treatment of hypersexual patients with pharmacologic interventions, such as selective serotonin reuptake inhibitors,[29] or opioid antagonists, such as naltrexone.[30] Nonmedication strategies suggest a vast array of interventions, including cognitive behavior therapy,[31] acceptance and commitment therapy,[32] 12-step programs, and couples therapy.[31,33-35]

Currently, the preferred treatment plan includes individual cognitive-behavioral or experiential psychotherapy, attendance at a treatment group or 12-step support meeting, and concurrent pharmacologic interventions to address both co-occurring psychopathology and hypersexual disorders.[35] Collectively, the goal of these treatments is to arrest hypersexual behaviors and address underlying issues that precipitate or perpetuate them. Given the DSM-V proposed classification criteria for HD,

> **Box 2**
> **CASE STUDY: Hypersexual disorder with pornography subtype**
>
> John is a 45-year-old traveling consultant who presents for an evaluation related to difficulties with anxiety and depression. He reports that his job has been stressful because of potential layoffs, which he states has also led to relationship difficulties with his wife. Although he denies current drug and alcohol problems, he admits to using marijuana in college as a way of coping during difficult semesters. When asked about sexual behaviors, he reports being faithful to his wife and denies any problems with erectile dysfunction or premature ejaculation. After starting him on an antidepressant and 4 weeks of individual therapy, his symptoms have not improved. Instead, he indicates that his wife recently caught him masturbating to online pornography and feels betrayed and upset because a year ago he had promised to discontinue this behavior. Upon further inquiry, John confides that although he has intended to stop consuming pornography in the past because it leaves him feeling empty inside, he has been unable to do so despite multiple attempts. He states "I've been using pornography the same way I used marijuana in college to cope with stress or distract myself from feeling discouraged about work." John further states that he has been staying up until 2 or 3 am masturbating to pornography several nights a week and was also reprimanded a month ago for downloading pornography at work in violation of corporate policies. After having John sign a release, the wife is contacted to discuss the situation. She reports that John's pornography issue has been a chronic problem during the marriage, has diminished their sexual intimacy, and that while doing a school assignment on their home computer, their 9-year-old son was exposed to pornography while clicking on an Internet "bookmark" than John had created. She is worried that John might lose his job over this issue because "this recent warning is the second time John has been caught at work."

interventions that help enhance emotional regulation and stress coping strategies such as mindfulness meditation are also likely to be beneficial (**Box 2**).

Brief Case Discussion

Because of high levels of shame, patients like John are often reluctant to disclose various manifestations of hypersexual behavior. Estimating the severity of hypersexual behavior can be difficult, as it is often minimized. In this regard, gathering information from collateral sources can provide further insight. In the case of John, his pornography consumption appears problematic from several perspectives. John continues to use pornography despite the risk of marital conflict and potential for loss of employment; he has even prematurely exposed his son to sexually explicit materials (which may have reporting implications in some demographic locations). He self-reports using pornography like a drug to cope with stress and distract himself from uncomfortable emotions. It is not possible from the information given ascertain whether John is compulsively masturbating to pornography. Generally, many patients with pornography issues also experience excessive masturbation problems. Although it is unclear to what extent his pornography problem may be contributing to his anxiety and depression, the consequences of his choices are likely exacerbating his mental health issues and should be considered in the case conceptualization of this patient.

PATHOLOGICAL GAMBLING

Gambling in the United States is a socially acceptable and widespread activity. Although most adults gamble without incurring problems, nearly 4% of the adult US population currently have a gambling disorder, and 6% will experience harm from gambling during their lifetime.[36] Pathological gamblers are those who gamble despite serious social and personal consequences and who meet 5 of 10 criteria encompassing:

Box 3
Criteria for diagnosis of pathological gambling, according to DSM-IV TR

A. Persistent and recurrent maladaptive gambling behavior as indicated by at least 5 of the following

1. Is preoccupied with gambling (eg, preoccupied with reliving past gambling experiences, handicapping or planning the next venture, or thinking of ways to get money with which to gamble

2. Needs to gamble with increasing amounts of money to achieve the desired excitement

3. Has repeated unsuccessful efforts to control, cut back, or stop gambling

4. Is restless or irritable when attempting to cut down or stop gambling

5. Gambles as a way of escaping from problems or of relieving a dysphoric mood (eg, feelings of helplessness, guilt, anxiety, depression)

6. After losing money gambling, often returns another day to get even ("chasing" one's losses)

7. Lies to family members, therapist, or others to conceal the extent of involvement with gambling

8. Has committed illegal acts, such as forgery, fraud, theft, or embezzlement, to finance gambling

9. Has jeopardized or lost a significant relationship, job, or educational or career opportunity because of gambling

10. Relies on others to provide money to relieve a desperate financial situation caused by gambling

B. The gambling behavior is not better accounted for by a manic episode

---

- Withdrawal (restful or irritable when attempting to cut down or stop gambling
- Tolerance (needs to gamble with increasing amounts of money to achieve the desired excitement)
- Preoccupation with gambling (preoccupied with reliving past gambling experiences, handicapping or planning the next venture, or thinking of ways to get money with which to gamble).[37]

The full list of criteria for pathological gambling is shown in **Box 3**.

Problem gamblers, who are at increased risk for the development of pathological gambling, have less severe gambling issues and meet 1 to 4 criteria.[38] Experts in the field use the term *disordered gambling* to refer jointly to problem and pathological gambling.[39] Other terms, such as *gambling addiction*, *compulsive gambling*, and *compulsive betting*, have also been used to describe problem gambling behaviors.

Clinical Characteristics

Pathological gambling has been described as a hidden addiction[40] because there are minimal signs and symptoms associated with this condition. **Box 4** presents a scenario of 2 gamblers, 1 recreational gambler and 1 pathological gambler, to demonstrate the difference between a gambler with and without a problem. Compared with the first gambler (1-Recreational), the second gambler (2-pathological) cannot control his gambling and experiences significant consequences from his gambling behavior.

Box 4
Two cases of gamblers: recreational versus pathological

Gambler 1: Recreational Gambler

- 67 year-old retired physician who plays poker at the local casino 5 times per week and up to 5 hours per session
- Not increased gambling limits for the past 20 years
- Never stayed at the casino for more than time planned
- Allocates appropriate time for exercise and family
- Financially comfortable with retirement account
- Family is aware of gambling behavior

Gambler 2: Pathological Gambler

- 20-year-old college student who gambles whenever he has money
- Skips courses and assignments to gamble
- Engages in bank fraud and steals from girlfriend to finance gambling
- Has attempted to quit or reduce gambling 10 times in the last 2 years
- Conceals gambling behavior to family and friends
- Used money from financial aid and scholarships to gamble
- About to get kicked out of college for poor grades and financial status

---

Given the possible concealment of this disorder, specific screening questions are important to determine pathology. This is usually accomplished with questions corresponding to the DSM-IV criteria for pathological gambling[41] that query about patterns of preoccupation, tolerance, withdrawal, loss of control, escapism, dishonesty, and risk-taking behaviors related to gambling.[37] These criteria are assessed through clinical interviews or self-report questionnaires and are considered valid and reliable methods to diagnose gambling disorders.[42,43] As an example, urges and cravings for gambling (ie, desires to gamble) alone are not enough to meet criteria for pathological gambling. It is the presence of an excessive amount, frequency, or intensity of preoccupation with gambling that reflects the core symptoms of the disease.

Pathological gambling must also be distinguished from excessive gambling secondary to dopamine agonists or during the course of a manic episode. Emerging literature shows that dopamine agonists used in Parkinson's disease is associated with an higher risk of gambling disorder development.[44] In bipolar affective disorder patients, when excessive gambling behavior is exhibited during the manic phase only, then true pathological gambling is not considered to be evident.

Etiology

Two integrative models have been proposed to explain the cause of pathological gambling.[39] The biopsychosocial model suggests that predisposing factors (ie, poor coping and problem-solving skills, personality, and genetic variability) interact with early gambling wins to create a cognitive-behavioral and diathesis-stress pathway that raises the risk for pathological gambling.[45] A more recent model suggests that this path is not homogeneous, as there may exist 3 pathways leading to 3 subtypes of pathological gamblers (behaviorally conditioned, emotionally vulnerable, and antisocial impulsivist).[46]

Researchers have also found numerous biological associated factors that may act as predictive risk factors for the development of pathological gambling. The involvement of the ventral tegmental-orbitofrontal cortex[47] and a variety of neurotransmitters (noradrenaline, serotonin, glutamate, dopamine, and endorphins) have also been implicated.[48]

Social factors, such as childhood exposure to gambling, may increase the risk for pathological gambling development. Children who learn and maintain observed gambling behaviors may find them more appealing and reinforcing[49,50] and may have higher rates of gambling pathology themselves.[51,52] Moreover, culture or ethnicity may play a role in the development of pathological gambling.[53] For example, pathological gambling may be more prevalent in the Chinese population because it is the preferred form of entertainment,[54] or Iranian-Americans may be more prone to pathological gambling behavior because gambling is a commonly practiced social family activity.[55]

Assessment and Diagnostic Considerations

It is important to assess the seriousness or severity of the gambling disorder to provide the appropriate treatment setting (eg, brief intervention, ongoing outpatient care, intensive outpatient treatment, or residential treatment). For some pathological gamblers, admission to an inpatient unit is necessary because of suicidal ideations. Most important in assessment of severity is remembering the increased risk for suicide that pathological gamblers have, especially when they "hit rock bottom" or have lost everything including financial assets and social relationships.[56] Providers should be vigilant for suicidal thoughts, especially at intake and during relapse because several studies have found that the risk for suicide attempts or ideations is notably higher in this population compared with those with other disorders.[57–60] A recent study found that 81% of pathological gamblers in treatment showed some suicidal ideation, and 30% reported 1 or more suicide attempts in the preceding 12 months (n = 43).[61]

A quick and straightforward method to assess severity is to consider the number of criteria endorsed by a patient,[62,63] but this approach limits information about duration, frequency, or the context of symptoms exhibited. Acquisition of information about the client's gambling behavior, including how often (frequency), how long (duration), and how much (amount) they gamble relative to what they can afford to lose, is also an important indication of severity. However, some argue that such information is insufficient to comprehensively assess gambling severity.[64-66] For example, reductions in gambling behavior may be influenced by extrinsic factors, such as exhaustion of funds, incarceration, and ultimatums from family members.[67] Furthermore, patterns of episodic gambling, such as binge gambling, may be difficult to assess using these 3 criteria alone.[68]

Severity might also be conceptualized by the extent of self-control and disregard of negative associated consequences. These consequences include an increased risk to experience financial problems (eg, bankruptcy, lost job, sizeable debt),[69-72] legal problems (eg, crime, arrests),[73,74] relational problems (eg, divorce, domestic violence, child abuse),[75-77] and health problems (eg, increased stress, sleep disturbances).[78-83]

Intervention and Treatment Approaches

There are no approved pharmacologic treatments for pathological gambling, but several studies carried out in the last 10 years examined the impact of antidepressants, mood stabilizers, and antipsychotic agents on pathological gambling.[84] The most promising pharmacologic treatments include opioid receptor antagonists and amino acid and glutamate modulators (*N*-acetyl cysteine).[39,84] However, studies of these agents are small, are of short duration, have high placebo effects, and do not directly compare against manualized psychotherapy.[39]

Nonpharmacologic treatment approaches for pathological gamblers include self-help manuals, brief interventions, short-term therapy, psychodynamic therapy, and cognitive behavioral treatments. Self-help manuals are an inexpensive and quick therapy for individuals with gambling problems, and evidence suggests that online self-guided interventions are helpful for individuals with gambling-related problems.[85] This becomes especially useful for those not interested in receiving formal treatment, possibly because of shame, denial, concerns over privacy, and financial problems. Other brief interventions that have had positive results include a single 10-minute informational session or a single 1-hour motivational enhancement interview.[86]

A recent meta-analysis reported that several types of therapy (cognitive therapy, motivational interviewing, and imaginal desensitization) were significantly effective in treating gambling disorders, but cognitive-behavioral therapies have an added advantage.[87] Specifically, behavioral strategies include reducing the patterns of reinforcement after exposure to high-risk situations that invoke gambling urges. Also, the development of healthy coping skills, such as assertiveness, problem solving, and relaxation, are critical to recovery. Finally, cognitive strategies modify distorted notions associated with gambling, such as overestimation of gambling skills, false beliefs in the probability of winning, or having inadequate loss aversion.[39]

Twelve-step support groups, such as Gamblers Anonymous (GA), offer peer support, fellowship, and a confidential network to support recovery. Although it is likely that such support group meetings may be especially beneficial for those with severe gambling desires (cravings and urges) as a frequent reminder of the negative repercussions associated with gambling, more empirical studies are needed to determine the impact of these meetings.

COMPULSIVE SHOPPING

Compulsive shopping is characterized by excessive or poorly controlled preoccupations, urges, or behaviors regarding shopping and spending that lead to subjective distress or impaired functioning.[88] This behavior has been given a wide range of labels such as *oniomania, shopaholism, compulsive spending, compulsive buying*, and *shopping addiction*, demonstrating the lack of clarity in this disorder. The term *shopping* refers to the process of seeking or examining good for sales while the term *buying* refers to acquiring an item through purchasing. The term *compulsive shopping* is preferred because it encompasses the different components including browsing, buying, and returning items for sale.

There is ongoing debate as to whether compulsive shopping is a separate psychiatric disorder or if it is a sign or symptom of another psychiatric disorder, such as obsessive-compulsive disorder, bipolar disorder, or major depressive disorder.[89] Current scientific literature on compulsive shopping is small compared with pathological gambling and hypersexual disorders, but the prevalence of this disorder is not rare. A national survey of compulsive shopping patterns found that nearly 6% of Americans might meet criteria for compulsive shopping.[90] In a more recent national survey in Germany, the prevalence rate of compulsive shopping was reported as 6.9%, highlighting that this disorder may be a global condition.[91] In an adolescent population, Grant and coworkers[92] found that nearly 3.5% of a representative population reported problems controlling their shopping and that this group had higher rates of depression, antisocial behaviors, and elevated risk of substance abuse. What is not for debate is the fact that persons affected by compulsive shopping present with significant harm or consequences to their personal, family, and work lives. Individual and family financial suffering can be devastating in terms of credit cards, store credit, and personal loans.

Etiology

There are several different models to explain compulsive shopping, including viewing it as an addictive disorder, as an impulse-control disorder, as an obsessive-compulsive spectrum disorder, or as part of a larger psychiatric disorder such as bipolar disorder.[93,94] Neurobiological models of compulsive shopping have not been conducted, but given the shared clinical symptoms of loss of control in the face of pathological urges and impulses, it is possible that the same brain regions involved in addictive disorders are involved here. Psychologically, compulsive shoppers present with themes of soothing conflict and tension through acquiring material possession that are thought to "make themselves whole." Compulsive shopping oftentimes serves as a stress response to depression and anxiety, particularly when patients have positive experiences with shopping at an early age.

No one model can comprehensively explain compulsive shopping, but a recent, well-designed survey found that compulsive shoppers appear to be more "impulsive acquirers" rather than bipolar or obsessive-compulsive.[95]

Clinical Characteristics

Similar to substance-related disorders, compulsive shopping is characterized by intense, frequent preoccupations with shopping, loss of control, and inability to stop despite negative consequences.[96] Compulsive shoppers report that the rewarding aspects of shopping are not just buying items but also, the planning, the hunting, the bargaining, and the returning of items for future credit.[97] This creates a situation of escape and avoidance, which leads to more shopping and subsequent harm.[89]

Scientific criteria for compulsive shopping have been proposed, but none are currently listed in the American Psychiatric Association's Diagnostic and Statistical Manual. Proposed criteria are listed in **Box 5** and represent similarities to substance dependence and pathological gambling. Up to now, this disorder has not been widely accepted because of a lack of recognition of the symptoms and a presumption that the behavior is deliberate and willful. In addition, harmful consequences (debt, depression, anxiety, impaired relationships) are often distal from the compulsive shopping behavior, making it difficult to recognize or identify the true source of the problem. Finally, because shopping is part of every day, it is not considered a deviant or abnormal behavior like gambling or drug use. Furthermore, as society celebrates material wealth and promotes obtaining items for form and not function, this normalizes nonessential spending behaviors.

Differentiating compulsive shoppers from those who love to shop and have a passion for it can be determined based on clinical characteristics. The hallmark of compulsive shopping is continued shopping despite adverse consequences caused by the shopping. The urges to shop can be intense, frequent, and similar in quality to cravings for food, drugs, or sex. Compulsive shoppers report an insatiable drive to shop and obtain items, not out of necessity or anxiety (ie, what if they run out of the item I want?) but instead by a need to stay in "action" with the shopping process.

The consequences from compulsive shopping can be variable and hidden.[98] No one "overdoses" from shopping, nor do they appear intoxicated, and the presence of

> **Box 5**
> **CASE STUDY: The depressed shopper**
>
> Jenny is a 32-year-old white female with a history of borderline personality disorder, major depressive disorder, and generalized anxiety disorder. She presents to the office for management of depressive symptoms triggered by a recent divorce. During the intake process, she denies drug or alcohol abuse but reports large financial debts and not having any time to "work on herself." When asked what she likes to do for relaxation, she states nothing, other than shopping. Ever since she was a teenager, she enjoyed shopping, especially trying on new clothes, browsing new products, and talking to retail salespeople. On further history, she reported that over the last 4 years, concurrent with her worsening mood, she reports shopping daily, oftentimes for 4 to 5 hours in search of material goods that she wants and often classifies as "needs." Her parents no longer are able to support her, which has led to increasing tension and her resorting to criminal behaviors to finance her shopping. She has taken loans out, committed insurance fraud, and turned to prostitution to obtain money to shop with. She describes shopping as the only activity that makes her feel "normal" and that when she doesn't have the money or time to shop, she gets irritated and anxious and has trouble sleeping. She uses the clothes she buys once or twice and then throws them into public storage. At this time, she has also fallen into a pattern of buying things, returning them for store credit, and then buying newer items. Treatment for the shopping behaviors initially focused on helping her to accept her diagnosis and recognize that reducing her shopping would significantly improve her life. Behavioral strategies such as identifying internal and external triggers to shop, reducing time spent alone, cutting up all forms of credit, and liquidating her possessions and assets were accomplished in the next 6 to 8 weeks. To reduce urges to shop, Jenny was encouraged to attend Debtor's Anonymous and to seek out additional socialization. After 12 weeks, Jenny felt considerably better but still struggled with the urges/cravings to shop, particularly around advertised specials or whenever she would get a courtesy call from one of her stores.

purchases, large or small, is not a telltale sign of compulsive behavior. As one of our patients simply stated "It's not how much you spend but that you spend it."

Compulsive shoppers incur significant harm in psychological and social domains, whereas normal shoppers do not. Examples of the more common consequences include financial, lost time and productivity, and negative impact on personal relationships. Psychologically, compulsive shoppers report intense and long-lasting feelings of guilt and shame related to their shopping.[97] They hide their purchases and, often, never use them or do not even take them out of the packaging. Even when they want to return their purchases, overwhelming guilt and shame can prevent that from happening, further deepening the impact of an unwanted purchase. 80% of patients are female; however, this apparent gender discrepancy is not well understood and may be a function of sociocultural factors, bias pertaining to treatment seekers, or other characteristics of this disorder.[93] Consistent with gender stereotypes, men tend to acquire electronics, gadgets, and tickets to concerts or sporting events, whereas women have been known to seek out clothing, accessories, and household items.[99]

Very little is known about the clinical course of compulsive shoppers, but based on the clinical experience of the patients from the UCLA Impulse Control Disorders Clinic, this appears to be a chronic, relapsing condition. The onset appears to be during the 18- to 25-year-old period, and the advent of online shopping, liberal return policies, and the flooding of retail marketing and advertising create a 24-hour access and availability issue for compulsive shoppers.

Co-occurring mood and anxiety disorders, substance use disorders, eating disorders, and other disorders of impulse control are common, as are Axis II disorders. Investigators have found that compulsive shopping in bipolar disorder is associated with exacerbation of both disorders but that they are separate.[100] In another study,

---

Box 6
Proposed criteria for compulsive shopping[29]

- Frequent preoccupation with buying
- Irresistible, intrusive, and/or senseless impulses to buy
- Frequently buying unneeded items or more than can be afforded
- Shopping for periods longer than intended
- Experiencing adverse consequences, such as marked distress, impaired social or occupational functioning, and/or financial problems
- Shopping behaviors not due to a manic episode[118]

---

researchers found that female compulsive shoppers were much more likely to also be suffering from mood, anxiety, and eating disorders compared with the general population.[101] Personality traits, such as emphasis on materialism and impulsivity, have also been shown to be associated with compulsive shoppers compared with healthy controls.[102]

Assessment and Diagnostic Considerations

At this time, there are no formal criteria for compulsive shopping, nor is this condition listed in the DSM-IV. Proposed criteria are similar to those of substance-related disorders and impulse control disorders (**Box 6**). Screening and assessments instruments, such as the Compulsive Buying Scale, are available to guide assessment.[103] Before making a diagnosis of compulsive shopping, other diagnoses must be excluded, such as bipolar disorder, obsessive-compulsive disorder, depression, or Axis II conditions.

Although there is overlap between obsessive-compulsive disorder, hoarding, and compulsive shopping, there are a few important distinguishing characteristics.[104] Compulsive shoppers describe an ego-syntonic quality to the shopping process. The shopping brings psychic relief, even if it is momentary, and there is an initial phase of shopping that is rewarding and emotionally positive.[105] In contrast, hoarding disorders or obsessive-compulsive disorders are about relieving tension or minimizing anxiety caused by the perceived possibility that something undesired will happen.

Medical conditions that have been associated with the development of compulsive shopping, and therefore must be ruled out during the assessment, include frontal lobe injuries, degenerative neurologic conditions such as progressive supranuclear palsy, traumatic brain injuries, and associations with dopamine agonists used for Parkinson's disease and restless leg syndromes.[106-109]

Interventions and Treatment Approaches

Pharmacological treatment

There have been several case reports and open-labeled trials of antidepressants and mood stabilizers to address the signs and symptoms of this condition.[110,111] Grant reported on a case series of naltrexone to block the associated urges and cravings for compulsive shopping.[112] One case report of topiramate suggests potential therapeutic benefit.[113] Double-blind placebo, controlled trials are lacking primarily because of a lack of funding support for these trials.[114]

Psychological treatment

Expert consensus has suggested that a combination of therapies effective for addiction or anxiety disorders may also be effective for these patients.[115] Cognitive-behavioral therapy and cognitive restructuring have also been shown to be helpful under controlled conditions.[116,117] The emphasis of these treatment approaches is establishing healthy purchasing patterns, restructuring maladaptive thoughts and negative feelings associated with shopping and buying, and developing healthy coping skills.

Debtor's Anonymous is a 12-step support group targeting those who feel that they have lost control over spending (called *debting*) and that through the power of 12-step fellowship and support they can overcome this. No empirical data on the effectiveness of Debtor's Anonymous exists, although nearly 500 chapters are active in the United States. Furthermore, it does not stipulate a difference between compulsive purchasing and compulsive shopping, thereby clouding the picture of whether this is a helpful intervention.

SUMMARY

Behavioral addictions can present in a variety of subtle and deceptive patterns. Because of the intense shame, guilt, and embarrassment felt by patients, it may fall to providers to utilize screening tools and deeper interviewing techniques to uncover the extent of these behaviors. Identifying when the line is crossed from recreation/ habit to psychopathology relies on understanding current diagnostic criteria and consideration of cultural, ethnic, and local community standards. Individuals are also likely to cross back and forth between this line of pathology and habit, further clouding provider's opinions of diagnosis; therefore, tracking and monitoring these symptoms over time is critical to establishing patterns of use and documenting ongoing consequences. Treatment for these conditions is emerging slowly, and treatment outcomes for these conditions appear to be similar to those with other addictive disorders.

REFERENCES

1. Mudry TE, Hodgins DC, el-Guebaly N, et al. Conceptualizing excessive behaviour syndromes: a systematic review. Current Psychiatry Reviews 2011;7:138–51.
2. Grant JE, Potenza MN, Weinstein A, et al. Introduction to behavioral addictions. Am J Drug Alcohol Abuse 2010;36(5):233–41.
3. Marshall LE, Briken P. Assessment, diagnosis, and management of hypersexual disorders. Curr Opin Psychiatry 2010;23(6):570–3.
4. Bancroft J. Sexual behavior that is "out of control": a theoretical conceptual approach. Psychiatr Clin North Am 2008;31(4):593–601.
5. Kafka MP. "What is sexual addiction?" A response to Stephen Levine. J Sex Marital Ther 2010;36(3): 276–81.
6. Kafka MP. Hypersexual disorder: a proposed diagnosis for DSM-V. Arch Sex Behav 2010;39(2):377–400.
7. Bancroft J, Vukadinovic Z. Sexual addiction, sexual compulsivity, sexual impulsivity, or what? Toward a theoretical model. J Sex Res 2004;41(3):225–34.
8. Dodge B, Reece M, Herbenick D, et al. Relations between sexually transmitted infection diagnosis and sexual compulsivity in a community-based sample of men who have sex with men. Sex Transm Infect 2008;84(4):324–7.
9. Coleman E, Horvath KJ, Miner M, et al. Compulsive sexual behavior and risk for unsafe sex among internet using men who have sex with men. Arch Sex Behav 2010;39(5):1045–53.
10. Garcia FD, Thibaut F. Sexual addictions. Am J Drug Alcohol Abuse 2010;36(5): 254–60.
11. Dodge B, Reece M, Cole SL, et al. Sexual compulsivity among heterosexual college students. J Sex Res 2004;41(4):343–50.

12. Raymond NC, Coleman E, Miner MH. Psychiatric comorbidity and compulsive/impulsive traits in compulsive sexual behavior. Compr Psychiatry 2003;44(5):370–80.

13. Kafka MP, Prentky RA. Preliminary observations of DSM-III-R axis I comorbidity in men with paraphilias and paraphilia-related disorders. J Clin Psychiatry 1994;55(11):481–7.

14. Black DW, Kehrberg LL, Flumerfelt DL, et al. Characteristics of 36 subjects reporting compulsive sexual behavior. Am J Psychiatry 1997;154(2):243–9.

15. Reid RC, Carpenter BN, Gilliland R, et al. Problems of self-concept in a patient sample of hypersexual men with attention-deficit disorder. J Addict Med 2011;5(2):134–40.

16. Reid RC, Harper JM, Anderson EH. Coping strategies used by hypersexual patients to defend against the painful effects of shame. Clin Psychol Psychother 2009;16(2):125–38.

17. Reid RC, Garos S, Carpenter BN, et al. A surprising finding related to executive control in a patient sample of hypersexual men. J Sex Med 2011;8(8):2227–36.

18. Reid RC, Carpenter BN, Spackman M, et al. Alexithymia, emotional instability, and vulnerability to stress proneness in patients seeking help for hypersexual behavior. J Sex Marital Ther 2008;34(2):133–49.

19. Chaney MP, Blalock AC. Boredom proneness, social connectedness, and sexual addiction among men who have sex with male internet users. Journal of Addictions and Offender Counseling 2006;26(2):111–22.

20. Albright JM. Sex in America online: an exploration of sex, marital status, and sexual identity in internet sex seeking and its impacts. J Sex Res 2008;45(2):175–86.

21. Coleman E. Is your patient suffering from compulsive sexual behavior? Psychiatric Annals 1992;22:320–5.

22. Carnes PJ, Green BA, Merlo LJ, et al. PATHOS: a brief screening application for assessing sexual addiction. J Addict Med 2012;6(1):29–34.

23. Skegg K, Nada-Raja S, Dickson N, et al. Perceived "out of control" sexual behavior in a cohort of young adults from the Dunedin Multidisciplinary Health and Development Study. Arch Sex Behav 2010;39(4):968–78.

24. Winters J, Christoff K. Gorzalka BB. Dysregulated sexuality and high sexual desire: distinct constructs? Arch Sex Behav 2010;39(5):1029–43.

25. Parsons JT, Kelly BC, Bimbi DS, et al. Explanations for the origins of sexual compulsivity among gay and bisexual men. Arch Sex Behav 2008;37(5):817–26.

26. Miner MH, Raymond N, Mueller BA, et al. Preliminary investigation of the impulsive and neuroanatomical characteristics of compulsive sexual behavior. Psychiatry Res, 2009;174(2):146–51.

27. Reid RC, Karim R, McCrory E, et al. Self-reported differences on measures of executive function and hypersexual behavior in a patient and community sample of men. Int J Neurosci 2010;120(2):120–7.

28. Hook JN, Hook JP, Davis DE, et al. Measuring sexual addiction and compulsivity: a critical review of instruments. J Sex Marital Ther 2010;36(3):227–60.

29. Kafka M. Psychopharmacologic treatments for nonparaphilic compulsive sexual behaviors. CNS Spectr 2000;5(1):49–59.

30. Grant JE, Kim SW. A case of kleptomania and compulsive sexual behavior treated with naltrexone. Ann Clin Psychiatry 2001;13(4):229–31.

31. Goodman A, Diagnosis and treatment of sexual addiction. J Sex Marital Ther 1993;19(3):225–51.

32. Reid RC, Woolley SR. Using emotionally focused therapy for couples to resolve attachment ruptures created by hypersexual behavior. Journal of Sexual Addiction and Compulsivity 2006;13:219–39.

33. Carnes PJ. Sexual addiction and compulsion: recognition, treatment, and recovery. CNS Spectr 2000;5(10):63–72.

34. Bird MH. Sexual addiction and marriage and family therapy: facilitating individual and relationship healing through couple therapy. J Marital Fam Ther 2006;32(3):297–311.

35. Parker J, Guest D. The integration of psychotherapy and 12-step programs in sexual addiction treatment. In: Carnes PJ, Adams KM, Editors. Clinical management of sex addiction. New York: Brunner-Routledge; 2002. p. 115–24.

36. Shaffer H, Hall M. Updating and refining prevalence estimates of disordered gambling behaviour in the United States and Canada. Can J Public Health Revue canadienne de santé publique 2002;92(3):168–72.

37. American Psychiatric Association. Diagnostic and statistical manual of mental disorders DSM-IV-TR (Text-Revision). Washington, DC: American Psychiatric Association Publishing; 2000.

38. Shaffer HJ, Hall MN, Vander Bilt J. Estimating the prevalence of disordered gambling behavior in the United States and Canada: a research synthesis. Am J Public Health 1999;89(9):1369–76.

39. Hodgins DC, Stea JN, Grant JE. Gambling disorders. Lancet 2011;378(9806):1874–84.

40. Ladouceur R. Gambling: the hidden addiction. Can J Psychiatry 2004;49(8):501–3.

41. Lorains FK, Cowlishaw S, Thomas SA. Prevalence of comorbid disorders in problem and pathological gambling: systematic review and meta analysis of population surveys. Addiction 2011;106(3):490–8.

42. Zimmerman M, Chelminski I, Young D. A psychometric evaluation of the DSM-IV pathological gambling diagnostic criteria. J Gambl Stud 2006;22(3):329–37.

43. Stinchfield R. Reliability, validity, and classification accuracy of a measure of DSM-IV diagnostic criteria for pathological gambling. Am J Psychiatry 2003;160(1):180.

44. Djamshidian A, Cardoso F, Grosset D, et al. Pathological gambling in Parkinson's disease—a review of the literature. Mov Disord 2011;26(11):1976–84.

45. Sharpe L. A reformulated cognitive-behavioral model of problem gambling: a biopsychosocial perspective. Clinl Psychol Rev 2002;22(1):1–25.

46. Blaszczynski A, Nower L. A pathways model of problem and pathological gambling. Addiction 2002;97(5):487–99.

47. Van Hols RJ, van dan Brink W, Veltman DJ, et al. Why gamblers fail to win: a review of cognitive and neuroimaging findings in pathological gambling. Neuroscience & Biobehavioral Reviews 2010;34(1):87–107.

48. Mamikonyan E, Siderowf AD, Duda JE, et al. Long-term follow-up of impulse control disorders in Parkinson's disease. Mov Disord 2008;23(1):75–80.

49. Gupta R, Derevensky J. Familial and social influences on juvenile gambling behavior. J Gamble Stud 1997;13(3):179–92.

50. Gupta R, Derevensky JL. Adolescent gambling behavior: a prevalence study and examination of the correlates associated with problem gambling. J Gamb Stud 1998;14(4):319–45.

51. Dickson L, Derevensky J, Gupta R. Youth gambling problems: examining risk and protective factors. International Gambling Studies 2008;8(1):25–47.

52. Jacobs DF. Juvenile gambling in North America: an analysis of long term trends and future prospects. J Gambl Stud 2000;16(2):119–52.

53. Raylu N, Oei T.P.Role of culture in gambling and problem gambling. Clinical Psychology Review 2004;23(8):1087–114.
54. Loo JMY, Raylu N, Oei TPS. Gambling among the Chinese: a comprehensive review. Clinical Psychol Rev 2008;28(7):1152–66.
55. Parhami I, Siani A, Campos MD, et al. Gambling in the Iranian-American community and an assessment of motives: a Case Study. Int J Ment Health Addict 2012. [Epub ahead of print].
56. Pulford J, Bellringer M, Abbott M, et al. Reasons for seeking help for a gambling problem: the experiences of gamblers who have sought specialist assistance and the perceptions of those who have not. J Gambl Stud 2009;25(1):19–32.
57. Blaszczynski A, Farrell E. A case series of 44 completed gambling-related suicides. J Gambl Stud 1998;14(2):93–109.
58. Zangeneh M. Suicide and gambling. Australian e-Journal for the Advancement of Mental Health 2005;4(1):1–3.
59. Ledgerwood DM, Petry NM. Gambling and suicidality in treatment-seeking pathological gamblers. J Nerv Ment Dis 2004;192(10):711.
60. Petry NM, Kiluk BD. Suicidal ideation and suicide attempts in treatment-seeking pathological gamblers. J Nerv Ment Dis 2002;190(7):462–9.
61. Battersby M, Tolchard B, Scurrah M, et al. Suicide ideation and behaviour in people with pathological gambling attending a treatment service. Int J Ment Health Addict 2006;4(3):233–46.
62. Toce Gerstein M, Gerstein DR, Volberg RA. A hierarchy of gambling disorders in the community. Addiction 2003;98(12):1661–72.
63. Strong DR, Kahler CW. Evaluation of the continuum of gambling problems using the DSM IV. Addiction 2007;102(5):713–21.
64. Blaszczynski A. Problem gambling: we should measure harm rather than 'cases'. Addiction 2009;104(7):1072–4.
65. Rodgers B, Caldwell T, Butterworth P. Measuring gambling participation. Addiction 2009;104(7):1065–9.
66. Namrata R, Oei TPS. Factors associated with the severity of gambling problems in a community gambling treatment agency. Int J Ment Health Addict 2009;7(1):124–37.
67. Hodgins D, El-Guebaly N. Natural and treatment-assisted recovery from gambling problems: a comparison of resolved and active gamblers. Addiction 2000;95(5):777–89.
68. Nower L, Blaszczynski A. Binge gambling: a neglected concept. Internat Gambl Stud 2003;3(1):23–35.
69. Gerstein DR, Murphy S, Toce M, et al. Gambling impact and behavior study: report to the National Gambling Impact Study Commission. Chicago (IL): National Opinion Research Center, University of Chicago; 1999.
70. De La Vina L, Bernstein D. The impact of gambling on personal bankruptcy rates. J Socio-Econ 2002;31(5):503–9.
71. Boardman B, Perry JJ. Access to gambling and declaring personal bankruptcy. J Socio Econ 2007;36(5):789–801.
72. Grant JE, et al. Pathologic gambling and bankruptcy. Compr Psychiatry 2010;51(2):115–20.
73. Folino JO, Abait PE. Pathological gambling and criminality. Curr Opin Psychiatry 2009;22(5):477–81.
74. Potenza MN, Steinberg MA, McLaughlin SD, et al. Illegal behaviors in problem gambling: analysis of data from a gambling helpline. J Am Acad Psychiatry Law 2000;28(4):389–403.

75. Shaw M, Forbush KT, Schlinder J, et al. The effect of pathological gambling on families, marriages, and children. CNS Spectrums 2007;12(8):615–22.
76. Korman LM, Collins J, Dutton D, et al. Problem gambling and intimate partner violence. J Gambl Stud 2008;24(1):13–23.
77. Afifi TO, Brownridge DA, MacMillan H, et al. The relationship of gambling to intimate partner violence and child maltreatment in a nationally representative sample. J Psychiatric Res 2010;44(5):331–7.
78. Goudriaan AE, Oosterlaan J, de Beurs E, et al. Pathological gambling: a comprehensive review of biobehavioral findings. Neurosci Biobehav Rev 2004;28(2):123–41.
79. Morasco BJ, Petry NM. Gambling problems and health functioning in individuals receiving disability. Disabil Rehab 2006;28(10):619–23.
80. Morasco BJ, Pietrzak RH, Blanco C, et al. Health problems and medical utilization associated with gambling disorders: results from the National Epidemiologic Survey on Alcohol and Related Conditions. Psychosom Med 2006;68(6):976–81.
81. Potenza MN, Fiellin DA, Heninger GR, et al. Gambling: an addictive behavior with health and primary care implications. J Gen Intern Med 2002;17(9):721–32.
82. Parhami I, Siani A, Rosenthal RJ, et al. Sleep and gambling severity in a community sample of gamblers. J Addict Dis 2012;31(1):67–79.
83. Parhami I, Siani A, Rosenthal RJ, et al. Pathological gambling, problem gambling and sleep complaints: an analysis of the National Comorbidity Survey: Replication (NCS-r). J Gambl Stud 2012. [Epub ahead of print].
84. Achab S, Khazaal Y. Psychopharmacological treatment in pathological gambling: a critical review. Curr Pharm Des 2011;17(14):1389–95.
85. Gainsbury S, Blaszczynski A. Online self-guided interventions for the treatment of problem gambling. International Gambling Studies 2011;11(3):289–308.
86. Petry NM, Weinstock J, Ledgerwood DM, et al. A randomized trial of brief interventions for problem and pathological gamblers. J Consult Clin Psychol 2008;76:318–28.
87. Gooding P, Tarrier N. A systematic review and meta-analysis of cognitive-behavioural interventions to reduce problem gambling: hedging our bets? Behav Res Ther 2009;47(7):592–607.
88. Lejoyeux M, Weinstein A. Compulsive buying. Am J Drug Alcohol Abuse 2010;36(5):248–53.
89. Tavares H, Lobo DS, Fuentes D, et al. [Compulsive buying disorder: a review and a case vignette]. Rev Bras Psiquiatr 2008;30(Suppl 1):S16–23.
90. Koran LM, Faber RJ, Aboujaoude E, et al. Estimated prevalence of compulsive buying behavior in the United States. Am J Psychiatry 2006;163(10):1806–12.
91. Mueller A, Mitchell JE, Crosby RD, et al. Estimated prevalence of compulsive buying in Germany and its association with sociodemographic characteristics and depressive symptoms. Psychiatry Res 2010;180(2–3):137–42.
92. Grant JE, Potenza MN, Krishnan-Sarin S, et al. Shopping problems among high school students. Compr Psychiatry 2011;52(3):247–52.
93. Black DW, Shaw M, Blum N. Pathological gambling and compulsive buying: do they fall within an obsessive-compulsive spectrum? Dialogues Clin Neurosci 2010;12(2):175–85.
94. Kellett S, Bolton JV. Compulsive buying: a cognitive-behavioural model. Clin Psychol Psychother 2009;16(2):83–99.
95. Filomensky TZ, Almeida KM, Castro Nogueira MC, et al. Neither bipolar nor obsessive-compulsive disorder: compulsive buyers are impulsive acquirers. Compr Psychiatry 2012. [Epub ahead of print].
96. Boermans JA, Egger JI. [Compulsive buying or oniomania: an overview]. Tijdschr Psychiatr 2010;52(1):29–39.

97. Lejoyeux M, Mathieu K, Embouazza H, et al. Prevalence of compulsive buying among customers of a Parisian general store. Compr Psychiatry 2007;48(1):42–6.
98. Black DW. A review of compulsive buying disorder. World Psychiatry 2007;6(1): 14–8.
99. Black DW. Compulsive buying disorder: definition, assessment, epidemiology and clinical management. CNS Drugs 2001;15(1):17–27.
100. Kesebir S, Isitmez S, Gundogar D. Compulsive buying in bipolar disorder: Is it a comorbidity or a complication? J Affect Disord 2012;136(3):797–802.
101. Mueller A, Muhlhans B, Silbermann A, et al. [Compulsive buying and psychiatric comorbidity]. Psychother Psychosom Med Psychol 2009;59(8):291–9.
102. Mueller A, Mitchell JE, Peterson LA, et al. Depression, materialism, and excessive Internet use in relation to compulsive buying. Compr Psychiatry 2011;52(4):420–4.
103. Manolis C, Roberts JA, Kashyap V. A critique and comparison of two scales from fifteen years of studying compulsive buying. Psychol Rep 2008;102(1):153–65.
104. Frost RO, Steketee G, Tolin DF. Comorbidity in hoarding disorder. Depress Anxiety 2011;28(10):876–84.
105. Dell'Osso B, Allen A, Altamura AC, et al. Impulsive-compulsive buying disorder: clinical overview. Aust N Z J Psychiatry 2008;42(4):259–66.
106. Rochat L, Beni C, Billieux J, et al. How impulsivity relates to compulsive buying and the burden perceived by caregivers after moderate-to-severe traumatic brain injury. Psychopathology 2011;44(3):158–64.
107. Reiff J, Jost WH. Drug-induced impulse control disorders in Parkinson's disease. J Neurol 2011;258(Suppl 2):S323–7.
108. O'Sullivan SS, Djamshidian A, Ahmed Z, et al. Impulsive-compulsive spectrum behaviors in pathologically confirmed progressive supranuclear palsy. Mov Disord 2010;25(5):638–42.
109. Schreglmann SR, Gantenbein AR, Eisele G, et al. Transdermal rotigotine causes impulse control disorders in patients with restless legs syndrome. Parkinsonism Relat Disord 2012;18(2):207–9.
110. Koran LM, Bullock KD, Hartston HJ, et al. Citalopram treatment of compulsive shopping: an open-label study. J Clin Psychiatry 2002;63(8):704–8.
111. Koran LM, Aboujaoude EN, Solvason B, et al. Escitalopram for compulsive buying disorder: a double-blind discontinuation study. J Clin Psychopharmacol 2007;27(2): 225–7.
112. Bullock K, Koran L. Psychopharmacology of compulsive buying. Drugs Today (Barc) 2003;39(9):695–700.
113. Guzman CS, Filomensky T, Tavares H. Compulsive buying treatment with topiramate, a case report. Rev Bras Psiquiatr 2007;29(4):383–4.
114. Di Nicola M, Martinotti G, Mazza M, et al. Quetiapine as add-on treatment for bipolar I disorder with comorbid compulsive buying and physical exercise addiction. Prog Neuropsychopharmacol Biol Psychiatry 2010;34(4):713–4.
115. Donahue CB, Odlaug BL, Grant JE. Compulsive buying treated with motivational interviewing and imaginal desensitization. Ann Clin Psychiatry 2011;23(3):226–7.
116. Filomensky TZ, Tavares H. Cognitive restructuring for compulsive buying. Rev Bras Psiquiatr 2009;31(1):77–8.
117. Mueller A, Mueller U, Silbermann A, et al. A randomized, controlled trial of group cognitive-behavioral therapy for compulsive buying disorder: posttreatment and 6-month follow-up results. J Clin Psychiatry 2008;69(7):1131–8.
118. McElroy SL, Keck PE, Pope HG, et al. Compulsive buying: a report of 20 cases. J Clin Psychiatry 1994;55(6): 242–8.

Advances in Opioid Antagonist Treatment for Opioid Addiction

Walter Ling, MD[a],*, Larissa Mooney, MD[a], Li-Tzy Wu, ScD[b]

KEYWORDS

- Addiction treatment • Depot naltrexone • Opioid dependence • Relapse

KEY POINTS

- The major problem with oral naltrexone is noncompliance. Administration of naltrexone as an intramuscular injection may be less onerous and improve compliance because it occurs only once a month (ie, extended-release depot naltrexone).
- To initiate treatment with extended-release depot naltrexone, steps should be taken to ensure that the patient is sufficiently free from physical dependence on opioids (eg, detoxification).
- Research on naltrexone in combination with other medications suggests many opportunities for studying mixed receptor activities in the treatment of opioid and other drug addictions.

PERSPECTIVE ON OPIOID ANTAGONIST TREATMENT FOR ADDICTION

Naltrexone, an opioid antagonist derived from the analgesic oxymorphone, was synthesized as EN-1639A by Blumberg and colleagues in 1967. Four years later, in 1971, naltrexone was selected for high-priority development as a treatment for opioid addiction by the Special Action Office for Drug Abuse Prevention, an office created by President Nixon and put under the leadership of Dr Jerome Jaffe.

Extinction Model

The rationale for the antagonist approach to treating opioid addiction had been advanced by Dr Abraham Wikler a decade earlier, based largely on the extinction model explored in animal behavioral studies. It was believed that by blocking the euphorogenic effects of opioids at the opioid receptors, opiate use would become

Disclosures: Dr Ling has served as a consultant to Reckitt Benckiser Pharmaceuticals and to Alkermes, Inc. Dr Mooney and Dr Wu report no relationships with commercial companies with any interest in the article's subject matters.
[a] UCLA Department of Psychiatry and Biobehavioral Sciences, UCLA Integrated Substance Abuse Programs, 1640 South Sepulveda, Suite 120, Los Angeles, CA 90025, USA; [b] Duke University School of Medicine, Duke University Medical Center, PO 3419, Durham, NC 27710, USA
* Corresponding author.
E-mail address: lwalter@ucla.edu

Psychiatr Clin N Am 35 (2012) 297–308
doi:10.1016/j.psc.2012.03.002
0193-953X/12/$ – see front matter © 2012 Elsevier Inc. All rights reserved.

less rewarding and less desirable and, in time, opiate users—animals and humans—would learn to stop.

Unfortunately humans do not always behave like animals. When an animal keeps pressing a lever and gets no rewarding drugs, it stops pressing the lever; however, when human addicts discover that their medication keeps them from getting high, they stop taking their medication instead. It seems that human beings make decisions to use or not use drugs based on a cognitive process. Even the worst of compulsive gamblers will not put money into a slot machine that has an "out of order" sign on it. The decision and action are not from a gradual process—as in extinction—but are immediate; it is a matter of cognition, not extinction. Even though the compulsive gambler may claim to have no control over his gambling habit, it is obvious that he does have control; he stops putting money into the machine the instant he learns that there is no payoff; extinction does not apply here.

NALTREXONE
Properties

Pharmacologically, naltrexone is almost an ideal medication and it was once regarded as such.

- It completely blocks the euphoric effects of opioids.
- It has no reinforcing effects of its own.
- It is relatively safe and easy to take, with few side effects.

Unfortunately, these favorable clinical properties did not translate into clinical success.

Clinical Experience

A major reason for its lack of clinical success was poor medication compliance, so much so that the pharmacologically "perfect drug" was becoming a "victimless cure." Dr Richard Resnick, a psychiatrist and an early clinical investigator, noted that naltrexone is ego-dystonic to an addict. Dr David Smith, who founded the Haight-Ashbury Free Clinic, said "addicts do not take naltrexone because they can't get high." My old friend and colleague Don Wesson simply notes that addicts do not like to take naltrexone because it ruins their lives.

Still, it is probably too pessimistic to say that the early clinical experience with naltrexone was a complete failure; there were certain special groups of patients who did very well with oral naltrexone treatments: Physicians, nurses, pharmacists, and lawyers who were under threat of losing their professional licenses. Prisoners on work release and parolees also seemed to do well. A common thread among these groups includes their having something to lose, the immediacy of the consequences of failure to comply with treatment, and, for the professionals at least, their knowledge that life could be quite different.

Agonist Versus Antagonist

Our enthusiasm for naltrexone despite early clinical failure can be explained, in part, by the treatment success in select subgroups of patients as noted; additional support for naltrexone development came from societal attitude toward addicts and addiction. The US social structure of authorities, policymakers, funding agencies, the public, and even clinicians had all been ambivalent about full agonist pharmacotherapy (methadone) from the very beginning, and the antagonist option held great appeal. Methadone treatment in the United States is the most regulated medical practice. We were never comfortable with giving our addicted patients something so close to their drug of abuse, clinical benefit and lives saved notwithstanding. We were determined to wean our patients off their drug of abuse or at least treat them with something they could not use to get high. Naltrexone looked like the answer.

Noncompliance with Naltrexone and Subsequent Opioid Overdose

The major problem with oral naltrexone is noncompliance, and that noncompliance and patient-initiated termination of naltrexone therapy have been linked with opioid overdose at a rate higher than occurs with methadone treatment,[1,2] possibly because of the decreased tolerance or receptor supersensitivity after ongoing opioid receptor blockade. So, although the antagonist approach is certainly plausible and has worked to treat addiction in controlled experimental conditions and in limited practice with select patient groups, the fact remains that oral naltrexone did not work for most opioid addicts, especially because of poor medication adherence. The answer to poor adherence to oral naltrexone was, therefore, an extended-release formulation as depot naltrexone.

DEPOT NALTREXONE
Development

Despite naltrexone's lack of early clinical success, investigators and policymakers as well as funding agencies reasoned that what was needed was a long-acting formulation of the medication that can be given to patients and, once administered, remains in effect regardless of patients' desires or behaviors; hence, the development of depot naltrexone, with the first attempts dating back to the 1970s. The idea was to produce a preparation that would last from weeks to months, thus relieving the addicted patients of their need to make daily decisions to take an antagonist medication that keeps them from getting high. In addition to the fact that patients are generally not keen on taking the medication, developing a reliable extended-release product was not technologically simple. It took nearly 30 years to get the first US Food and Drug Administration (FDA)-approved form of extended-release naltrexone to the market.

While the scientists were busy developing a more ideal formulation of naltrexone for opioid addicts, no one seems to have figured that perhaps we should ask our patients whether they would like to have such a medication. Patient compliance was poor in the early clinical trials with naltrexone as a liquid, which was very bitter. A tablet formulation did not improve compliance. Administration of naltrexone as an intramuscular injection may be less onerous because it occurs only once a month. Early-phase clinical experience with depot naltrexone has not wholly resolved the question about patients' acceptance of or disinclination toward extended-release naltrexone by injection, because we are seeing limited uptake in practice.

Studies for the Treatment of Opioid Addiction

Research on depot naltrexone formulations has found positive results. As demonstrated by Comer and others,[3–5] 384 mg naltrexone delivered in extended-release depot formulation blocked the reinforcing, subjective, and physiologic effects of up to 25 mg of heroin, and provided consistent plasma levels for approximately 30 days.[6–8] Importantly, at this dose, naltrexone resulted in retention of more than 80% of patients in treatment at 6 weeks versus 40% for placebo.[4] In comparison with the oral formulation, patients on depot naltrexone showed significantly higher rates of abstinence and better treatment outcomes at 12-month follow-up.[9] Adverse events were minimal and limited to local responses at the injection site.[10]

Extended-release naltrexone preparation was approved by the FDA in October 2010, based predominantly on data from a large trial set in Russia, where no agonist pharmacotherapy is available for treatment of opioid addiction. In the approved formulation (XR-NTX [Vivitrol]; Alkermes, Inc., Waltham, MA, USA), naltrexone is slowly released from microspheres composed of a polymer, poly-(D, L-lactide-co-glycolide), which is also used in dissolvable surgical sutures. With its approval came a surge of interest in antagonist treatment for opioid addiction because the medication offered an alternative to the mainstay of methadone maintenance and the rapidly increasing popularity of buprenorphine, a partial agonist. XR-NTX has not yet commanded a staunch following, although its use is perhaps on a modest upswing. The focus of this article is on the use of XR-NTX, the only approved depot naltrexone medication available for addiction treatment; the basic information will be generally applicable to other extended-release depot forms as they come to market in North America and internationally.

Lessons from the Large-Scale Trial of XR-NTX for Opioid Addiction

Study data from the industry-sponsored trial in Russia were provided to the FDA in the summer of 2010. These data formed the foundation for the FDA approval of XR-NTX to treat opioid addiction and prevent relapse in patients who have been detoxified from opioids. The study results were published in August 2011,[11] and the article provided limited guidance for clinicians who would bring XR-NTX into clinical practice. However, clinicians interested in using XR-NTX in treating opioid addiction still face a steep learning curve. The Russian study and findings from previous work made evident the following:

- XR-NTX improves treatment retention and substance use outcomes (eg, more weeks abstinent, fewer opioid-positive urine analyses) relative to placebo, which may be partially attributable to better engagement in behavioral therapies via more attendance.
- The 6-month regimen may not suit everybody; only 57.9% of the XR-NTX patients and 41.9% of the placebo patients received all 6 monthly injections.
- The placebo group did not fare so poorly, notwithstanding the significant difference in outcomes; of the 250 participants (126 in the active condition, 124 in the placebo condition), 45 patients on XR-NTX had "total confirmed abstinence" (all urine tests negative for opioids) compared with 28 in the placebo group. One could argue for a strong placebo effect or a strong counseling condition that helped the placebo group to remain somewhat free of opioids; however, XR-NTX was superior to placebo in its ability to prevent relapse to opioid use.
- XR-NTX has an anti-craving effect; opioid craving scores were significantly reduced over the 24-week course of treatment relative to placebo, beginning at week 8 and persisting for the duration of the trial.

A larger trial with more comprehensive measures of patient characteristics conceivably would be able to tease outpatient typologies that may be most suited to XR-NTX and whose outcomes might be expected to be optimized as a result of engaging in depot antagonist pharmacotherapy. The Russian study found "no significant relation . . . between age, sex, or duration of opioid dependence and the rate of opioid-free urine tests" with a stable treatment effect across baseline variables. No notable findings emerged regarding safety or tolerability, although more information on the reason for many participants declining XR-NTX injections would have been helpful to inform future clinical use; perhaps the dataset can be reanalyzed to reveal possible associated characteristics to inform practice. For now, other research and clinical reports must stand as the source of limited information on the use of XR-NTX.

EXTENDED-RELEASE DEPOT NALTREXONE IN CURRENT PRACTICE
Primary Pharmacotherapy for Opioid Addiction

Detoxification required
Unlike methadone and buprenorphine, which with certain precautions can be given to opioid-addicted patients who are actively using illicit opioids, an antagonist can only be administered to patients who are not physically opioid dependent. This means most patients need to be "detoxified" to become opioid free before inducting them onto naltrexone. Unfortunately, many patients fail to complete detoxification and cannot begin antagonist treatment. The problem is troublesome enough with oral naltrexone, but it is much more serious an issue with the extended-release depot formulation because of its long duration of action and potential to precipitate prolonged opioid withdrawal.

Clinicians interested in using depot naltrexone in their practice need to learn to safely induct patients onto the medication. Detoxification can be done either in outpatient or inpatient settings, and a number of conventional methods are available. Although practiced by some clinicians, ultra-rapid detoxification under anesthesia is not recommended given the added risks of serious adverse events and lack of demonstrated benefit over other naltrexone induction methods.[12]

To initiate treatment with XR-NTX, steps should be taken to ensure that the patient is sufficiently free from physical dependence on opioids. These steps typically include confirmation of (1) absence of recent self-reported opioid use, (2) opioid-negative urine drug screen, and (3) tolerance of naloxone challenge test. According to package insert guidelines, patients should be opioid-free for at least 7 to 10 days before commencing XR-NTX treatment. However, rapid induction strategies have been utilized that incorporate the use of buprenorphine, clonidine, benzodiazepines, and other supportive medications; escalating doses of oral naltrexone may be incorporated to ensure absence of opioid withdrawal and facilitate initiation of XR-NTX treatment.

Administration Challenges for Psychiatrists
The administration of XR-NTX to patients, although not particularly complicated, is time consuming and not a routine part of the practice for psychiatrists. The medication has to be kept refrigerated until ready for use, then prepared and shaken as instructed and administered. This usually requires the medication to be taken out of the refrigerator about 1 to 2 hours before the patient's appointment. If the patient fails to keep the appointment, the medication needs to be promptly returned to refrigeration, within a few hours. Moreover, clinicians are reminded about the need for careful preparation of the patient. Because many psychiatric clinicians find the detoxification/pre-induction procedures difficult or impossible to perform, most refer the process to colleagues of other specialties.

Outcomes of Depot Naltrexone
It is intuitively tempting to want to compare treatment outcomes of depot naltrexone to agonist or partial agonist treatment (methadone or buprenorphine), even though they may serve very different patient populations. If one were to combine retention and abstinence as a composite outcome measure, depot naltrexone may yet compare favorably to agonist treatment; only time can tell. Such comparisons are not always useful or even fair; agonist treatment is not always available to certain patient

groups, such as opioid-dependent physicians or nurses, who can do well with an antagonist medication.

Side Effects of Naltrexone

The potential side effects of naltrexone include nausea, vomiting, worsening of depression, and suicidal thinking. When given in excessive doses, naltrexone carries a risk of hepatocellular injury, which is listed as a black box warning, though XR-NTX does not seem to have hepatotoxic effects at recommended doses. Still, it should be used cautiously in patients with active liver disease and is contraindicated in patients with acute hepatitis or liver failure. Injection site reactions may occur and may be characterized by pain, tenderness, erythema, induration, swelling, bruising, and pruritus. In some cases, reactions may be severe and may rarely require operative intervention.

XR-NTX blocks the effects of opioids for 28 days and, after cessation of treatment, patients may have reduced tolerance to opioids. Opioid use after treatment with XR-NTX, or the use of large amounts of opioids in an attempt to overcome the blockade, could result in opioid toxicity or potentially fatal overdose; however, these outcomes have not been observed in clinical trials of XR-NTX to date. Case reports have documented the potential to overcome mu blockade with opioids towards the end of the dosing interval, causing precipitated withdrawal upon subsequent administration of XR-NTX.[13]

COMBINATIONS WITH OTHER MEDICATIONS

Research on naltrexone in combination with other medications suggests many opportunities for studying mixed receptor activities in the treatment of opioid and other drug addictions (eg, increasing retention, relapse prevention, treatment for polysubstance abuse, pain management). Such combinations require careful evaluation by well-designed controlled clinical studies to understand the added therapeutic effects as well as safety issues.[14] The availability of XR-NTX represents a potentially valuable approach for replicating and improving studies done with oral naltrexone, because XR-NTX is likely to eliminate concern about medication compliance the adherence issue. Meanwhile, clinicians must balance the potential benefit against the added side effects and the potential for abuse of the added medications. Some of the most promising classes of medications that could be used in combination with XR-NTX are presented below.

Antidepressants

Depression is among the most prevalent comorbid mental health condition among opioid-addicted individuals,[15] which provides rationale to combine depot naltrexone with antidepressants. Landabaso and associates[16] conducted a randomized trial of 112 heroin addicts in Spain to test whether fluoxetine would enhance retention in a naltrexone treatment program. The investigators found that the combination of fluoxetine and naltrexone (n = 56) produced significantly greater retention than in patients given only naltrexone (n = 56). The findings show that placebo-controlled trials are warranted to assess further specific pharmacologic effects.

In Russia, Krupitsky and colleagues[17] used a randomized, placebo-controlled design to test the efficacy of oral naltrexone with or without fluoxetine for preventing relapse to heroin addiction and for reducing HIV risk, psychiatric symptoms, and outcome (n = 280). All patients received drug counseling with parental or significant-other involvement to encourage adherence. At the end of 6 months, 43% of subjects in the naltrexone/fluoxetine group, 36% in the naltrexone/placebo–fluoxetine group, 21% in the placebo–naltrexone/fluoxetine group, and 10% in the placebo–naltrexone/placebo–fluoxetine group remained in treatment and had not relapsed. Although adding fluoxetine did not improve the overall outcomes, women receiving naltrexone/fluoxetine showed a trend toward an advantage when compared with women receiving naltrexone/placebo–fluoxetine. Like other studies, dropout is a concern, which calls for randomized trials of long-acting depot naltrexone to determine whether it would improve retention.[17]

γ-Aminobutyric Acid Agonists

One factor that may contribute to noncompliance or relapse among opioid-dependent individuals undergoing naltrexone treatment has been reported to be related to stress, drug cue–induced cravings, and arousal responses or insomnia. Therefore, pharmacologic interventions that specifically target the negative affectivity, which co-occurs with drug cue– and stress–induced craving, could be of benefit in improving naltrexone treatment outcomes for opioid dependence.[18,19] Stella and co-workers[19] evaluated whether naltrexone combined with the benzodiazepine prazepam was more effective than naltrexone alone in keeping patients opioid free. Relapse rates over 6 months in 56 opioid-dependent subjects were compared among 4 groups with an equal sample size. Group 1 did not receive pharmacologic treatment (control), group 2 received naltrexone alone, group 3 received naltrexone plus placebo, and group 4 received naltrexone plus prazepam. Ten patients in group 1 relapsed within 3 months, 1 after 6 months, and 3 remained opioid free. Six patients in group 2 relapsed within 3 months, 2 after 6 months, and 6 remained opioid free. Seven patients from group 3 relapsed within 3 months, 1 after 6 months, and 6 remained opioid free. In group 4, 1 patient relapsed within 3 months and 1 patient after 6 months; 12 patients of this group remained opioid free. More patients in the naltrexone plus prazepam group also remained cannabis free than the other groups. The authors concluded that combination treatments seem to be a promising strategy in naltrexone long-term treatment of opioid addiction.

α-Adrenergic Agents

One approach with naltrexone aims to enhance the therapeutic effect for treating opioid addiction by the additive or synergistic effects of the drug combination. Naltrexone has, for instance, been combined with the α-adrenergic agents (eg, lofexidine and guanfacine) to take advantage of the latter medications' ability to reduce symptoms of opioid withdrawal.[20,21]

Sinha and colleagues[22] examined whether lofexidine would decrease stress- and cue-induced opioid craving and improve opioid abstinence in naltrexone-treated, opioid-dependent individuals. Eighteen opioid-dependent patients were stabilized for 4 weeks with naltrexone (50 mg daily) and lofexidine (2.4 mg bid) before entering a 4-week randomized, double-blind, placebo-controlled discontinuation study where 1 group continued on lofexidine for an additional 4 weeks, and the second was tapered to placebo (lofexidine–naltrexone vs placebo–naltrexone). Results indicated that the lofexidine–naltrexone group had higher opioid abstinence rates and improved relapse outcomes than the placebo–naltrexone group, and that lofexidine–naltrexone patients had significantly lower heart rates and an attenuated stress and drug cue-induced opioid craving response in the laboratory compared with the Placebo-naltrexone group. Sinha and associates concluded that combination therapies targeting both drug-related reinforcement (naltrexone) and stress- and cue-related aspects of drug seeking could be beneficial in reducing relapse in addictive disorders.

In Russia, a large, randomized, double-blind, double-dummy, placebo-controlled, 4-cell study of naltrexone and guanfacine among 300 opioid-dependent patients is being conducted to examine the additive effect of guanfacine on preventing relapse among opioid-dependent patients.[23] When completed, results should provide information useful for informing naltrexone research.

Opioid Agonists

Opioid addiction is frequently comorbid with other substance abuse, particularly with alcohol and cocaine use disorders.[24] Buprenorphine has been found to reduce cocaine use in opioid-dependent patients.[25] Preclinical evidence suggests possible beneficial effects of κ-opioid receptor antagonist in treating cocaine addiction, and Rothman and co-workers[26] proposed and explored the combination of naltrexone and buprenorphine as a functional κ-opioid receptor antagonist to reduce dysphoric symptoms associated with opioid withdrawal and cocaine use in a sample of 15 opioid-dependent individuals. Five patients (33%) completed the 3-month study; 4 were abstinent from opioids and cocaine for the entire study and 1 was abstinent from opioids and cocaine for the last 9 weeks. Rothman and colleagues[26] concluded that the positive response to treatment exceeded that expected from naltrexone alone (90% dropout).

Subsequently, Gerra and co-workers[27] examined naltrexone and buprenorphine combination in the treatment of opioid dependence in a nonrandomized, 3-month, observational study. The buprenorphine/naltrexone group showed a lower rate of positive urines for opioids and cocaine metabolites and more improvement in psychological symptoms (irritability, depression, tiredness, psychosomatic symptoms, and craving) than the naltrexone-only group.

These findings suggest a theoretical rationale for further investigation of the efficacy of the naltrexone and buprenorphine combination in treating opioid and cocaine addictions. Additionally, oral naltrexone and XR-NTX have been approved by the Food and Drug Administration for the treatment of alcoholism. The beneficial effects of mixed receptor activities of the buprenorphine plus naltrexone combination on opioid and alcohol addictions may warrant research.[28] Given that availability of XR-NTX, these studies lend some support for evaluating the combination of buprenorphine and long-acting depot naltrexone in treatment for polysubstance addictions.

Opioids and Low Doses of Opioid Receptor Antagonists

Preclinical and clinical studies have shown that co-treatments of opioids and ultra-low doses of opioid receptor antagonists (eg, naltrexone, naloxone) may enhance the efficacy of opioid analgesics and simultaneously attenuate opioid tolerance and dependence.[29] Findings from a study of 60 patients showed that a low-dose infusion of naloxone in patient-administered morphine sulfate was associated with fewer morphine-related side effects and reduced postoperative opioid requirements.[30] However, application of such co-treatment procedures with low-dose opioid antagonist plus morphine to chronic pain patients who are also dependent on prior use of opioid analgesics requires careful monitoring to avoid possible transitory opioid withdrawal symptoms, which might be elicited by administration of low doses of opioid antagonists.[29]

Of note, oxycodone plus an ultra-low dose of naltrexone (Oxytrex; Pain Therapeutics, Inc., Austin, TX, USA) was developed as an alternative to oxycodone to treat moderate to severe chronic pain without increasing side effects. Using an animal model, Largent-Milnes and associates[31] proposed that Oxytrex presents a novel approach to neuropathic pain therapy. Chindalore and co-workers[32] conducted a phase II clinical trial to evaluate the safety and efficacy of Oxytrex in 360 patients with moderate to severe chronic pain caused by osteoarthritis of the knee or hip. Four treatment conditions were examined: Placebo, oxycodone 4 times a day (qid), Oxytrex qid, and Oxytrex twice a day (bid). Results indicated that the Oxytrex bid group received a lower daily dose of naltrexone than the Oxytrex qid group and that the Oxytrex bid group produced a 39% reduction in pain intensity, which was significantly greater than that of the placebo, oxycodone qid, and Oxytrex qid groups. The Oxytrex bid group was also superior to the placebo group in quality of analgesia, duration of pain control each day, and patients' global assessments.

Additionally, the potential effects that ultra-low doses of naltrexone may reduce abuse or dependence liability (or decrease the reinforcing effects of opioids) were examined in human subjects. Tompkins and colleagues[33] conducted a double-blind, placebo-controlled study to investigate the subjective and physiologic effects of combining oral oxycodone and ultra-low naltrexone doses in 14 experienced opioid abusers. Seven acute drug conditions given at least 5 days apart were compared in a within-subject crossover design: placebo, oxycodone 20 mg, oxycodone 40 mg, plus each of the active oxycodone doses combined with 0.0001 and 0.001 mg naltrexone. Results showed no significant differences or evident trends associated with the addition of either naltrexone dose on any abuse liability indices. They thus suggest that the addition of ultra–low-dose naltrexone to oxycodone does not decrease abuse liability of acutely administered oxycodone in experienced opioid abusers.

Considered jointly, well-designed randomized trials of chronic pain patients co-treated with morphine plus low-dose naltrexone or other opioid receptor antagonists are required to elucidate the degree to which selective antagonists of excitatory opioid receptor functions can reliably attenuate opioid tolerance and dependence liability.[29]

BEHAVIORAL THERAPIES WITH NALTREXONE

Contingency management (CM) and significant other involvement were evaluated as strategies to enhance treatment retention, medication compliance, and outcome for naltrexone treatment of opioid dependence in a randomized trial of 127 opioid-dependent patients.[34] Results showed that CM was associated with significant improvements in treatment retention and reduction in opioid use compared with standard naltrexone treatment. Additionally, assignment to significant other involvement did not improve retention, compliance, or substance abuse outcomes compared with CM. Significant effects for the significant other involvement condition over CM on retention, compliance, and drug use outcomes were seen only for the subgroup who attended at least 1 family counseling session. The use of CM with XR-NTX would seem a likely combination to enhance outcomes. In an approach known as behavioral naltrexone therapy, voucher incentives have been integrated with the community reinforcement approach and involvement of significant others to support abstinence from opioids and improve adherence.[35]

Although the relevant literature remains sparse, studies to date suggest that XR-NTX is superior to the oral form in reducing drug use and retaining patients in treatment.[23] Similarly, although the injectable formulation, once successfully administered, does ensure medication adherence for the 30-day period, it is still "short term" considering the need for long-term treatment for most opioid-addicted patients. Research is clearly needed to evaluate compliance issues of long-acting depot naltrexone over an extended period of time and to determine whether behavioral therapies, such as CM, can be targeted to address compliance issues that may remain even with long-acting depot naltrexone.

THE FUTURE OF EXTENDED-RELEASE DEPOT NALTREXONE TREATMENT FOR ADDICTION
Depot Naltrexone for Other Indications

Alcohol dependence was the original indication for which FDA approval of XR-NTX (as Vivitrol) was obtained in April 2006. Opioid addiction was the logical next application of the medication, and the use of XR-NTX for other drug use disorders seems promising based on work that has examined naltrexone in oral form in research settings. For example, Swedish researchers have found positive results for naltrexone used in treating individuals dependent on amphetamine,[36] and subsequent research is seeking to confirm efficacy and safety in methamphetamine-dependent individuals.

Naltrexone could be effective for treatment of cocaine use disorder, cannabis use disorder, gambling disorder, eating disorder, and other behavioral conditions. Underlying the presumed efficacy are mechanistic arguments based on the opioid system; naltrexone's ability to reduce the reinforcing effects of alcohol, opioids, and other drugs appears to derive from a blockade of effects of endogenous opioid peptides by occupation and binding of opioid receptors. In a study of combination opioid and stimulant abusers, Comer and colleagues[3] found that cocaine use was reduced among the portion of the sample randomized to 384 mg of extended-release naltrexone.

Combining naltrexone with the partial agonist buprenorphine may reduce cocaine use; a multicenter trial is currently underway in an effort of the National Institute on Drug Abuse Clinical Trial Network, to examine buprenorphine for treatment of cocaine dependence in opioid-experienced individuals who are also receiving XR-NTX to blunt the reinforcing effects from the partial agonist action of buprenorphine. This is yet another example of the range of potential clinical applications of XR-NTX.

REFERENCES

1. Digiusto E, Shakeshaft A, Ritter A, et al; NEPOD Research Group. Serious adverse events in the Australian National Evaluation of Pharmacotherapies for Opioid Dependence (NEPOD). Addiction 2004;99:450-60 [Erratum in: Addiction 2005;100:139].
2. Gibson AE, Degenhardt LJ, Hall WD. Opioid overdose deaths can occur in patients with naltrexone implants. Med J Aust 2007;186:152-3.
3. Comer SD, Collins ED, Kleber HD, et al. Depot naltrexone: long-lasting antagonism of the effects of heroin in humans. Psychopharmacology (Berl) 2002;159:351-60.
4. Comer SD, Sullivan MA, Yu E, et al. Injectable, sustained-release naltrexone for the treatment of opioid dependence. Arch Gen Psychiatry 2006;63:210-8.
5. Hulse GK, Tait RJ, Comer SD, et al. Reducing hospital presentations for opioid overdose in patients treated with sustained release naltrexone implants. Drug Alcohol Dependence 2005;79;351-7.
6. Hulse GK, Arnold-Reed DE, O'Neil G, et al. Blood naltrexone and 6-beta-naltrexol levels following naltrexone implant: comparing two naltrexone implants. Addict Biol 2004;9:59-65.
7. Hulse GK, Arnold-Reed DE, O'Neil G, et al. Achieving long-term continuous blood naltrexone and 6-beta-naltrexol coverage following sequential naltrexone implants. Addict Biol 2004;9:67-72.
8. Olsen L, Christophersen AS, Frogopsahl G, et al. Plasma concentrations during naltrexone implant treatment of opiate-dependent patients. Br J Clin Pharmacol 2004;58:219-22

9. Colquhoun R, Tan DY, Hull S. A comparison of oral and implant naltrexone outcomes at 12 months. J Opioid Manag 2005;1:249–56.

10. Carreño JE, Alvarez CE, Narciso GI, et al. Maintenance treatment with depot opioid antagonists in subcutaneous implants: an alternative in the treatment of opioid dependence. Addict Biol 2003;8:429–38.

11. Krupitsky E, Nunes E, Ling W, et al. Injectable extended-release naltrexone for opioid dependence: a double-blind, placebo-controlled, multicentre randomised trial. Lancet 2011;377:1506–13.

12. Collins E. Anesthesia-assisted vs buprenorphine- or clonidine-assisted heroin detoxification and naltrexone induction. JAMA 2005;294:903–13.

13. Fishman M. Precipitated withdrawal during maintenance opioid blockade with XR-NTX. Addiction 2008;103:1399–401.

14. Mannelli P, Peindl KS, Wu LT. Pharmacological enhancement of naltrexone treatment for opioid dependence: a review. Subst Abuse Rehabil 2011;2011:113–23.

15. Wu LT, Woody GE, Yang C, et al. How do prescription opioid users differ from users of heroin or other drugs in psychopathology: results from the National Epidemiologic Survey on Alcohol and Related Conditions. J Addict Med 2011;5:28–35.

16. Landabaso MA, Iraurgi I, Jimanez-Lerma JM, et al. A randomized trial of adding fluoxetine to a naltrexone treatment programme for heroin addicts. Addiction 1998; 93:739–44.

17. Krupitsky EM, Zvartau EE, Masalov DV, et al. Naltrexone with or without fluoxetine for preventing relapse to heroin addiction in St. Petersburg, Russia. J Subst Abuse Treat 2006;31:319–28.

18. Hyman SM, Fox H, Hong KI, et al. Stress and drug-cue-induced craving in opioid-dependent individuals in naltrexone treatment. Exp Clin Psychopharmacol 2007;15: 134–43.

19. Stella L, D'Ambra C, Mazzeo F, et al. Naltrexone plus benzodiazepine aids abstinence in opioid-dependent patients. Life Sci 2005;77:2717–22.

20. Gerra G, Zaimovic A, Giusti F, et al. Lofexidine versus clonidine in rapid opiate detoxification. J Subst Abuse Treat 2001;21:11–7.

21. Yu E, Miotto K, Akerele E, et al. A Phase 3 placebo-controlled, double-blind, multi-site trial of the alpha-2-adrenergic agonist, lofexidine, for opioid withdrawal. Drug Alcohol Depend 2008;97:158–68.

22. Sinha R, Kimmerling A, Doebrick C, et al. Effects of lofexidine on stress-induced and cue-induced opioid craving and opioid abstinence rates: preliminary findings. Psychopharmacology (Berl) 2007;190:569–74.

23. Krupitsky E, Zvartau E, Woody G. Use of naltrexone to treat opioid addiction in a country in which methadone and buprenorphine are not available. Curr Psychiatry Rep 2010;12:448–53.

24. Wu LT, Ling W, Burchett B, et al. Use of item response theory and latent class analysis to link poly-substance use disorders with addiction severity, HIV risk, and quality of life among opioid-dependent patients in the Clinical Trials Network. Drug Alcohol Depend 2011;118:186–93.

25. Montoya ID, Gorelick DA, Preston KL, et al. Randomized trial of buprenorphine for treatment of concurrent opiate and cocaine dependence. Clin Pharmacol Ther 2004;75:34–48.

26. Rothman RB, Gorelick DA, Heishman SJ, et al. An open-label study of a functional opioid kappa antagonist in the treatment of opioid dependence. J Substance Abuse Treat 2000;18:277–81.

27. Gerra G, Fantoma A, Zaimovic A. Naltrexone and buprenorphine combination in the treatment of opioid dependence. J Psychopharmacol 2006;20:806–14.

28. McCann DJ. Potential of buprenorphine/naltrexone in treating polydrug addiction and co-occurring psychiatric disorders. Clin Pharmacol Ther 2008;83:627–30.

29. Crain SM, Shen KF. Antagonists of excitatory opioid receptor functions enhance morphine's analgesic potency and attenuate opioid tolerance/dependence liability. Pain 2000;84:121–31.

30. Gan T, Ginsberg B, Glass P, et al. Opioid-sparing effects of a low-dose infusion of naloxone in patient-administered morphone sulfate. Anesthesiology 1997;87:1075–81.

31. Largent-Milnes TM, Guo W, Wang HY, et al. Oxycodone plus ultra-low-dose naltrexone attenuates neuropathic pain and associated mu-opioid receptor-Gs coupling. J Pain 2008;9:700–13.

32. Chindalore VL, Craven RA, Yu KP, et al. Adding ultralow-dose naltrexone to oxycodone enhances and prolongs analgesia: a randomized, controlled trial of Oxytrex. J Pain 2005;6:392–9.

33. Tompkins DA, Lanier RK, Harrison JA, et al. Human abuse liability assessment of oxycodone combined with ultra-low-dose naltrexone. Psychopharmacology (Berl) 2010;210:471–80.

34. Carroll KM, Ball SA, Nich C, et al. Targeting behavioral therapies to enhance naltrexone treatment of opioid dependence: efficacy of contingency management and significant other involvement. Arch Gen Psychiatry 2001;58:755–61.

35. Rothenberg J, Sullivan M, Church S, et al. Behavioral naltrexone therapy: an integrated treatment for opiate dependence. J Subst Abuse Treat 2002;23:351–60.

36. Jayaram-Lindström N, Hammarberg A, Beck O, et al. Naltrexone for the treatment of amphetamine dependence: a randomized, placebo-controlled trial. Am J Psychiatry 2008;165:1442–8.

State of the Art Treatments for Cannabis Dependence

Itai Danovitch, MD[a],*, David A. Gorelick, MD, PhD, DFAPA[b,c]

KEYWORDS

- Cannabis • Dependence • Endocannabinoids • Marijuana • Therapy
- Treatment • Withdrawal

KEY POINTS

- The high prevalence of cannabis dependence, its strong association with comorbid mental health problems, and the difficulty of achieving cannabis cessation ensure that many psychiatrists will face patients with cannabis dependence.
- The comparatively lower "severity" of cannabis-associated consequences compared with other drugs of abuse creates a challenge for treatment providers since consensus has not been established about the value of nonabstinence goals, such as moderation and harm reduction.
- Cannabis intoxication is a syndrome recognized in DSM-IV and ICD-10, with psychological/behavioral and physical manifestations.
- Although no medication has been shown broadly effective in the treatment of cannabis dependence, evaluation is ongoing for 3 major strategies for treatment: agonist substitution, antagonist, and modulation of other neurotransmitter systems.
- A number of evidence-based psychotherapies have been shown to be efficacious for cannabis dependence, and efforts are underway to determine optimal combinations.

Worldwide, cannabis is the most commonly used illicit substance.[1] In the United States, 42% of persons over age 12 have used cannabis at least once in their lifetime, 11.5% have used within the past year, and 1.8% have met diagnostic criteria for cannabis abuse or dependence within the past year.[2,3] Among individuals who have

Disclosures: Dr Gorelick is supported by the Intramural Research Program, National Institutes of Health, National Institute on Drug Abuse. He has participated in NIH research sponsored by a Collaborative Research and Development Agreement with Sanofi-aventis, the maker of rimonabant.
[a] Department of Psychiatry and Behavioral Neurosciences, Cedars-Sinai Medical Center, 8730 Alden Drive, Suite 301, Los Angeles, CA 90048, USA; [b] Chemistry and Drug Metabolism Section, Intramural Research Program, National Institute on Drug Abuse, National Institutes of Health, 251 Bayview Boulevard, Suite 200, Baltimore, MD 21224, USA; [c] Department of Psychiatry, University of Maryland School of Medicine, Baltimore, MD 21201, USA
* Corresponding author.
E-mail address: itai.danovitch@cshs.org

Psychiatr Clin N Am 35 (2012) 309–326
doi:10.1016/j.psc.2012.03.003
0193-953X/12/$ – see front matter © 2012 Elsevier Inc. All rights reserved.

ever used cannabis, conditional dependence (the proportion who go on to develop dependence) is 9%.[4] This rate is lower than many other drugs of abuse, but it is nonetheless significant considering the high prevalence of cannabis use across the population. Children and young adults have substantially higher rates of conditional dependence, a concerning notion given the fact that in recent years a decade-long trend of decreasing cannabis use has reversed. Between 2007 and 2010, past month use among youth aged 12 to 17 increased from 6.7 to 7.4%, corresponding with a decrease in perception of risk over that same period.[2,5] Altogether, there are 6600 new users of cannabis every day in the United States.[2]

Initial Characterization of Cannabis Addiction

Before the 1980s, cannabis was not thought to produce significant dependence.[6] Physical dependence, particularly the presence of a withdrawal syndrome, was not well characterized, animal models had not convincingly demonstrated reinforcing effects, and the neurobiology of cannabis was not well understood. Further, cannabis use did not seem to cause the dramatic harms typified by other drugs of abuse, such as alcohol, cocaine, and heroin. Discussion of adverse effects often focused on the "amotivational" syndrome,[7] a syndrome that was never fully disentangled from cannabis intoxication itself.

The primary psychoactive component of cannabis, tetrahydrocannabinol (THC), was identified in 1965,[8] but it was not until the 1990s, when the first cannabinoid receptor (CB1) was described, that researchers began to characterize the endocannabinoid system.[9] CB1 receptors were found to be localized throughout the brain, and although their purpose was not well-understood, cannabis exposure was shown to alter them.[10] The development of cannabinoid receptor antagonists permitted studies of precipitated withdrawal, which added to the mounting evidence of a clinically significant and specific cannabis withdrawal syndrome.[11] Cannabis was also shown to promote release of dopamine in the nucleus accumbens, one of the cornerstone features of reinforcing drugs.[12]

Broadening of Addiction Concept

Simultaneously, in the late 1970s and early 1980s, the conceptualization of addiction began to change. Rather than focusing on physical dependence, the phenomenology of addiction broadened to include such constructs as compulsivity, loss of control, consequences, salience, and relapse.[13] The DSM-III codified a view of substance dependence for which symptoms of physical dependence were neither necessary nor sufficient for establishing a diagnosis.[14] Among regular cannabis users, a dependence syndrome very similar to that described for other drugs of abuse was reliably described.[15] Users described unsuccessful attempts to cut down, use despite knowledge of persistent psychological or physical problems, excessive time spent buying, using or recovering from cannabis effects, and loss of control over use.[16] Perhaps the most important factor demonstrating the validity and clinical significance of cannabis dependence was that many heavy users sought help with problems related to cannabis use. Cannabis was the most common illicit drug responsible for substance abuse treatment admissions in the United States in 2007, and among youth under the age of 19, primary cannabis abuse accounted for over half of all admissions.[17]

Adverse Effects of Cannabis

Epidemiologic surveys revealed subtle but significant adverse outcomes associated with cannabis dependence. Chronic heavy use was associated with poor educational attainment among youth,[18] an unsurprising association given the fact that cannabis intoxication directly impairs cognition, and some studies,[19–21] but not all,[22,23] pointed to subtle but persistent long-term impairments. Cannabis use during adolescence may be distinct in that, alongside the putative neurobiological consequences of heavy cannabinoid exposure,[24] chronic intoxication may fundamentally alter developmental trajectories.[25,26] Heavy cannabis use has been linked to school failure, early pregnancy, crime, and progression to further drug use.[18,27,28] Even where these associations are demonstrated in prospective, longitudinal studies that control for baseline (ie, precannabis use) presence of the adverse outcome and known common risk factors (eg, other substance use, psychiatric comorbidity), it remains possible that the observed associations result from convergent risks and common predisposing factors, as much as direct effects of cannabis use.

Cannabis Dependence and Other Disorders

With regard to mental health, individuals with cannabis dependence were found to be 6-fold more likely to have mood or anxiety disorders,[29] and cannabis use was repeatedly correlated with poor clinical outcomes and exacerbation of symptoms across many psychiatric disorders.[30–33] A causal relationship between cannabis use and affective disorders has not been established. However, the link between cannabis use and risk of psychotic disorders has now been replicated across at least 6 well-controlled prospective longitudinal studies,[34] and specific genetic factors are emerging as plausible explanations for increased risk among subsets of users.[30,35,36] Demonstrating causality with epidemiologic or association studies is impossible because of the inability to ever completely exclude the presence of unmeasured shared predisposing or risk factors (common antecedent causality) or subtle presence of the adverse outcome at baseline (reverse causality),[37,38] but the consistency of the associations described above has fundamentally changed the appraisal of "hazard" associated with heavy cannabis use.

Cannabis dependence poses some distinct challenges for treatment providers. The evolving sociocultural context of use for medical (as opposed to recreational) purposes, policy liberalization, and societal normalization has contributed to decreased perceived risk and increased acceptability of use.[39–43] Simultaneously, the comparatively lower "severity" of cannabis-associated consequences (compared with other drugs of abuse)[44] makes it more difficult for some users to recognize the impact of their use and establish an enduring commitment to change. As a result, many treatment seekers are reluctant to accept traditional abstinence-based goals.[45] Among treatment providers, consensus has not been established about the value of nonabstinence goals, such as moderation and harm reduction.

Models and Approaches for Cannabis Dependence Treatment

Notwithstanding these challenges, the high prevalence of cannabis dependence, its strong association with comorbid mental health problems, and the difficulty of achieving cannabis cessation ensure that many psychiatrists will face patients with cannabis dependence. Although no pharmacotherapy has been approved for cannabis dependence, a number of promising approaches are in development. Psychotherapy studies are establishing a number of evidence-based models and techniques in the armamentarium of treatment resources for patients in need. This article reviews established and emerging treatment options for cannabis dependence.

Table 1	
Manifestations of Cannabis intoxication	
Psychological and Behavioral	**Physical**
Euphoria	Motor incoordination
Relaxation	Tachycardia
Increased appetite	Orthostatic hypotension
Impaired memory and concentration	
Anxiety, panic attack, psychosis	

PHARMACOTHERAPY FOR CANNABIS DEPENDENCE
Cannabis Intoxication

Cannabis intoxication is a syndrome recognized in DSM-IV and ICD-10, with psychological/behavioral and physical manifestations (**Table 1**). Intoxication is usually mild and self-limiting, not requiring pharmacologic treatment.[46] The most severe effects (anxiety, panic attack, psychosis) are best treated with a benzodiazepine or second-generation (atypical) antipsychotic medication, as appropriate to acutely control symptoms.[46] No medication is approved specifically for treatment of cannabis intoxication.

Cannabis Withdrawal

Increasing evidence from human laboratory and clinical studies indicates that there is a true cannabis withdrawal syndrome,[11] which has been proposed for inclusion in DSM-V.[47] The commonest symptoms of cannabis withdrawal are dysphoric mood (anxiety, irritability, depressed mood, restlessness), disturbed sleep, gastrointestinal symptoms, and decreased appetite. Most symptoms begin during the first week of abstinence and resolve after a few weeks. Up to one half of patients in treatment for cannabis use disorders report symptoms of a withdrawal syndrome.[11,48–50] Although not medically serious, cannabis withdrawal should be a focus of treatment, because it may serve as negative reinforcement for relapse to cannabis use in individuals trying to abstain.[48,51]

Treatment approaches for cannabis withdrawal

No medications are approved for the treatment of cannabis withdrawal, but several medications have been evaluated in small clinical studies.[52,53] One approach is cross-tolerant (cannabinoid CB1 receptor) agonist substitution to suppress the withdrawal syndrome (analogous to using an opiate to suppress heroin withdrawal). This approach can be implemented using synthetic THC (dronabinol), which is legally marketed in many countries, including the United States (Marinol, Solvay Pharmaceuticals, Marietta, GA, USA), as an oral medication for appetite stimulation and suppression of nausea and vomiting owing to chemotherapy. Dronabinol has shown efficacy in several human laboratory studies and open-label case series, at doses up to 30 mg tid, with minimal side effects.[54–56] A controlled, clinical trial of dronabinol (20 mg bid), although not showing efficacy for reducing cannabis use (see below), did significantly reduce cannabis withdrawal symptoms.[57]

Lithium, a mood stabilizer used primarily in the treatment of bipolar disorder, has been evaluated in 2 small open-label clinical studies. In the first study, lithium (600–900 mg/d for 6 days) reduced withdrawal symptoms in 4 of the 9 participants, although 1 of the 4 continued to smoke some cannabis.[58] Abstinence was not verified in the other 8 participants. In the second study, lithium (500 mg bid for 7 days) was given to 20 cannabis-dependent in-patients undergoing detoxification.[59] Twelve patients completed the 7-day detoxification program. Over 90 days of follow-up, participants reported being abstinent on 88% of days, with 64% abstinence on day 10, 65% on day 24, and 41% on day 90. Five participants reported continuous abstinence, with cannabis-negative urine tests on day 90. These results suggest a possible persisting therapeutic effect of lithium given during the withdrawal (detoxification) period.

Another approach, which has been evaluated in human laboratory studies, tries to alleviate symptoms of cannabis withdrawal (e.g., dysphoric mood, disturbed sleep) by influencing the brain circuits that mediate these symptoms, using medications already approved for other psychiatric conditions. Human laboratory studies found that the anticonvulsant and mood stabilizer divalproex (1500 mg/d for 29 days) and the antidepressant buproprion (300 mg/d sustained release for 17 days) worsened, rather than improved, some withdrawal symptoms and had no positive effects.[55,60] A single dose of the antidepressant nefazodone (450 mg/d) decreased some, but not the majority, of cannabis withdrawal symptoms.[61] The combination of lofexidine (2.4 mg/d), an alpha2-adrenergic receptor agonist used to treat opiate withdrawal, and THC (60 mg/d) produced more improvement over 3 days in symptoms of cannabis withdrawal than either medication alone.[62]

Cannabis Dependence

No medication has been shown broadly effective in the treatment of cannabis dependence, nor is any medication approved for this condition by any regulatory authority. Ongoing research is evaluating 3 major strategies for treatment: Agonist substitution, antagonist, and modulation of other neurotransmitter systems.

Agonist substitution with antagonist

One treatment strategy is substitution with a cross-tolerant agonist drug to suppress withdrawal and drug craving, analogous to using nicotine itself to treat tobacco dependence or methadone for heroin dependence. For treatment of cannabis dependence, this strategy can be implemented using the legally available agonist, dronabinol. Oral dronabinol (10–50 mg/d) successfully reduced cannabis use and suppressed cannabis withdrawal in several outpatient cases.[54] Controlled clinical trials of oral THC are currently underway. In a controlled clinical trial, dronabinol (20 mg bid for 8 weeks) significantly improved treatment retention and reduced cannabis withdrawal symptoms, but did not improve rates of abstinence.[57]

Neuromodulation

Another strategy is modulation of other neurotransmitter systems to reduce the reinforcing effects of and craving for cannabis. This strategy has been implemented using a variety of medications approved for other psychiatric conditions.

Entacapone inhibits catechol-O-methyl transferase, an enzyme that metabolizes catecholamine neurotransmitters and regulates dopamine levels in the synapse. In an open-label trial in 36 patients with cannabis dependence (DSM-IV), entacapone (up to 2000 mg/d for 12 weeks) significantly decreased craving for cannabis in 52.7% of the patients (no data on cannabis use was reported).[63] The medication was well tolerated; there were no serious adverse events.

N-acetylcysteine reverses the down-regulation of the cystine-glutamate exchanger associated with chronic drug exposure in animals, thereby restoring normal regulation of glutamate release and reducing compulsive drug-seeking behaviors.[64] In an open-label trial in 24 cannabis-dependent outpatients, N-acetylcysteine (1200 mg twice daily for 4 weeks) significantly decreased self-reported cannabis use and craving, with no significant change in semiquantitative urine cannabinoid levels.[65] The medication was well tolerated.

Atomoxetine is a selective norepinephrine reuptake inhibitor used in the treatment of attention deficit/hyperactivity disorder, and considered to have low abuse potential. In an 11-week, open-label study in 13 cannabis-dependent outpatients, atomoxetine (25, 40, or 80 mg/d) showed a trend toward reduction in cannabis use and increase in proportion of abstinent days only in the 8 patients who completed the trial.[66] The majority of patients experienced gastrointestinal adverse events. In a double-blind, placebo-controlled clinical trial in 38 cannabis-dependent outpatients with comorbid attention deficit/hyperactivity disorder, atomoxetine (25–100 mg/d escalating doses over 12 weeks) produced no significant change in cannabis use, although there was some improvement in attention deficit/hyperactivity disorder symptoms.[67]

Buspirone is a 5-HT$_{(1A)}$ receptor agonist and a D$_2$ receptor antagonist that is used as an anxiolytic. In an open-label trial in 10 cannabis-dependent men, buspirone (up to 60 mg/d for 12 weeks) significantly reduced frequency and duration of cannabis craving and use and reduced irritability and depression.[68] In a placebo-controlled clinical trial in 50 cannabis-dependent outpatients, buspirone (up to 60 mg/d for 12 weeks) in conjunction with motivational interviewing significantly increased the proportion of cannabis-negative urine samples (95% confidence interval for increase, 7%–63%; $P<.05$) among the 24 patients who completed the entire trial.[69] There was a trend toward faster initiation of abstinence (first cannabis-negative urine) among those receiving buspirone. These findings support the promise of buspirone as a treatment for cannabis dependence.

Divalproex is an anticonvulsant used as a mood stabilizer in the treatment of bipolar disorder. In a 6-week, placebo-controlled clinical trial in 25 cannabis-dependent outpatients, divalproex (1500–2000 mg/d for 6 weeks, with target plasma concentration of 50–120 ng/mL) in conjunction with weekly relapse prevention psychotherapy was not significantly more effective than placebo in reducing cannabis use and was poorly tolerated by participants.[70]

In a 13-week, placebo-controlled clinical trial in 106 cannabis-dependent outpatients, the antidepressants nefazodone (300 mg/d) or bupropion (150 mg sustained release per day) in conjunction with weekly, individual coping skills therapy were not significantly better than placebo in reducing cannabis use or symptoms of cannabis withdrawal.[71]

Treatment of Comorbid Symptoms in Cannabis Users

Cannabis users frequently have comorbid mood symptoms, especially depression.[29] Two studies evaluated the selective serotonin reuptake inhibitor antidepressant fluoxetine in such a population. A post hoc analysis of 13 cannabis-using patients among a larger sample of alcohol-abusing, depressed adolescents treated with fluoxetine (20–40 mg/d) showed reduction in both cannabis and alcohol use and depressive symptoms.[72] Five-year follow-up of 10 patients showed that cannabis and alcohol dependence were reduced and academic ability improved, but clinical depression remained problematic. In a placebo-controlled clinical trial in 70 adolescents and young adults with comorbid major depression and cannabis use disorder, fluoxetine (20 mg/d for 12 weeks) in conjunction with cognitive behavioral/motivational enhancement psychotherapy was no better than placebo in reducing either depressive symptoms or cannabis-related symptoms.[73]

Emerging Pharmacologic Targets for Cannabis Dependence

Growing knowledge about the endogenous cannabinoid (endocannabinoid) system in the brain and its role in mediating behavior offers potential new targets for the treatment of cannabis use disorders. The endocannabinoid system includes the cannabinoid (CB1) receptor, a G-protein–coupled receptor located on neuronal membranes in several brain regions, and several endogenous cannabinoids (endocannabinoids) which act as agonists at this receptor.[74,75] These endocannabinoids are primarily phospholipid esters, including anandamide and 2-arachidonoylglycerol (2-AG). Plant-derived cannabinoids such as THC are also ligands at this receptor, which mediates their actions. The synthetic and metabolic pathways for endocannabinoids are being worked out, and compounds that modulate these pathways or bind to the CB1 receptor have been developed.

Studies with the selective CB1 receptor antagonist/inverse agonist rimonabant suggest that CB1 receptors mediate many of the acute effects of cannabis in humans. In human laboratory studies, a single, double-blind oral dose of rimonabant (90 mg) produced significant dose-dependent attenuation of the subjective intoxication and tachycardia caused by an active (2.64% THC) cannabis cigarette smoked (double-blind) 2 hours later.[76] Subacute (2-week) treatment with rimonabant (40 mg/d) also attenuated the subjective intoxication and tachycardia caused by an active cannabis cigarette (2.78% THC) smoked double-blind.[77] Rimonabant alone did not significantly affect THC pharmacokinetics or produce significant physiologic or psychological effects, suggesting that the observed effects were owing to CB1 receptor blockade and not reduced brain THC concentrations. This pattern of findings suggests that CB1 receptor blockade might be beneficial acutely in the treatment of cannabis intoxication or overdose (analogous to the use of the mu-opiate receptor antagonist naloxone in the treatment of opiate overdose), and beneficial as a chronic treatment for cannabis dependence (analogous to the use of the long-acting mu-opiate receptor antagonist naltrexone in the treatment of opiate dependence).

Several CB1 receptor antagonists/inverse agonists were in clinical development by major multinational pharmaceutical companies, albeit for the treatment of obesity (activation of the CB1 receptor mediates increased appetite and weight gain). Rimonabant earned regulatory approval in more than 50 countries (but not the United States). However, its clinical use was associated with significant psychiatric side effects (anxiety, depression, suicidality), leading to suspension of marketing in the European Union in November 2008.[78] Further clinical development of rimonabant and other CB1 receptor antagonists/inverse agonists was subsequently halted worldwide. Thus, no such medication is currently available for human use.

An alternative approach to receptor blockade is modulation of brain concentrations of endocannabinoids. The enzyme fatty acid amide hydrolase catalyzes the breakdown of anandamide. Inhibitors of fatty acid amide hydrolase inhibitor, such as URB597, selectively increase brain anandamide concentrations in rodents and primates. In rodent studies, URB597 produced analgesic, anxiolytic-like, and antidepressant-like effects, but had no effects suggestive of abuse liability, such as self-administration. These findings suggest that enhancing brain endocannabinoid activity with a fatty acid amide hydrolase inhibitor might offer benefit for the treatment of acute cannabis withdrawal.[79]

Animal studies show that mu-opiate receptor antagonists block acute effects of THC, suggesting that such medications might be useful in the treatment of cannabis intoxication or overdose. Several human laboratory studies have explored this possibility by evaluating whether naltrexone reduces the subjective effects of cannabinoids in humans. Most findings to date have been disappointing. Pretreatment with high doses of naltrexone (50–200 mg) failed to attenuate or enhanced the subjective effects of THC.[80–82] A lower, more mu-selective dose of naltrexone (12 mg) decreased the intoxicating effects of 20 mg, but not 40 mg, of THC.[83] A recent placebo-controlled study in 29 heavy cannabis smokers found that opioid receptor blockade by naltrexone (12, 25, 50, or 100 mg/d) enhanced the subjective and cardiovascular effects of cannabis.[84] This pattern of human experimental findings suggests that naltrexone would not be an effective treatment for cannabis dependence.

PSYCHOTHERAPY FOR CANNABIS DEPENDENCE

Psychotherapy for cannabis dependence has its origins in psychotherapy for substance dependence in general. Randomized studies of psychotherapy for cannabis dependence have manualized and studied various iterations of motivational enhancement therapy (MET), cognitive–behavioral therapy (CBT), and contingency management, as well as community and family interventions. Because the underpinnings of these therapeutic models are complementary, researchers have been less focused on treatment superiority and more on identifying effective combinations.

Motivational Enhancement Therapy

MET is a patient-centered therapy that seeks to help individuals resolve ambivalence to generate commitment to change.[85] MET views readiness to change as a dynamic process involving multiple stages: Precontemplation, contemplation, preparation, action, and maintenance (consider using a figure to demonstrate these), and proposes that the role of the therapist is to create the conditions that promote the patient's intrinsic motivation.[86] Five core tenets characterize the motivational "style"[85]:

1. Maintain empathy and create a respectful, nonjudgmental therapeutic frame through the use of open-ended questions and validation.
2. Develop cognitive discrepancy by identifying goals that are meaningful to the patient and incrementally linking them to contrary behaviors.
3. Avoid arguments that cause patients to become defensive by letting the patient lead and working from within their perspective.
4. Roll with resistance by using reflective interpretations and reframing rather than confrontations.
5. Support self-efficacy to engender confidence in the ability to make and sustain change by utilizing support and validation.

Whereas in clinical practice MET may be used repeatedly over time as the targets for behavioral change evolve, in clinical studies, MET sessions are typically 60 to 90 minutes long, with treatment occurring over 1 to 4 sessions. MET has been shown to improve cannabis related outcomes among treatment-seeking adults,[87] non-treatment seekers,[88] and individuals with co-occurring disorders.[89] There have been efforts to computerize motivational interventions,[90,91] simplify them for use in community settings and busy primary practices, and utilize them in inpatient settings for patients with significant co-occurring disorders.[92] Studies of brief motivational interventions in adolescents show only minimal impact on cannabis use outcomes.[93,94] However, these studies have reinforced the feasibility of brief motivational interventions for moderating use and improving education.[95] It remains to be seen whether brief interventions for non–treatment-seeking cannabis users will increase the possibility of self-directed change by facilitating openness to education and consideration of future intervention.[93]

Cognitive–Behavioral Therapy

CBT views drug use as a learned behavior. CBT posits that by identifying the associative links and chain of events precipitating use, patients can identify opportunities to alter their behavioral repertoire and use alternative, healthy coping mechanisms.[96] CBT begins by establishing a therapeutic framework and teaching self-monitoring of underlying triggers. The therapy then moves to the development of relapse prevention skills, such as relaxation techniques, mindfulness, cognitive restructuring, positive self-talk, and assertiveness. The therapist may impart these skills through instruction, modeling, and role playing, but eventually the patient is encouraged to practice those skills outside of therapy, such that they develop the skills to adaptively deal with high-risk situations without relapsing.

CBT is typically provided over 6 to 12 individual or group sessions. The earliest randomized psychotherapy studies for cannabis dependence showed small but significant benefits.[97,98] CBT was not superior to MET,[49] but the synergies offered compelling rationale to integrate them.[99] Subsequent studies have demonstrated efficacy for CBT in the context of brief interventions,[97] combination with motivational techniques and contingency management,[100,101] and for individuals with co-occurring disorders.[89,92,102]

Contingency Management

Contingency management posits that behaviors will increase or decrease as a function of immediate and directly associated consequences. By manipulating the quality and immediacy of external consequences, contingency management attempts to systematically increase the likelihood of desired behaviors, and minimize undesired behaviors. Studies of CM show that rewards are generally more effective than punishments and that they do not have to be large or monetary to substantially alter behaviors.[103] For goals such as abstinence, that require continuous behavior, escalating values of reward can be very effective (i.e., longer periods of continuous abstinence increase the value of the reinforcer, whereas relapse resets the reinforcer back to a minimal level).[103,104] Rewards are most effective when they are provided in close proximity to the desired behavior, and frequency of reinforcement increases efficacy.[104] Whereas traditionally CM links rewards with abstinence confirmed by urine monitoring, CM can be effectively tied to a broader set of therapeutic goals, including attendance of counseling sessions, completion of therapy-related assignments, and adherence to medications.

The first randomized study of CM for cannabis dependence demonstrated that adding voucher-based incentives could improve responses to a motivational behavioral coping skills intervention.[100] CM is not a replacement for motivational enhancement or skill building, but can be used to augment the decisional balance among patients who would not otherwise be ready to address their substance use. In accordance with this, studies consistently show that, although not effective in isolation, CM reliably augments treatment outcomes of other effective psychotherapies.[105,106] CM also improves engagement among non–treatment-seeking adults with cannabis dependence, such as those referred by probation,[107] and young adults referred by the criminal justice system.[101] At least 1 study showed promise for utilization of CM among adolescents,[108] as well as for individuals with severe persistent mental illness.[109]

Supportive-Expressive Psychotherapy

Supportive-expressive psychotherapy has many characteristics similar to motivational and skills-based treatment. The supportive element of the therapy involves establishing a helpful, optimistic, encouraging, and empathic relationship between the patient and therapist. The development of a strong therapeutic alliance enables an expressive component, in which the therapist utilizes reflective listening and interpretation to explore the patient's subjective experience, point out patterns that manifest within the therapeutic relationship, and facilitate development of self-awareness, insight, and adaptive coping.[110] Through self-understanding, supportive-expressive psychotherapy aims to help patients achieve greater mastery over problem behavior and improved personal well-being.[111]

Supportive-expressive psychotherapy is typically delivered in hour-long sessions, once or twice each week, over at least 4 months. In contrast with the other therapies, supportive-expressive psychotherapy has not been studied in well-controlled randomized trials, but is worth mention because it is a commonly utilized technique among community providers of psychotherapy. One poorly controlled study compared a 16-week supportive-expressive intervention to a single session self-help intervention for cannabis dependence—significant abstinence—was achieved at the close of therapy, but significant gains were not maintained over the subsequent year.[112]

Family and Systems Interventions

Recognizing the complex interplay of psychosocial factors for many cannabis-dependent youth, system-based interventions have been established to involve family, utilize case managers to decrease obstacles, incorporate community supports to navigate environmental challenges, and collaborate with other stakeholders such as schools. Three manualized "systems" interventions have been studied among cannabis-using adolescents. Family therapy views the family as the patient, taking a family systems approach to resolving problems, by enhancing intrafamily communication, improving parental limit setting, and facilitating collaborative recovery work.[113] The Adolescent Community Reinforcement Approach is a multisystem behavioral therapy that seeks to integrate cognitive behavioral skills training with collaborative community support, and contingency management.[114] Multidimensional family therapy (MDFT) is a comprehensive systems therapy that targets the functioning of the individual within the context of his or her environment by integrating individual therapy, parent coaching, family systems therapy, and engagement of key community stakeholders, such as school, medical supports, juvenile justice, and social services.[115]

In small, randomized trials, MDFT has shown greater and more sustainable gains than CBT,[116] group therapy, and MET interventions alone.[117] However, MDFT was not significantly better when compared with other high-quality treatment interventions in the Cannabis Youth Treatment study, which randomized 600 adolescents to 5 different treatment approaches across multiple sites.[118,119] The treatment interventions included Adolescent Community Reinforcement Approach, Family Support Network, MDFT, and a 5-session and 12-session version of combined MET and CBT. The Cannabis Youth Treatment study had good retention rates, acceptability of manual-based interventions to therapists, treatment efficacy (across all arms), and economic feasibility (costs were comparable to national outpatient program costs). Long-term follow-up data are anticipated, as are initial findings from a large international study of MDFT, which is currently under way.[115]

Twelve-Step Facilitation

Twelve-step programs are an integral part of the treatment of substance dependence,[120] and manualized protocols for 12-step facilitation have been developed and implemented for alcohol and many substance use disorders.[121] However, 12-step programs are notably absent from the literature on psychosocial interventions for cannabis dependence. In 2008, the Marijuana Anonymous World Service published a 12-step workbook.[122] The extent to which 12-step programs are utilized, long-term efficacy and potential role as an integrated component of psychosocial interventions for cannabis dependence has not been examined.

SUMMARY

The treatment of cannabis dependence can be viewed as a cup half empty or half full. On the one hand, few people who might benefit from treatment actually receive it. Among those who undergo treatment in randomized trials, long-term abstinence is achieved by fewer than 20%.[123] Moderate use goals have been associated with decreases in consequences, but the differential impact of such goals on the long-term course of cannabis dependence is unknown. Optimal duration of treatment is unclear, and certain populations, particularly patients with co-occurring disorders, have not been studied adequately.[92] Twelve-step programs are low cost, effective for other substance use disorders, and readily available in most regions of the world. However, their role and efficacy in cannabis dependence has not been examined. Finally, effective pharmacologic treatments are under development, but none have yet been firmly established.

On the other hand, psychotherapeutic strategies used to treat other substance use disorders can be effective for cannabis dependence. A recent meta-analysis of psychosocial interventions for illicit substance use disorders found that treatments for cannabis dependence had comparatively larger effect sizes than treatments for other substance use disorders.[124] Combination therapies have proven most effective, particularly those that begin with a motivational intervention, utilize incentives to enhance the commitment to change, and teach behavioral and cognitive copings skills to prevent relapse. Among adolescents, family engagement and collaboration with community stakeholders adds substantial value.

Although only 9% of cannabis users develop cannabis dependence, the volume of people who smoke cannabis ensures that the total number of people in need of help is larger than the capacity of substance abuse specialty services. Thus, although efforts to refine and improve the efficacy of treatment interventions continue, innovations that increase the availability and accessibility of treatment are also needed. Computer- and phone-based interventions, social media, and brief interventions that can be implemented in primary care settings are areas that may hold promise for reaching at-risk populations. Adolescents and persons with co-occurring mental illness are at particularly high risk of cannabis dependence, and may suffer disproportionately from cannabis's adverse effects. As in the treatment of other substance use disorders, there is a need for a continuing care model with long-term follow-up that extends past the periods typically evaluated in treatment studies.[125] Additionally, there is a need for further investigation of genetic underpinnings and endophenotypes underlying cannabis dependence to identify neurobiological mechanisms for targeted intervention.[126] One benefit of the societal focus on cannabis has been a prominent increase in research covering everything from the basic science to public health impact of cannabis. Over the next decade, physicians who provide treatment for individuals with cannabis dependence are likely to see their armamentarium of effective interventions expand, to the ultimate betterment of patients, their families, and society at large.

REFERENCES

1. United Nations Office on Drugs and Crime. World drug report 2011. Sales No. E.11.XI.10. Vienna (Austria): United Nations Publication; 2011.
2. Substance Abuse and Mental Health Services Administration. Results from the 2010 National Survey on Drug Use and Health: summary of national findings, NSDUH Series H-41, HHS Publication No. (SMA) 11-4658. Rockville (MD): Substance Abuse and Mental Health Services Administration; 2011.
3. Degenhardt L, Chiu WT, Sampson N, et al. Toward a global view of alcohol, tobacco, cannabis, and cocaine use: findings from the WHO World Mental Health Surveys. PLoS Med 2008;5:e141.
4. Swift W, Hall W, Teesson M. Characteristics of DSM-IV and ICD-10 cannabis dependence among Australian adults: results from the National Survey of Mental Health and Wellbeing. Drug Alcohol Depend 2001;63:147–53.
5. Johnston LD, O'Malley PM, Bachman JG, et al. Monitoring the future national survey results on drug use, 1975-2010. Volume I: secondary school students. Ann Arbor: Institute for Social Research, The University of Michigan; 2011.
6. Dennis M, Babor TF, Rebuck MC, et al. Changing the focus: the case for recognizing and treating cannabis use disorders. Addiction 2002;97(Suppl 1):4–15.
7. McGlothlin WH, West LJ. The marihuana problem: an overview. Am J Psychiatry 1968;125:126–34.
8. Mechoulam R, Gaoni Y. A total synthesis of Dl-delta-1-tetrahydrocannabinol, the active constituent of hashish. J Am Chem Soc 1965;87:3273–5.
9. Howlett AC, Barth F, Bonner TI, et al. International Union of Pharmacology. XXVII. Classification of cannabinoid receptors. Pharmacol Rev 2002;54:161–202.
10. Cooper ZD, Haney M. Cannabis reinforcement and dependence: role of the cannabinoid CB1 receptor. Addict Biol 2008;13:188–95.
11. Budney AJ, Hughes JR, Moore BA, et al. Review of the validity and significance of cannabis withdrawal syndrome. Am J Psychiatry 2004;161:1967–77.
12. Tanda G, Loddo P, Di Chiara G. Dependence of mesolimbic dopamine transmission on delta9-tetrahydrocannabinol. Eur J Pharmacol 1999;376:23–6.
13. Edwards G, Gross MM. Alcohol dependence: provisional description of a clinical syndrome. Br Med J 1976;1:1058–61.
14. American Psychiatric Association. Diagnostic and statistical manual of mental disorders. 3rd edition (DSM-III). Washington, DC: American Psychiatric Association; 1981.
15. Teesson M, Lynskey M, Manor B, et al. The structure of cannabis dependence in the community. Drug Alcohol Depend 2002;68:255–62.
16. Stephens RS, Babor TF, Kadden R, et al. The Marijuana Treatment Project: rationale, design and participant characteristics. Addiction 2002;97(Suppl 1):109–24.
17. DHHS Office of Applied Studies. Treatment episode data set (TEDS) highlights-2007: national admissions to substance abuse treatment services (DASIS Series: S-45, DHHS Publication No. SMA 09-4360). Rockville (MD): Author; 2008.
18. Fergusson DM, Horwood LJ, Beautrais AL. Cannabis and educational achievement. Addiction 2003;98:1681–92.
19. Crean RD, Crane NA, Mason BJ. An evidence based review of acute and long-term effects of cannabis use on executive cognitive functions. J Addict Med 2011;5:1–8.
20. Solowij N, Stephens RS, Roffman RA, et al. Cognitive functioning of long-term heavy cannabis users seeking treatment. JAMA 2002;287:1123–31.

21. Solowij N, Battisti R. The chronic effects of cannabis on memory in humans: a review. Curr Drug Abuse Rev 2008;1:81–98.
22. Dregan A, Gulliford MC. Is illicit drug use harmful to cognitive functioning in the midadult years? A cohort-based investigation. Am J Epidemiol 2012;175:218–27.
23. Pope HG Jr, Gruber AJ, Hudson JI, et al. Neuropsychological performance in long-term cannabis users. Arch Gen Psychiatry 2001;58:909–15.
24. Medina KL, Hanson KL, Schweinsburg AD, et al. Neuropsychological functioning in adolescent marijuana users: subtle deficits detectable after a month of abstinence. J Int Neuropsychol Soc 2007;13:807–20.
25. Brook JS, Lee JY, Brown EN, et al. Developmental trajectories of marijuana use from adolescence to adulthood: personality and social role outcomes. Psychol Rep 2011;108:339–57.
26. Fontes MA, Bolla KI, Cunha PJ, et al. Cannabis use before age 15 and subsequent executive functioning. Br J Psychiatry 2011;198:442–7.
27. Fergusson DM, Boden JM. Cannabis use and later life outcomes. Addiction 2008; 103:969–76.
28. Macleod J, Oakes R, Copello A, et al. Psychological and social sequelae of cannabis and other illicit drug use by young people: a systematic review of longitudinal, general population studies. Lancet 2004;363:1579–88.
29. Stinson FS, Ruan WJ, Pickering R, et al. Cannabis use disorders in the USA: prevalence, correlates and co-morbidity. Psychol Med 2006;36:1447–60.
30. Genetic Risk in Outcomes in Psychosis (GROUP) Investigators. Evidence that familial liability for psychosis is expressed as differential sensitivity to cannabis: an analysis of patient-sibling and sibling-control pairs. Arch Gen Psychiatry 2011;68:138–47.
31. Bovasso GB. Cannabis abuse as a risk factor for depressive symptoms. Am J Psychiatry 2001;158:2033–7.
32. de Graaf R, Radovanovic M, van Laar M, et al. Early cannabis use and estimated risk of later onset of depression spells: epidemiologic evidence from the population-based World Health Organization World Mental Health Survey Initiative. Am J Epidemiol 2010;172:149–59.
33. Kuepper R, van Os J, Lieb R, et al. Continued cannabis use and risk of incidence and persistence of psychotic symptoms: 10 year follow-up cohort study. BMJ 2011;342: d738.
34. Moore TH, Zammit S, Lingford-Hughes A, et al. Cannabis use and risk of psychotic or affective mental health outcomes: a systematic review. Lancet 2007;370:319–28.
35. Verweij KJ, Zietsch BP, Lynskey MT, et al. Genetic and environmental influences on cannabis use initiation and problematic use: a meta-analysis of twin studies. Addiction 2010;105:417–30.
36. van Winkel R; Genetic Risk and Outcome of Psychosis (GROUP) Investigators. Family-based analysis of genetic variation underlying psychosis-inducing effects of cannabis: sibling analysis and proband follow-up. Arch Gen Psychiatry 2011;68: 148–57.
37. Arseneault L, Cannon M, Witton J, et al. Causal association between cannabis and psychosis: examination of the evidence. Br J Psychiatry 2004;184:110–7.
38. Harder VS, Morral AR, Arkes J. Marijuana use and depression among adults: testing for causal associations. Addiction 2006;101:1463–72.
39. Aggarwal SK, Carter GT, Sullivan MD, et al. Medicinal use of cannabis in the United States: historical perspectives, current trends, and future directions. J Opioid Manag 2009;5:153–68.

40. Arbour-Nicitopoulos KP, Kwan MY, Lowe D, et al. Social norms of alcohol, smoking, and marijuana use within a Canadian university setting. J Am Coll Health 2011;59: 191–6.

41. Gates P, Copeland J, Swift W, et al. Barriers and facilitators to cannabis treatment. Drug Alcohol Rev 2011. [Epub ahead of print].

42. Hoffmann DE, Weber E. Medical marijuana and the law. N Engl J Med 2010;362: 1453–7.

43. Lewis TF, Mobley AK. Substance abuse and dependency risk: the role of peer perceptions, marijuana involvement, and attitudes toward substance use among college students. J Drug Educ 2010;40:299–314.

44. Nutt D, King LA, Saulsbury W, et al. Development of a rational scale to assess the harm of drugs of potential misuse. Lancet 2007;369:1047–53.

45. Lozano BE, Stephens RS, Roffman RA. Abstinence and moderate use goals in the treatment of marijuana dependence. Addiction 2006;101:1589–97.

46. Wilkins JN, Gorelick DA. Management of stimulant, hallucinogen, marijuana, phencyclidine, and club drug intoxication and withdrawal. In: Ries FD, Miller SC, Saitz R, editors. Principles of addiction medicine. 4th edition. Philadelphia: Lippincott Williams & Wilkins; 2009. p. 607–28.

47. Diagnostic and statistical manual of mental disorders (DSM-5), 2011. Available at: http://www.dsm5.org/. Accessed March 7, 2012.

48. Budney AJ, Hughes JR. The cannabis withdrawal syndrome. Curr Opin Psychiatry 2006;19:233–8.

49. Stephens RS, Roffman RA, Curtin L. Comparison of extended versus brief treatments for marijuana use. J Consult Clin Psychol 2000;68:898–908.

50. Budney AJ, Moore BA. Development and consequences of cannabis dependence. J Clin Pharmacol 2002;42(Suppl 11):28S–33S.

51. Levin KH, Copersino ML, Heishman SJ, et al. Cannabis withdrawal symptoms in non-treatment-seeking adult cannabis smokers. Drug Alcohol Depend 2010;111: 120–7.

52. Weinstein AM, Gorelick DA. Pharmacological treatment of cannabis dependence. Curr Pharm Des 2011;17:1351–8.

53. Vandrey R, Haney M. Pharmacotherapy for cannabis dependence: how close are we? CNS Drugs 2009;23:543–53.

54. Levin FR, Kleber HD. Use of dronabinol for cannabis dependence: two case reports and review. Am J Addict 2008;17:161–4.

55. Haney M, Hart CL, Vocburg SK, et al. Marijuana withdrawal in humans: effects of oral THC or divalproex. Neuropsychopharmacology 2004;29:158–70.

56. Budney AJ, Vandrey RG, Hughes JR, et al. Oral delta-9-tetrahydrocannabinol suppresses cannabis withdrawal symptoms. Drug Alcohol Depend 2007;86:22–9.

57. Levin FR, Mariani JJ, Brooks DJ, et al. Dronabinol for the treatment of cannabis dependence: a randomized, double-blind, placebo-controlled trial. Drug Alcohol Depend 2011;116:142–50.

58. Bowen R, McIlwrick J, Baetz M, et al. Lithium and marijuana withdrawal. Can J Psychiatry 2005;50:240–1.

59. Winstock AR, Lea T, Copeland J. Lithium carbonate in the management of cannabis withdrawal in humans: an open-label study. J Psychopharmacol 2009;23:84–93.

60. Haney M, Ward S, Comer SD, et al. Bupropion SR worsens mood during marijuana withdrawal in humans. Psychopharmacology (Berl) 2001;155:171–9.

61. Haney M, Hart CL, Ward AS, et al. Nefazodone decreases anxiety during marijuana withdrawal in humans. Psychopharmacology (Berl) 2003;165:157–65.

62. Haney M, Hart CL, Vosburg SK, et al. Effects of THC and lofexidine in a human laboratory model of marijuana withdrawal and relapse. Psychopharmacology (Berl) 2008;197:157–68.

63. Shafa R. COMT-inhibitors may be a promising tool in treatment of marijuana addiction. Am J Addict 2009;18(AAAP 19th Annual Meeting Poster Abstracts):322.

64. Kau KS, Madayag A, Mantsch JR, et al. Blunted cystine-glutamate antiporter function in the nucleus accumbens promotes cocaine-induced drug seeking. Neuroscience 2008;155:530–7.

65. Gray KM, Watson NL, Carpenter MJ, et al. N-acetylcysteine (NAC) in young marijuana users: an open-label pilot study. Am J Addict 2010;19:187–9.

66. Tirado CF, Goldman M, Lynch K, et al. Atomoxetine for treatment of marijuana dependence: a report on the efficacy and high incidence of gastrointestinal adverse events in a pilot study. Drug Alcohol Depend 2008;94:254–7.

67. McRae-Clark AL, Carter RE, Killeen TK, et al. A placebo-controlled trial of atomoxetine in marijuana-dependent individuals with attention deficit hyperactivity disorder. Am J Addict 2010;19:481–9.

68. McRae AL, Brady KT, Carter RE. Buspirone for treatment of marijuana dependence: a pilot study. Am J Addict 2006;15:404.

69. McRae-Clark AL, Carter RE, Killeen TK, et al. A placebo-controlled trial of buspirone for the treatment of marijuana dependence. Drug Alcohol Depend 2009;105:132–8.

70. Levin FR, McDowell D, Evans SM, et al. Pharmacotherapy for marijuana dependence: a double-blind, placebo-controlled pilot study of divalproex sodium. Am J Addict 2004;13:21–32.

71. Carpenter KM, McDowell D, Brooks DJ, et al. A preliminary trial: double-blind comparison of nefazodone, bupropion-SR, and placebo in the treatment of cannabis dependence. Am J Addict 2009;18:53–64.

72. Cornelius JR, Clark DB, Bukstein OG, et al. Acute phase and five-year follow-up study of fluoxetine in adolescents with major depression and a comorbid substance use disorder: a review. Addict Behav 2005;30:1824–33.

73. Cornelius JR, Buksten OG, Douaihy AB, et al. Double-blind fluoxetine trial in comorbid MDD-CUD youth and young adults. Drug Alcohol Depend 2010;112: 39–45.

74. Kano M, Ohno-Shosaku T, Hashimotodani Y, et al. Endocannabinoid-mediated control of synaptic transmission. Physiol Rev 2009;89:309–80.

75. Parolaro D, Realini N, Vigano D, et al. The endocannabinoid system and psychiatric disorders. Exp Neurol 2010;224:3–14.

76. Huestis MA, Gorelick DA, Heishman SJ, et al. Blockade of effects of smoked marijuana by the CB1-selective cannabinoid receptor antagonist SR141716. Arch Gen Psychiatry 2001;58:322–8.

77. Huestis MA, Boyd SJ, Heishman SJ, et al. Single and multiple doses of rimonabant antagonize acute effects of smoked cannabis in male cannabis users. Psychopharmacology (Berl) 2007;194:505–15.

78. Le Foll B, Gorelick DA, Goldberg SR. The future of endocannabinoid-oriented clinical research after CB1 antagonists. Psychopharmacology (Berl) 2009;205:171–4.

79. Clapper JR, Mangieri RA, Piomelli D. The endocannabinoid system as a target for the treatment of cannabis dependence. Neuropharmacology 2009;56(Suppl 1): 235–43.

80. Greenwald MK, Stitzer ML. Antinociceptive, subjective and behavioral effects of smoked marijuana in humans. Drug Alcohol Depend 2000;59:261–75.

81. Wachtel SR, de Wit H. Naltrexone does not block the subjective effects of oral Delta(9)-tetrahydrocannabinol in humans. Drug Alcohol Depend 2000;59:251–60.

82. Haney M, Bisaga A, Foltin RW. Interaction between naltrexone and oral THC in heavy marijuana smokers. Psychopharmacology (Berl) 2003;166:77–85.

83. Haney M. Opioid antagonism of cannabinoid effects: differences between marijuana smokers and nonmarijuana smokers. Neuropsychopharmacology 2007;32:1391–403.

84. Cooper ZD, Haney M. Opioid antagonism enhances marijuana's effects in heavy marijuana smokers. Psychopharmacology (Berl) 2010;211:141–8.

85. Miller W, Rollnick S. Motivational interviewing: preparing people for change. 2nd edition. New York: The Guilford Press; 2002.

86. Prochaska JO, DiClemente CC, Norcross JC. In search of how people change. Applications to addictive behaviors. Am Psychol 1992;47:1102–14.

87. Babor TF. Brief treatments for cannabis dependence: findings from a randomized multisite trial. J Consult Clin Psychol 2004;72:455–66.

88. Stein LA, Lebeau R, Colby SM, et al. Motivational interviewing for incarcerated adolescents: effects of depressive symptoms on reducing alcohol and marijuana use after release. J Stud Alcohol Drugs 2011;72:497–506.

89. Baker A, Turner A, Kay-Lambkin FJ, et al. The long and the short of treatments for alcohol or cannabis misuse among people with severe mental disorders. Addict Behav 2009;34:852–8.

90. Kay-Lambkin FJ, Baker AL, Lewin TJ, et al. Computer-based psychological treatment for comorbid depression and problematic alcohol and/or cannabis use: a randomized controlled trial of clinical efficacy. Addiction 2009;104:378–88.

91. Walker DD, Roffman RA, Picciano JF, et al. The check-up: in-person, computerized, and telephone adaptations of motivational enhancement treatment to elicit voluntary participation by the contemplator. Subst Abuse Treat Prev Policy 2007;2:2.

92. Baker AL, Hides L, Lubman DI. Treatment of cannabis use among people with psychotic or depressive disorders: a systematic review. J Clin Psychiatry 2010;71:247–54.

93. Martin G, Copeland J. The adolescent cannabis check-up: randomized trial of a brief intervention for young cannabis users. J Subst Abuse Treat 2008;34:407–14.

94. Walker DD, Roffman RA, Stephens RS, et al. Motivational enhancement therapy for adolescent marijuana users: a preliminary randomized controlled trial. J Consult Clin Psychol 2006;74:628–32.

95. Stephens RS, Roffman RA, Fearer SA, et al. The Marijuana Check-up: promoting change in ambivalent marijuana users. Addiction 2007;102:947–57.

96. Beck AT, Wright FD, Newman CF, et al. Cognitive therapy of substance abuse. New York: The Guilford Press; 2001.

97. Copeland J, Swift W, Roffman R, et al. A randomized controlled trial of brief cognitive-behavioral interventions for cannabis use disorder. J Subst Abuse Treat 2001;21:55–64.

98. Stephens RS, Roffman RA, Simpson EE. Treating adult marijuana dependence: a test of the relapse prevention model. J Consult Clin Psychol 1994;62:92–9.

99. Stephens RS, Roffman RA, Copeland J, et al. Cognitive-behavioral and motivational enhancement treatments for cannabis dependence. In: Roffman R, Stephens R, editors. Cannabis dependence: its nature, consequences and treatment. Cambridge: Cambridge University Press; 2006. p. 131–53.

100. Budney AJ, Higgins ST, Radonovich KJ, et al. Adding voucher-based incentives to coping skills and motivational enhancement improves outcomes during treatment for marijuana dependence. J Consult Clin Psychol 2000;68:1051–61.

101. Carroll KM, Easton CJ, Nich C, et al. The use of contingency management and motivational/skills-building therapy to treat young adults with marijuana dependence. J Consult Clin Psychol 2006;74:955–66.

102. Baker A, Bucci S, Lewin TJ, et al. Cognitive-behavioural therapy for substance use disorders in people with psychotic disorders: randomised controlled trial. Br J Psychiatry 2006;188:439–48.

103. Budney AJ, Moore BA, Sigmon SC, et al. Contingency-management interventions for cannabis dependence. In: Roffman R, Stephens R, editors. Cannabis dependence: its nature, consequences, and treatment. Cambridge: Cambridge University Press; 2006. p. 154–76.

104. Petry NM. A comprehensive guide to the application of contingency management procedures in clinical settings. Drug Alcohol Depend 2000;58:9–25.

105. Budney AJ, Moore BA, Rocha HL, et al. Clinical trial of abstinence-based vouchers and cognitive-behavioral therapy for cannabis dependence. J Consult Clin Psychol 2006;74:307–16.

106. Kadden RM, Litt MD, Kabela-Cormier E, et al. Abstinence rates following behavioral treatments for marijuana dependence. Addict Behav 2007;32:1220–36.

107. Sinha R, Easton C, Renee-Aubin L, et al. Engaging young probation-referred marijuana-abusing individuals in treatment: a pilot trial. Am J Addict 2003;12: 314–23.

108. Stanger C, Budney AJ, Kamon JL, et al. A randomized trial of contingency management for adolescent marijuana abuse and dependence. Drug Alcohol Depend 2009;105:240–7.

109. Sigmon SC, Steingard S, Badger GJ, et al. Contingent reinforcement of marijuana abstinence among individuals with serious mental illness: a feasibility study. Exp Clin Psychopharmacol 2000;8:509–17.

110. Misch DA. Basic strategies of dynamic supportive therapy. J Psychother Pract Res 2000;9:173–89.

111. Grenyer BFS, Luborsky L, Solowij N. Treatment manual for supportive-expressive dynamic psychotherapy: special adaptation for treatment of cannabis (marijuana) dependence. Sydney (Australia): National Drug and Alcohol Research Centre; 1995.

112. Grenyer B, Solowij N, Peters R. A comparison of brief versus intensive treatment for cannabis dependence. Aust J Psychol 1996;48(Suppl 106).

113. Diamond G, Leckrone J, Dennis ML, et al. The Cannabis Youth Treatment Study: the treatment models and preliminary findings. In: Roffman R, Stephens RS, editors. Cannabis dependence; its nature, consequences and treatment. Cambridge: Cambridge University Press; 2006. p. 247–74.

114. Waldron HB, Kern-Jones S, Turner CW, et al. Engaging resistant adolescents in drug abuse treatment. J Subst Abuse Treat 2007;32:133–42.

115. Rigter H, Pelc I, Tossmann P, et al. INCANT: a transnational randomized trial of multidimensional family therapy versus treatment as usual for adolescents with cannabis use disorder. BMC Psychiatry 2010;10:28.

116. Liddle HA, Dakof GA, Turner RM, et al. Treating adolescent drug abuse: a randomized trial comparing multidimensional family therapy and cognitive behavior therapy. Addiction 2008;103:1660–70.

117. Liddle HA, Dakof GA, Parker K, et al. Multidimensional family therapy for adolescent drug abuse: results of a randomized clinical trial. Am J Drug Alcohol Abuse 2001; 27:651–88.

118. Dennis M, Titus JC, Diamond G, et al. The Cannabis Youth Treatment (CYT) experiment: rationale, study design and analysis plans. Addiction 2002;97(Suppl 1): 16–34.

119. Diamond G, Godley SH, Liddle HA, et al. Five outpatient treatment models for adolescent marijuana use: a description of the Cannabis Youth Treatment Interventions. Addiction 2002;97(Suppl 1):70–83.

120. Brigham GS. 12-step participation as a pathway to recovery: the Maryhaven experience and implications for treatment and research. Sci Pract Perspect 2003; 2:43–51.

121. Humphreys K. Professional interventions that facilitate 12-step self-help group involvement. Alcohol Res Health 1999;23:93–8.

122. Marijuana 12 step workbook, 2008. Available at: http://www.marijuana-anonymous. org/ma12stepworkbook.shtml. Accessed October 21, 2011.

123. Stephens R, Roffman A. The nature, consequences and treatment of cannabis dependence: implications for future research and policy. In: Roffman A, Stephens R, editors. Cannabis dependence: its nature, consequences and treatment. Cambridge: Cambridge University Press; 2006. p. 343–56.

124. Dutra L, Stathopoulous G, Basden SL, et al. A meta-analytic review of psychosocial interventions for substance use disorders. Am J Psychiatry 2008;165:179–87.

125. McLellan AT, Lewis DC, O'Brien CP, et al. Drug dependence, a chronic medical illness: implications for treatment, insurance, and outcomes evaluation. JAMA 2000;284:1689–95.

126. Solowij N, Michie PT. Cannabis and cognitive dysfunction: parallels with endophenotypes of schizophrenia? J Psychiatry Neurosci 2007;32:30–52.

New Systems of Care for Substance Use Disorders
Treatment, Finance, and Technology Under Health Care Reform

David R. Pating, MD[a,b,]*, Michael M. Miller, MD[c,d],
Eric Goplerud, PhD, MA[e], Judith Martin, MD[f],
Douglas M. Ziedonis, MD[g]

KEYWORDS

- Substance abuse • Addiction treatment • Health care reform • Brief intervention

KEY POINTS

- Approximately 23.5 million American adults have a substance use disorder, but only 10.4% receive the addiction treatment they need.
- Few patients with addiction receive continuity care, despite the fact that the course of illness is often characterized by acute exacerbations followed by periods of remission and relapse.
- For persons with substance use disorders, integration with primary care may be the only hope for patients for whom stigma substantially impedes utilization of specific addiction care services.
- Within the world of addiction care, clinicians must move beyond their self-imposed "stigmatization" and sequestration of specialty addition treatment.
- Clinicians need to show exactly *how* addiction treatment works, and to what extent it works through metrics showing changes in symptom level or functional outcome, changes in health care utilization, or other measures.

Overall, persons in America with substance abuse disorders receive insufficient professional treatment and the frequency and duration of care they receive is

[a] Department of Psychiatry, University of California, San Francisco, San Francisco, CA, USA; [b] Kaiser Permanente San Francisco, 1201 Fillmore Street, San Francisco, CA 94115, USA; [c] Department of Psychiatry, University of Wisconsin School of Medicine and Public Health, Oconomowoc, WI, USA; [d] Herrington Recovery Center, Rogers Memorial Hospital, 34700 Valley Road, Oconomowoc, WI 53066, USA; [e] National Opinion Research Center (NORC) at the University of Chicago, 4350 East West Highway, 8th Floor, Bethesda, MD 20814, USA; [f] BAART Turk Street Clinic, 433 Turk Street, San Francisco, CA 94102, USA; [g] Department of Psychiatry, University of Massachusetts Medical School and UMass Memorial Health Care, 55 Lake Avenue North, Worcester, MA 01655, USA
* Corresponding author. Kaiser Permanente San Francisco, 1201 Fillmore Street, San Francisco, CA 94115.
E-mail address: david.pating@kp.org

Psychiatr Clin N Am 35 (2012) 327–356
http://dx.doi.org/10.1016/j.psc.2012.03.004
0193-953X/12/$ – see front matter © 2012 Elsevier Inc. All rights reserved.

psych.theclinics.com

inadequate to produce meaningful clinical results. Recent legislative reforms and policy initiatives will increase the accessibility and availability of clinically appropriate substance abuse treatment services. In this report, we review the current system of health care delivery for the treatment of substance use disorders as well as examine opportunities for the expansion and improvement of treatment under health care reform.

This 4-part report examines new systems of care for substance use conditions under health reform.

1. We briefly review the **prevailing general system** of care for the treatment for substance-related conditions.
2. We provide a **detailed exploration of the emerging systems** of publicly and privately funded substance use disorders treatment, which—driven by new insurance regulations and new mechanisms for payment reimbursement—will change significantly under health care reform.
3. We examine **3 case studies of expanded care** for clinically distinct subsets of patients—those with unhealthy substance use who do not yet have addiction (persons with hazardous use), those with the highest recent rate of increase in mortality among substance use disorders (persons with opioid addiction), and those with the highest overall incidence of substance-related deaths (persons with nicotine addiction)—to examine how persons with different disorders should be able to receive better, more frequent care through federally mandated health care reforms.
4. We examine **how health information technology systems will** drive substance use disorders treatment toward greater connectivity, accountability, and improved outcomes.

Embedded throughout this discussion are recommendations to transform the care for substance use disorders under health care reform. These recommendations are offered with a caveat: although the authors are all experts in their field, no amount of evidence-based forecasting can capture the enormous change and complexity that we anticipate will result from health care reform. Instead, we are humbled by the complex fabric of overlapping systems, which will form the new system of care for the treatment of substance use disorders as the US health care system evolves toward increased affordability and accountability.

PREVAILING SYSTEMS OF ADDICTION TREATMENT AND FUNDING

Roughly 23.5 million American adults have a substance use disorder, but only 10.4% receive the addiction treatment they need.[1,2] Stated differently, 20.9 million persons, totaling 8.3% of the US population age 12 years or older, needed treatment for an illicit drug or alcohol use problem but did not receive treatment at a specialty substance abuse facility in the last year. Although most persons with addiction see a physician at least once every 2 years,[3] it is most often for medical/surgical complications of their substance use, rather than for the addiction itself. Among those receiving treatment, only 20% are offered US Food and Drug Administration (FDA)-approved pharmacotherapies from which they may benefit.[4,5] The "treatment gap" experienced by persons with addiction results in substantial social burdens and is acknowledged by major health services researchers and federal policymakers.[6] According to the United States Preventive Services Task Force, reducing hazardous alcohol use through early screening and brief intervention is a more cost-efficient and effective prevention activity than breast or prostate cancer screenings, depression screening, or reduction of obesity. Hazardous alcohol use screening only narrowly falls behind tobacco cessation, immunizations, and taking daily aspirin in its positive public health impact; yet, its broad scale adoption grossly lags behind other public health priorities.[7]

Part of the complexity of adequately addressing substance use conditions has to do with the fact that addiction is essentially both an acute and chronic health problem. The course of illness is often characterized by acute exacerbations (intoxication and withdrawal requiring intervention and stabilization) followed by periods of remission and relapse, which may diminish in frequency over time with appropriate continuing care.[8,9] Few patients with addiction, however, receive continuity care, despite the fact that continuity is a standard of care for other chronic diseases (diabetes, heart disease, or cancer) in which disease management is a "mainstream" activity. When patients do receive addiction treatment, it is usually episodic and in specialty care delivery systems that are separate from general medical care.[10] Addiction services are rarely located in general medical hospitals or clinics. Instead, addiction treatment is usually offered in separate locations by staffs who specialize in addiction care but who interact infrequently with general medical providers or even the primary care physicians for the patients treated in their programs.

When patients do receive addiction treatment, it is generally paid for by payment systems separate from the ones that pay for general medical care. Things have likely not changed from a decade ago, when 82% of the addiction treatment in America was paid for by public funding systems, and 9% of addiction treatment was paid for by private health insurance (with the remaining costs paid for out of pocket).[11] Most public funding for addiction treatment does not come via Medicare or Medicaid but via unique Substance Abuse Prevention and Treatment Block Grants from the federal government to specific state agencies that administer receipt of those funds and distribution of dollars to local treatment agencies.[10] In the ensuing years, these trends did not see any increases in private sector (commercial insurance) contributions to payment for addiction services. With health care reform, major changes in insurance regulation and reimbursement will dramatically alter how addiction treatment is delivered in the United States and how it is paid for.

EMERGING SYSTEMS OF ADDICTION TREATMENT AND FUNDING

For the last decade, national quality agencies have recognized the need to transform the US health care system. Acknowledging inefficiencies in health care service delivery and deficiencies in overall health care quality, the Institute for Healthcare Improvement called for the simultaneous pursuit of 3 aims as part of a national vision to improve the US health care system: improving the experience of care, improving the health of populations, and reducing per-capita costs of health care.[12] Similar to this, recognizing the large "gaps" in the treatment of substance use disorders as well the significant imbalance in public versus private funding for addiction services, the Institute of Medicine called for a fundamental transformation in the system of care for substance use disorders to "cross the quality chasm."[6] Fundamental to both these general and specialty perspectives is the view underscored by the President's New Freedom Commission: "To achieve the promise of community living for everyone, new service delivery patterns and incentives must ensure that every American has easy and continuous access to the most current treatments and best support services."[13]

The Affordable Care Act

The Affordable Care Act of 2010 (ACA) brings new opportunity to transform the delivery of general medical and specialty addiction treatment to the United States.

Box 1
The Affordable Care Act: what is it?[a]

Coverage: Expands coverage to 32 million Americans who are currently uninsured.

Health Insurance Exchanges: Creates state-run exchanges, which create purchasing pools to offer insurance at reduced rate for individuals and small employer groups.

Subsidies: Available to individuals and families with income between the 133% and 400% of federal poverty level.

Medicaid: Expands Medicaid to include 133% of federal poverty level but excludes illegal immigrants as not eligible for Medicaid.

Medicare: Closes the Medicare prescription drug "donut hole" by 2020.

Insurance Reform: Coverage for children, regardless of a preexisting condition. Dependent care coverage for children younger than 26. Mandatory preventive care coverage for all new, private policies. Removal of annual and lifetime benefit limits. Elimination of policy cancellations. Guarantees coverage and renewal. Bans preexisting conditions. Mandates Essential Benefits Package, which includes benefitted treatment for mental health and substance use disorders.

Affordability: Reduces out-of-pocket costs (for lower-incomes). Limits small group plan deductibles. Requires copay and limits for mental health and substance abuse be comparable to those for medical and surgical disorders (parity).

Individual Mandate: (pending legal challenge as of 12/2011) Everyone must purchase health insurance or face a $695 annual fine. There are some exceptions for low-income people.

Employer Mandate: Employers with more than 50 employees must provide health insurance or pay a fine of $2000 per worker each year if any worker receives federal subsidies to purchase health insurance.

Immigration: Illegal immigrants will not be allowed to buy health insurance in the exchanges—even if they pay completely with their own money.

[a]**This is a partial list of key ACA provisions adapted from Henry J. Kaiser Family Foundation.**

Adapted from The Henry J Kaiser Family Foundation. Focus on health reform: summary of new health reform law. Updated April 15, 2011. Available at: http://www.kff.org/healthreform/upload/8061.pdf. Accessed December 18, 2011.

The ACA establishes new financing and insurance mechanisms to provide health insurance to more than 30 million persons currently uninsured, among which it is estimated that the rates of substance use disorders could be 2 or 3 times the rates in the population in general. The ACA and related legislation, collectively known as Health Care Reform, creates new governmental structures (health insurance and health technology exchanges), increases the availability of private insurance and Medicaid coverage, assures coverage for mental health and substance use disorders as essential health care benefits, protects patients from inappropriate denial of coverage for preexisting conditions, and directs payment incentives to improve quality of care, which includes addiction treatment (**Box 1**).[14]

Coverage expansion
Under the ACA, 4.3 million of 32 million newly insured persons are expected to become new users of mental health or substance abuse treatment services, either through expanded affordability for privately funded health insurance (2.0 million) or

expanded eligibility of publically sponsored Medicaid coverage (2.3 million).[15] The expansion in health care coverage embraces 3 financially distinct sectors of care comprising:

1. Individuals with private insurance
2. Those receiving Medicaid
3. Uninsured individuals who belong to the "Safety Net."

Individuals with private insurance
For individuals with higher incomes, capable of purchasing commercial insurance (especially sole proprietors and farmers who are not part of group health insurance plans), newly created state-run health insurance exchanges offer the opportunity to purchase health insurance at lower premiums through large purchasing pools, which leverage multiple sources of funding including individual contributions, subsidies from employers, and contributions from federal Medicare programs. These are combined with premium and cost-sharing subsidies, which further lower the cost of available insurance for citizens and legal immigrants with incomes between 133% and 400% of federal poverty level (FPL) (FPL in 2011 is $10,890 for an individual and $22,350 for a family of 4).[16]

Individuals receiving Medicaid
For those with lower incomes, eligibility for Medicaid will expand to include those with incomes up to 133% of FPL. In most states, these Medicaid changes will increase enrollment and increase Medicaid benefits for new Medicaid enrollees, whose coverage must be comparable to the essential benefits required for exchange-qualified health plans.

Uninsured individuals
For the remaining individuals who are uninsured, county and state "safety net" services will continue to provide the bulk of available care, which unfortunately may be subject to future reductions in direct federal funding.

The net effect of coverage expansion under this 3-tier financial system is the dominant position of health insurance as the backbone of US health care. In this system:

1. Dollars will follow patients with substance use disorders, rather than flow into prepurchased "block-grant" programs
2. States and counties will develop or expand Medicaid-eligible managed care health plans (a government-funded form of health insurance) to control population-based risks
3. Medicaid fee-for-service reimbursement will decrease
4. Local contracts for addiction treatment services, typically as county-purchased treatment beds or slots, will become less common (counties will receive less federal "block grant" funding funneled to them by state addiction agencies).

Significantly, substance abuse treatment programs incapable of billing insurance for their services may not survive if they are unable to adapt to these financial reforms.

Mental Health and Addiction Treatment Parity
While health care reform increases the affordability of health insurance, separate provisions of the ACA additionally mandate that all "qualified health plans" increase equity in coverage for substance use disorders. Under the ACA, not only will mental health and addiction treatment likely be included as "essential health benefits" in all plans, but benefit structures will have to incorporate provisions from the Mental Health Parity and Addiction Equity Act of 2008 (Parity Act).[17] The Parity Act mandates

that covered health benefits for the treatment of substance use disorders must be equal to or comparable (at par) with the benefits offered for medical and surgical conditions. More importantly, the Parity Act mandates that individual service copays and day or dollar limits for addiction treatment in a health plan must be "not substantially different" from the "predominant" level of copays, deductibles, and day/dollar limits for medical or surgical disorders offered by the same plan.

The benefits to be derived from addiction treatment parity are significant.[18] In a study of 6 Federal Employee Health Benefit Plans, which had mandates in place since 1996 to provide parity-level addiction treatment benefits, addiction treatment parity resulted in increased utilization that was paid for by medical cost offsets (reduced emergency room visits or hospitalizations).[19] The results were a minimal net increase in overall cost and a larger increase in quality because of greater utilization of appropriate treatment. Similar results have been reported for the states of Washington and Oregon, whose parity laws closely mirror the benefits mandated under the federal Parity Act.[20,21]

Despite the positive effects of parity-level benefits, prior experience from states in which broad-scale ACA-like universal coverage expansion has been mandated—including Massachusetts, Maine, and Vermont—demonstrated mixed results in the ability to promote access to care through expanded coverage alone. In these states, individuals with substance use disorders failed to meet enrollment expectations, despite the overall lowered cost to purchase insurance.[22] One possible explanation for this failure is that individuals with substance use disorders are medically disenfranchised; as a cohort, they do not access regular medical care or access the financial means (insurance) to pay for care, even when systemic barriers to enrollment are lowered.[22] As state health insurance exchanges roll out nationwide, it is necessary to ensure that outreach programs actively enroll individuals in needed substance use disorders care. Failure to repatriate individuals with substance use problems into the health care system will make it difficult to realize the social benefits (eg, reduced homelessness or crime) of improved health care.[13]

Delivery System Reform

Alongside the expansion in health insurance coverage, the ACA mandates reforms to health care service delivery. The ACA links reimbursement for addiction treatment to 6 quality aims for health care services outlined by the Institute of Medicine (IOM). According to the IOM, high quality care is[23]:

1. Safe
2. Effective
3. Patient-centered
4. Timely
5. Efficient
6. Equitable.

These aims prompted a nationwide movement to integrate behavioral health (mental health and substance use disorders treatment services) into primary care,[24] because the majority of patients with substance use disorders also have chronic medical or psychiatric conditions; yet, in the current pre-ACA environment, only 20% of adults with addiction and only 3% to 6% of older adults (over 65 years) with addiction actually receive treatment in specialty addiction treatment programs.[25] When we consider that the majority of individuals with substance use disorders present to primary care at some point during their illness, as well as the declaration by the World Health Organization that the comorbidity of mental and physical

---

Box 2
What are patient-centered health care homes?

In 2007, the American Academy of Family Physicians, American Academy of Pediatrics, American College of Physicians, and American Osteopathic Association released the Joint Principles of the Patient-Centered Medical Home. In a patient-centered medical home, key characteristics of health care should include:

1. Personal physicians

2. Physician-directed medical practice

3. Whole person orientation

4. Coordinated/integrated care

5. Quality and safety

6. Enhanced access

7. Payment for value-added

Adapted from Joint Principles of the Patient-Centered Medical Home March 2007, http://www.aafp.org/online/en/home/media/releases/2007/20070305pressrelease0.html.

---

disorders is the norm across the lifespan,[26] the failure to engage persons with substance use disorders presenting in the primary care setting is a tremendous "missed opportunity."[27] For persons with substance use disorders, integration with primary care may be the only hope for patients for whom stigma substantially impedes utilization of specific addiction care services.

Public sector reforms

In the public system of most states, the shift to primary care as the location in which people will receive care for their substance use conditions will be effected mostly via an expansion of Federally Qualified Health Centers (FQHC). FQHC and other Primary Care clinics designated as Patient Centered Health Care Homes (PCHCHs) are targeted to receive incentives for funding workforce development under the ACA (**Box 2**).[10,28] Financial incentives are also provided to FQHCs to bring mental health and addiction clinicians into those settings to work as full members of the clinical team[10] so that persons with these conditions will be able to be treated within FQHCs and PCHCHs and not have to be referred to separately located, separately staffed, separately funded clinics offering mental health and substance use disorders care. In the ACA, physician and nonphysician clinicians with psychiatric or addiction treatment expertise are envisioned to be teachers, mentors, clinical consultants, and direct caregivers for the benefit of persons with substance use disorders and the generalists who are caring for them. In a reformed health care system, this expanded and newly certified mental health and addiction treatment workforce will deliver care at the time and place requested by the patient, not when or where it is convenient for the provider (Roy K, Miller M. The medicalization of addiction treatment professionals. J Psychoactive Drug 2012. Submitted for publication). For patients with substance use disorders, there can be "no wrong door" to addiction treatment if we want to reduce the impact of substance abuse on their comorbid medical conditions. Similarly, there can be no effective health care without integrated behavioral health care.

Integrated behavioral health care

Several models of integrated care have proven feasible in demonstration proj-ects.[29,30] These include:

1. Fully integrated services in which primary care providers may provide medication-assisted therapy, such as buprenorphine, and coordinate care with onsite spe-cialty alcohol and drug counselors
2. Onsite colocation of substance use treatment services in primary care, or "reverse colocation" of primary care services into substance use treatment settings
3. Various sequential or coordinated care models by clinics that are not colocated.

Each of these models has strengths and weakness, and almost all must overcome implementation challenges including new costs, required staffing, establishment of infrastructure including health information sharing, and concrete needs, such as office space. Regardless, over the last half decade, the Substance Abuse and Mental Health Services Administration (SAMHSA), the Indian Health Service, and many national state mental health and alcohol and drug programs have committed to collaborative demonstration efforts (**Box 3**).[31]

Research studies on the effectiveness of behavioral health service integration within a large private-sector prepaid integrated health care system have been positive. When patients with medical or psychiatric problems (the majority of the patients) receive medical services in "reverse colocated" primary care clinics embed-ded in an outpatient addiction treatment setting (rather than with addiction services colocated in a primary care clinic), they are twice as likely to be sober at 6 months and have significantly reduced hospital and medical costs than a comparable cohort receiving nonintegrated care.[32–34] In a parallel study, patients who received coordi-nated (not-integrated) care consisting of routine physician screening for substance abuse in primary care, referral to specialty care when needed, and referral back to primary care when stabilized, also had reduced costs and improved outcomes.[35] Unfortunately, only 13% of patients studied received this level of coordination despite the availability of these services. This is a sobering caution to clinical administrators who must be aware of the complex systemic, provider, and culture changes that are required to effectively adopt integrated care strategies. Health care costs consumed by those who receive continuing care have been shown to approach other matched health plan members when tallied over a 9-year span.[36]

Private sector reforms

In the private sector—where 80% of patients receive their general medical and mental health care, mostly through employer-sponsored commercial insurance as the major source of funding for treatment—one of the major impediments to patients receiving adequate treatment for substance use disorders has been the discriminatory struc-ture of insurance benefits and utilization review processes for addiction treatment. Benefit structures limiting the number of lifetime encounters for intensive outpatient or inpatient addiction treatment, the number of outpatient visits for addiction treatment, the medications that would be covered under the formulary for the pharmacy benefit, and the specific providers who could see patients under behavioral health care "carve-out" plans, all restrict access to care and widen the "treatment gap."[37]

Systemically, large gaps in the continuum of services available to privately insured individuals with addiction are the norm.[10] Private sector organizations such as general hospitals and multispecialty medical clinics have not built capacity for treating patients with addiction like they have for treating persons with cancer or heart disease. In some cases, the private insurance industry has utilized treatment capacity

---

Box 3
Models of integrated behavioral health care

Integrated models of Behavioral Health Care incorporate an array of services elements to improve efficiency and effectiveness of patient-centered care. Common elements include:

- Use of a screening tool to identify mental health or substance use problems
- Presence of "warm hand-offs"
- Physical proximity of behavioral staff with medical staff
- Financial integration
- Use of outcome measures to assess effectiveness
- Case conferencing between primary and behavioral staff
- Use of psychiatrists and addiction specialists as service providers or consultants
- Degree of case management
- Length of therapy
- Therapeutic orientation
- Severity of substance use or mental health disorders the clinic is willing to treat
- Physician willing to prescribe anti-craving or psychiatric medication
- Involvement of primary care physicians in behavioral care
- Consolidation/separation of client's record
- Group or individual self-management sessions designed to help patients' compliance with medical treatment regimen
- Provision of cross-education: mental health training for primary care providers and medical training for behavioral staff
- Conjoint consultation
- "Ownership" and supervision of the behavioral staff
- Level of involvement of behavioral staff with medical issues
- Relationship with local mental health or addiction treatment program; and ease of referrals to that system
- Comprehensiveness of feedback provided to the primary care physician by behavioral staff
- Collaboration with colleges/universities to provide training for students
- Participation in collaboratives

The design of integrated programs varies widely—often they evolve in unique ways to match staffing, available funding, and system of care structure to meet the needs of populations served. There is no "one size fits all." Integrated services may be colocated or offered separately through coordinated (not colocated) programs that provide services either sequentially or concurrently.

Adapted from the Integrated Behavioral Health Project (IBHP) Models of Behavioral Health Integration. Available at: http://www.ibhp.org/index.php?section=pages&cid=91. Accessed December 19, 2011; with permission.

---

from public sector agencies, "piggy-backing" onto the publicly funded addiction treatment system, which would redirect its block grants to fund prepaid outpatient treatment slots or beds in residential treatment programs for privately insured individuals, making it even tougher for persons relying on the public system to receive treatment.

Another approach would see private insurers providing limited or "carved-out" benefits, which may also include limited counseling by individual therapists from a narrowly constructed network of approved providers, occasional use of office-based medication-assisted treatment (buprenorphine, injectable naltrexone), and referrals to self-help meetings[38] as substitutes for offering patients comprehensive drug and alcohol treatment administered by experienced and licensed addiction clinicians. At the other extreme of this spectrum, private fee-for-service specialty clinics and "luxury rehab" programs serve elite clients who have the capability to pay out of pocket. Often costing $10,000 to $50,000 per month of treatment, these programs represent a Cadillac-level of services without a broad demonstration of enhanced outcomes commensurate with the enhanced fees charged for these services.[39]

With the advent of the Mental Health Parity and Addiction Equity Act of 2008, some of these treatment gaps in privately funded services will narrow. Federal regulations will prohibit group health plans—even those offered via self-insured companies, unions, and municipalities to their employees, outside of a formal insurance policy— from having addiction treatment benefit limits that are more restrictive than the prevailing limits for medical/surgical care. Indeed, an early survey of employer-sponsored insurance coverage since 2008 indicates that most sponsored health plans have removed treatment limitations, such as the number of allowed office visits or inpatient days and slightly decreased required copayments for outpatient or in-network care, in response to the Parity Act.[37] Little is known, however, about how health plans use nonquantifiable treatment limits, such as pre-authorization requirements for mental health or substance use benefits, which must also remain comparable to the use of pre-authorization of medical/surgical benefits if they are to be in compliance with the Parity Act.[37] Continued vigilance will be needed by consumers, clinicians and policy makers to assure that insurers meet the medically necessary treatment needs of individuals with addiction.

Optimal health insurance benefits

We envision, when freed of utilization-based benefit limits, new models for office- and clinic-based services will permit the development of evidence-based continuums of care that are both appropriate and medically necessary to manage addiction as it manifests both as acute and chronic conditions. At the time of this article, the covered services under the federal ACA-mandated essential health benefits for substance use disorders treatment, to be incorporated into all plans purchased through state health insurance exchanges, are under review. Expert consensus supports optimal substance use disorder treatment benefits that provide at least 3 months of treatment initiation and stabilization per episode, provided as a graded continuum of age-appropriate outpatient or residential counseling, followed by up to 3 years of continuing care monitoring in either primary care or a specialty outpatient settings. Benefits must also include detoxification, hospitalization, and medical or psychiatric care as needed for co-occurring conditions; appropriate placement to achieve psychosocial stabilization through either outpatient or residential treatment; anticraving or anti-addiction medications (including methadone); and random drug/toxicology testing and other ongoing clinical monitoring.[40–42] Placement in care should be determined by professionally accepted tools such as the American Society of Addiction Medicine's *Patient Placement Criteria* (**Fig. 1**).[43] Also, as addiction treatment becomes more integrated into primary care, broader use of screening tools will require greater use of motivational interventions, perhaps offered by addiction treatment counselors working outside their usual work settings.

IMPLEMENTING AND EXPANDING SYSTEMS OF ADDICTION TREATMENT: CASE STUDIES

By now, it should be recognized that expansions in health insurance coverage and incentives to transform the delivery of services under health care reform, harbors the promise to develop a national system of care for the treatment of addiction that is both comprehensive and effective. Realizing this national promise, however, is fraught with uncertainty, arising from new regulations, financing, incentives and real-world implementation challenges, which all must be mastered to "put services on

Adolescent Criteria: Crosswalk of Levels 0.5 through IV

Criteria Dimensions	Levels of Service				
	Level 0.5 Early Intervention	Level I Outpatient Treatment	Level II Intensive Outpatient Treament	Level III Medically-Monitored Intensive Inpatient Treatment	Level IV Medically-Managed Intensive Inpatient Treatment
DIMENSION 1: Acute Intoxication and/or Withdrawal Potential	No withdrawal risk	No withdrawal risk	Manifests no overt symptoms of withdrawal risk	Risk of withdrawal syndrome is present but manageable in Level III	Severe withdrawal risk
DIMENSION 2: Biomedical Conditions and Complications	None or very stable	None or very stable	None or, if present, does not distract from addiction treatment; manageable at Level II	Require medical monitoring but not intensive treatment	Requires 24-hour medical and nursing care
DIMENSION 3: Emotional/Behavioral Conditions and Complications	None or very stable	None or manageable in an outpatient structured environment	Mild severity, with the potential to distract from recovery efforts	Moderate severity; requires a 24-hour structured setting	Severe problems require 24-hour psychiatric care, with concomitent addiction treatment
DIMENSION 4: Treatment Acceptance/ Resistance	Willing to understand how current use may affect personal goals	Willing to cooperate but needs motivating and monitoring strategies	Resistance high enough to require structured program but not so high as to render outpatient treatment ineffective	Resistance high despite negative consequences; needs intensive motivating strategies in a 24-hour structured setting	Problems in this dimension do not qualify patient for Level IV treatment
DIMENSION 5: Relapse/ Continued Use Potential	Needs understanding of, or skills to change, current use patterns	Able to maintain abstinence and recovery goals with minimal support	Intensification of addiction symptoms; high likelihood of relapse without close monitoring and support	Unable to control use despite active participation in less intensive care; needs 24-hour structure	Problems in this dimension do not qualify patient for Level IV treatment
DIMENSION 6: Recovery Environment	Social support system or significant others increase risk of personal conflict about alcohol/other drug use	Supportive recovery environment and/or patient has skills to cope	Environment unsupportive but, with structure or support, patient can cope	Environment dangerous for recovery, necessitating removal from the environment; logistical impediments to outpatient treatment	Problems in this dimension do not qualify patient for Level IV treatment

This overview of the Adolescent Admission Criteria is an approximate summary to illustrate the principal concepts and structure of the criteria.

Fig. 1. ASAM Patient Placement Criteria 2. (*Courtesy of* the American Society of Addiction Medicine, Chevy Chase, MD; with permission.)

the street." Additionally, Although integrating behavioral health care broadly into primary care theoretically improves overall health care quality, the actual delivery of care for specific substance use disorders remains complicated by intangibles, such as clinic culture, workforce competency, and the capacity of health information systems to meaningfully bridge programs.

We examine 3 case studies of clinically distinct subsets of patients to explore with higher resolution, how new systems of care for specific conditions may evolve under health care reform:

1. Those with unhealthy substance use who do not yet have addiction (persons with hazardous use)
2. Those with the highest recent rate of increase in mortality among substance use disorders (persons with opioid addiction)
3. Those with the highest overall incidence of substance-related deaths (persons with nicotine addiction).

In these examples, we (1) study the prevalent system of care for specific substance use disorders, (2) study variations on how health care reform may facilitate implementation of integrated services or the adoption of effective best-practices, and (3) provide recommendations to establish optimal systems of care.

Case Study: Expanding Preventive Care for the Person with Subsyndromal Unhealthy Alcohol and Other Drug Use

Historically, the emphasis of substance use–related intervention has been placed on either specialist treatment for the most severely affected individuals who have alcohol

---

Box 4
Screening and brief intervention: what is it?

Screening and Brief Intervention (SBI) is a set of therapeutic techniques and a clinical orientation toward preventive care designed to opportunistically assess individuals for possible unhealthy or dependent alcohol or drug use and to provide brief counseling with those who screen positive to assist them to reduce their harmful or hazardous use.

How does it work? Screening: Patients are screened for substance use with a brief, standardized tool. This tool should be simple enough to be administered by a wide range of health professionals. It should focus on the frequency and the quantity of substance use over a particular timeframe (generally 1 to 3 months). An online screening tool at www.alcoholscreening.org provides a demonstration of a basic screening tool, the Alcohol Use Disorder Identification Test (AUDIT). Brief Intervention: Brief intervention, which usually happens in a single session immediately after a positive screening test, consists of a motivational discussion with the patient. This discussion is focused on increasing the patient's understanding of the impact of substance use and motivating behavior change. If the patient needs more extensive treatment than a brief intervention, the provider can refer the patient to specialized substance use treatment. One mnemonic for organizing brief counseling, the 5As, includes:

1. **Assess:** Ask about/assess behavioral health risk(s) and factors affecting choice of behavior change goals/methods.
2. **Advise:** Give clear, specific, and personalized behavior change advice, including information about personal health harms and benefits.
3. **Agree:** Collaboratively select appropriate treatment goals and methods based on the patient's interest in and willingness to change the behavior.
4. **Assist:** Using behavior change techniques (self-help and/or counseling), aid the patient in achieving agreed-upon goals by acquiring the skills, confidence, and social/environmental supports for behavior change, supplemented with adjunctive medical treatments when appropriate.
5. **Arrange:** Schedule follow-up contacts (in person or by telephone) to provide ongoing assistance/support and to adjust the treatment plan as needed, including referral to more intensive or specialized treatment.

---

or other drug addiction[44,45] or on universal prevention strategies aimed at those who have never initiated use.[46] Until recently, little attention was paid to the large group of individuals who use alcohol and other drugs, are not dependent or addicted, and could successfully reduce their use through *early intervention.*[47] Providing universal screening combined with early intervention (screening and brief intervention [SBI]) to those demonstrating *hazardous levels of substance use*[48] leads to substantial reductions in the problems caused by hazardous substance use.[49,50]

For quite some time, research evidence has pointed to the effectiveness of opportunistic screening and brief counseling for alcohol and drug use (**Box 4**). In 1990, the IOM found that, "suitable methods of identification and readily learned brief intervention techniques with good evidence of efficacy are now available."[46] Fourteen years later, the US Preventive Services Task Force (USPTF) in 2004 recommended:

Screening and behavioral counseling for all adults, including pregnant women, in the primary care setting. . .can accurately identify those patients whose levels or patterns of alcohol consumption do not meet criteria for alcohol dependence, but place them at risk for increased morbidity or mortality and brief behavioral counseling interventions with follow-up produce small to moderate reductions in alcohol consumption that are sustained over 6 to 12 month periods or longer.[51]

In 2009, the federal Centers for Medicare and Medicaid Services (CMS) initiated payment for Screening and Brief Intervention delivered to Medicare beneficiaries, and in 2011, CMS officially determined that evidence of the effectiveness and cost effectiveness of SBI as a population health intervention was sufficiently strong that Medicare would cover SBI as a 100% Medicare reimbursable preventive service. Medicare will reimburse primary care physicians and other primary care practitioners to deliver annual alcohol screening; for those that screen positive, Medicare will reimburse up to 4 brief, face-to-face, behavioral counseling interventions per year for beneficiaries, including pregnant women. Finally, beginning mid-2102, under the ACA, all insurers must cover preventive services without copayment or coinsurance. This includes SBI for alcohol and drug misuse, as well as screening and counseling for depression, tobacco, and obesity and other prevention activities.

The evidence for screening and brief intervention
A comprehensive analysis of 361 controlled clinical trials of treatments for alcohol use disorders[49] found the evidence of effectiveness of SBI found in 31 controlled clinical trials of SBI was the strongest of more than 40 alcohol treatment modalities studied. For example, 1 randomized study that assessed effects of SBI after a 48-month follow-up found that the intervention group had, relative to controls[52]:

- 20% reduction in emergency department visits
- 33% reduction in nonfatal injuries
- 37% fewer hospitalizations
- 46% fewer arrests
- 50% fewer motor vehicle crashes.

The intervention group experienced, relative to controls:

- 20% reduction in binge drinking episodes
- 10% reduction in drinks per week
- 4% reduction in those reporting no binge drinking episodes.

And the impact of SBI on mortality and health care service utilization may exceed reductions in alcohol consumption itself.[53] Project TREAT (Trial for Early Alcohol Treatment), a 4-year randomized clinical trial of SBI in 64 primary care clinics in Wisconsin found a $4.30 cost savings towing to reductions in future health care costs for each $1.00 invested in the intervention for nondependent adults who used alcohol at unhealthy levels.[54]

Another randomized, control trial of SBI among hospitalized trauma patients[55] found $3.81 in savings in health care use over 3 years for each $1.00 spent on the intervention. Similar positive returns on investment in SBI have been reported for inpatient medical/surgical patients[56] and specialty substance use treatment. Those interested in health reform and reducing health care costs should take heed of such compelling data.

Opportunities for improved screening through accreditation processes
SBI shows up frequently among the clinical practice standards for primary care and specialty physicians. A compilation of the practice guidelines and performance measures develop by professional societies that recommend routine, opportunistic SBI has been assembled by the Agency for Healthcare Research and Quality (AHRQ www.guidelines.gov). Prominent among these are the guidelines of the Committee on Trauma of theAmerican College of Surgeons, which is responsible for accrediting the nation's trauma centers. Recognizing that alcohol is a significant associated factor

and contributor to injury, the ACS has decreed that it is vital that trauma centers have a mechanism to identify patients who are problem drinkers. Since January 2007, level I and level II trauma centers must demonstrate to accreditors that they can use the teachable moment generated by the injury to implement effective primary prevention, for example, alcohol counseling for problem drinkers. In addition, level I centers must demonstrate the capability to provide an intervention for patients identified as problem drinkers. Such steps have been found to reduce trauma recidivism by 50%.

Similarly, in 2011, The Joint Commission (formerly, the Joint Commission on Accreditation of Healthcare Organizations) adopted a set of 4 substance use screening and intervention performance measures for use with virtually all hospital inpatients[57]:

1. Inpatient screening for unhealthy alcohol use
2. Brief interventions for patients who screen positive for unhealthy alcohol use
3. Initiation of treatment while inpatient or immediately on discharge for patients with substance use disorders
4. Assessing response to the intervention or referral within 30 days after discharge.

These recommendations are now under review for endorsement by the National Quality Forum. Additionally, in 2008, the Physician Consortium on Performance Improvement of the American Medical Association developed and approved perfor-mance measures addressing "Unhealthy Alcohol Use: Screening" and "Unhealthy Alcohol Use: Screening & Brief Counseling" among its performance measure set on Preventive Care and Screening.[58] Despite this high-level support for SBI, opportuni-ties exist to increase the availability of SBI in general medical and specialty settings, facilitated by provisions of the ACA.

Primary care

In a nationally representative survey of general internal medicine physicians, family medicine physicians, obstetrician/gynecologists, and psychiatrists, Friedmann and his colleagues (2000) found that only 13% used standardized alcohol screening instruments. A survey of primary care patients with diagnosable substance use disorders found that more than half reported their physician did nothing about their substance abuse; 43% said their physicians never diagnosed their condition.[54] Only 10% to 20% of patients in primary care settings are screened for alcohol misuse,[59] making it one of the least commonly performed of the USPTF-recommended clinical preventive services.[60] In the absence of screening, clinicians cannot reliably identify those with alcohol misuse.[61] Millstein and Arik[62] found that between 23% and 43% of pediatricians and 14% to 27% of family physicians ask adolescents whether they use alcohol, but only 17% inquire more fully and systematically about alcohol use through a standardized screening instrument.

Emergency physicians and trauma surgeons

A nationally representative study of the quality of care delivered conducted by McGlynn and her colleagues at RAND[63] found that only 15.5% of hospitalized trauma or hepatitis patients have any indication in their medical records that alcohol or drug use was assessed, despite evidence that 40% to 60% of trauma admissions are caused by alcohol or drug use. In a self-report survey of emergency physicians, O'Rourke and colleagues[64] found that 29% assert that they routinely ask about alcohol quantity and frequency. A survey of trauma surgeons[65] reported that more than two-thirds of respondents asserted that they frequently check a blood alcohol concentration, with one-third of the group reporting that they always do. However, only one-fourth reported use of formal screening questionnaires. Just more than one-third (36%) reported that their trauma center was currently performing brief interventions with patients with alcohol problems.

General medical, surgical, and orthopedic inpatients

At least 2.5 million of the 35 million people admitted to US hospitals annually have serious alcohol and drug problems that go untreated. Opportunistic screening of medical/surgical inpatients by research teams finds between 20% or more of hospitalized adults drinking at moderate to high risk levels.[66] Fewer than half have any indication in their medical records that drinking or drug use was assessed, and only about half of hospitalized patients the research teams determine to have a diagnosable substance use disorder have any notation in their records. Only 1 in 5 patients with an alcohol use disorder received any inpatient alcohol intervention, and less than one-fourth were referred for alcohol treatment at discharge.[67]

Taken as a whole, these studies substantiate the meta-analysis conducted by The Partnership for Prevention, which ranked the clinical effectiveness and cost effectiveness of SBI among 1 of the top 5 public health prevention activities by the USPTF.[7,68] Although the ACA eliminates copayments for screening and brief intervention, clinical leaders must work diligently to train staff and modify clinic culture to assure adoption of SBI as an essential service in reformed health care systems.

Case Study: Expanding Behavioral Health Integration for the Person with Opioid Addiction

Persons in America with opioid addiction receive professional interventions for their heroin or prescription opioid problems—but not often enough and generally not using the modalities and durations of care that can produce the best clinical results. The rate of increase in opioid overdose deaths is accepted by the Centers for Disease Control and Prevention and others as a true epidemic.[69] In 2011, prescription drugs were the second-most abused category of drugs in the United States after marijuana.[70] Recently, annual prescription drug deaths in America reached almost 40,000, exceeding the annual deaths from motor vehicle crashes.[71] Although responsible prescribing and use of opioids for pain is a rational approach to this crisis, the need to treat opioid addiction is overlooked.[72] Opioid addiction is virtually never addressed in the general medical care setting, and treatment of persons with opioid addiction using maintenance pharmacotherapies is not even embraced in many specialty addiction treatment clinics.

Methadone maintenance treatment

The primary medical approach offered in the United States for chronic opiate addiction since the Narcotics Treatment Act of 1974 has been methadone maintenance treatment (MMT). The Narcotics Treatment Act of 1974 established the highly regulated system of specialty licensed facilities called Opioid Treatment Programs (OTPs), which are largely sequestered from mainstream medical care—and often considered as "last resort" by patients and practitioners. Payment for OTP care is usually not included in private health insurance plans, but some states allow Federal Substance Abuse Treatment Block Grant funds to be used for methadone maintenance treatment. MMT requires high levels of interdisciplinary care, with daily observed dosing by a nurse or pharmacist, mandated counseling, and medical monitoring, including random toxicology tests. In 1997, the National Institutes of Health declared MMT the most successful treatment option for heroin addiction of its time, calling for increased access and reduced regulatory restraints on methadone maintenance.[73] Since then, dramatic changes in patterns of opioid use, especially increases in the nonmedical use of prescription opioids, even in areas of the country where heroin use is rare, have underscored the need for new treatment alternatives for patients with opioid addiction. Epidemics of human immunodeficiency virus (HIV) and hepatitis C have furthered the public health mandate demanding that improved systems of care be implemented to reduce the impact of injection drug use, as is seen in many persons with heroin addiction, on infectious disease incidence in American communities, large and small.[74]

Throughout the 1990s, successful pilots of office-based methadone treatment proved equally as effective in reducing heroin use compared with OTP care, with positive experiences noted by both patients and providers.[75–77] Based on such pilots, changes in Federal Regulations in 2001 allowed monthly dispensing of methadone from OTPs; stable patients who are compliant with treatment can receive 1 observed dose per month at the OTP, taking home the remainder of the month's doses for unsupervised use. For these patients, the components of care for opioid dependence are similar to the those of the office-based treatment for chronic intractable pain, including use of opioid contracts or patient agreements, random call-back for medication monitoring ("pill counts") and toxicology tests, and psychosocial services as needed. Reimbursement for these treatment alternatives are different, and levels of oversight, including Drug Enforcement Agency rules, state regulations, and unique accreditation requirements, remain much higher for the OTP than for office-based physician who prescribes opioids for the treatment of pain or the treatment of addiction.

Office-based opioid treatment

Since 2001, office-based maintenance with sublingual buprenorphine/naloxone has been available, with fewer restrictions than those for methadone maintenance OTPs.[78] Contrary to OTP care, buprenorphine treatment under the Drug Abuse Treatment Act of 2000 does not require observed dosing and can be prescribed in a general medical office setting. In most locations, maintenance treatment with buprenorphine and maintenance treatment with methadone are in different venues and not equitably available. For many patients, the cost of sublingual buprenorphine preparations is prohibitive.

Under SAMHSA's strategy to address the wave of prescription drug abuse, office-based buprenorphine maintenance expanded in the last 10 years. The initial model for medication-assisted therapy utilizing buprenorphine, based on early evidence from US clinical trials, included an intense induction phase, which required observation over several hours, and was inconsistent with typical office-based practice scheduling patterns.[79] Observed induction was seen as a patient hurdle— patients were required to have withdrawal symptoms before induction—and scheduling for busy clinicians was difficult. Since then, more flexible induction algorithms have emerged, including home induction under various levels of clinical supervision.[80] Following induction, the need for frequent visits necessary to achieve stabilization still poses challenges; however, once patients are stabilized, treatment structure and patient agreements related to use of buprenorphine for opioid dependence can be similar to opioid medication agreements used in pain management. Bringing addiction care into primary care via office-based opioid treatment is an excellent example of the "colocation" of addiction care into general medical care that will become more prevalent with integration of addiction and general medical care via health care reform. As maintenance treatment with buprenorphine moves into general medical service delivery systems, a new challenge is to assure that patients will receive needed psychosocial treatments so that medication-assisted treatment of opioid addiction through office-based general medical physicians does not become medication-only treatment.

Relationship of opioid treatment to medical homes

Because of the prevalence of high medical comorbidity associated with opioid addiction (hepatitis C, HIV, chronic pain), there is great support under the ACA for the integration of medication-assisted therapy for opioid addiction into the primary care medical home, particularly for populations with high comorbid risks.[81] Protocols to coordinate office-based medication-assisted treatment include the association of buprenorphine "induction centers," which admit, evaluate, and stabilize patients on buprenorphine before transfer back to primary care for ongoing maintenance. Other models include integrating knowledgeable clinicians, who are capable of providing on-site buprenorphine maintenance, counseling, or drug testing, into the medical home team.[80] Lastly, the most common model remains primary care coordination with a "medical neighbor" that offers addiction treatment.

In the case of methadone maintenance at OTPs, several considerations make it reasonable to have OTPs themselves become medical homes (another example of "reverse colocation"). These clinics are especially effective in providing essential medical services to intravenous drug users, individuals who are homeless, or those with severe psychiatric impairment. Patients with these conditions often prioritize receiving their daily methadone dose ahead of receiving medical care. The presence of nurses, physicians, and counselors at embedded medical services in OTP clinics facilitates these patients obtaining medications for infections, chronic medical disorders, or psychiatric conditions[82] and provides a reliable setting to obtain blood tests, glucose checks, blood pressure monitoring—all under supervision at the methadone dosing window. Some OTPs even provide chronic medical care, for example, interferon therapy for needle-related illnesses such as hepatitis C or HIV. In these clinics, OTP-based individual and group counseling not only helps provide basic addiction recovery skills but can reinforce medical health, safety, and medication adherence.[83]

To make this level of integration commonplace, regulations impacting federal and state reimbursement for OTPs must allow greater flexibility to blend and braid funding to achieve optimally integrated medical and OTP care. Similarly, public policy directed by state health insurance exchanges must require the incorporation of methadone and other medication-assisted therapies into the essential health benefits of privately insured and Medicaid-eligible individuals, as well as require health plans to provide opioids-dependent patients with all medically necessary services to manage their many comorbid conditions. As is the case for all cases of addiction, the best results for opioid addiction derive from offering patients both medications and counseling, integrated and individualized to the patient's needs.[9] Maintenance therapies with opioid agonists (methadone and buprenorphine) or antagonists (naltrexone) lead to reduced craving and preoccupation and effectively prevent opioid overdose. The most important aspects of the ACA with respect to opioid addiction treatment involve the requirement that health plans abide by the provisions of the Mental Health Parity and Addiction Equity Act and not establish arbitrary a priori limitations on authorizations for referral to methadone maintenance treatment or formulary exclusions for methadone, buprenorphine, or long-acting injectable naltrexone.

Case Study: Expanding Chronic Care Management for the Person with Nicotine Addiction

Persons in America with nicotine (tobacco) addiction receive professional interventions for smoking and addiction to smokeless tobacco—but not often enough and not using the modalities and durations of care that can produce the best clinical results. Tobacco addiction is the leading cause of increased morbidity and mortality in the United States and the second most common cause of morbidity and mortality in the world. Almost 50% of smokers will die from a chronic medical disease caused or worsened by tobacco use.[84] Nicotine addiction negatively impacts the prognosis and treatment of most medical disorders, other addictions, mental illnesses, and common health problems such as obesity. Health care reform must address tobacco and expand access to the many excellent effective evidence-based pharmacotherapy and counseling approaches and guidelines, which must be better integrated into all health care settings and practices. In recent years, more individuals are receiving these interventions; however, most do not receive the full range of both modalities or durations of care that can produce the best clinical results, and some continue to receive no treatment.[85–88]

Despite numerous best practice examples from hospitals, health care networks, and outpatient practices,[89,90] there is continued need to train clinicians in all settings, disciplines, and specialties on how to better screen, assess, document treatment plans, refer for postdischarge treatment and community resources, and integrate tobacco addiction treatment and medications into provider's clinical practice. Currently, there are seven FDA-approved medications, including 5 nicotine replacements (patch, gum, spray, lozenge, and inhaler)—providing patient and provider education on use of these is important.[91] There are also effective evidence-based psychosocial treatments, including cognitive behavioral therapy and educational/motivational interventions for higher or lower motivated individuals.[92] Both pharmacotherapy and counseling achieve good outcomes, and better outcomes when both approaches are combined. Effective community-based interventions are also available, including quit lines (phone counseling often with medication support; 1-800-QUIT-NOW), internet-based counseling (eg, *www.becomeanex.org*), mobile technology applications, and community-based peer support such as Nicotine Anonymous (NicA). Of note, NicA has limited availability and even less research evaluation compared with other 12-step programs such as Alcoholics Anonymous or Narcotics Anonymous; however, 12-step facilitation has been shown to be effective for other addictions.[86,93]

Clinical care systems most effective in integrating tobacco addiction treatment utilize combined staff training with organizational change strategies by modifying the electronic health record to include reminders and clinical prompts, incentivizing or monitoring clinical practices, promoting employee and staff recovery from tobacco addiction, and developing tobacco-free campuses for both buildings and grounds.[94] Outstanding resources are available to help guide systems to better address tobacco and become tobacco free, including the following: Helping Patients Quit: Implementing The Joint Commission Tobacco Measure Set in Your Hospital (Partnership for Prevention)[89] Destination Tobacco-Free: A Practical Tool for Hospitals and Health Systems (Washington Health Foundation)[90] Becoming Tobacco-Free, A Guide for Healthcare Organizations (Maine Health).[95]

Changing incentives to better address tobacco, driven by the ACA, the 2011 Joint Commission on Tobacco Use and Cessation Measures, and improved reimbursement by the Centers for Medicare & Medicaid Services (CMS), will encourage and create incentives for private and public health care systems to implement sustainable tobacco addiction treatment programs. Health care reform policies, including electronic health record "meaningful use" requirements specific to tobacco use assessment, treatment, and follow-up, will encourage the development of registries and primary care network model practices for tobacco addiction. The Veterans Affairs Health Care system is an outstanding example of an Electronic Health Record system that includes many cues for tobacco assessment and treatment. The decision by CMS to improve Medicare and Medicaid reimbursements for tobacco counseling will financially incentivize programs of behavioral counseling and medication therapy for tobacco addiction. Soon, CMS may even align its tobacco measurements with the Joint Commission through the Inpatient Prospective Payment System. Yet, while Medicare provides medications and counseling coverage, most state Medicaid programs provide less than full treatment except for pregnant women, who are eligible for comprehensive tobacco addiction treatment.[90,96] Perhaps, specific ACA incentives to promote prevention services, which may include tobacco addiction treatment as prevention for many other medical diseases, may advance this cause.[97]

In 2011, Rigotti proposed that all tobacco care management systems include routine assessment of tobacco use, the development of tobacco user registries, provision of comprehensive treatment, "direct to smoker" outreach as supplement to visit-based care, centrally coordinated care across networks and plans, and requirements for reporting tobacco outcomes as proposed in "meaningful use" incentives.[96] This type of plan is within reach and requires organizational change, staff training, eliminating copayments for tobacco treatment, employee and staff recovery from nicotine addiction, and system incentives and monitoring. These are all possible under the ACA and are needed now.

EMERGING TECHNOLOGY AND INFORMATION MANAGEMENT IN ADDICTION TREATMENT

Supporting all the aforementioned advances in clinical care are parallel advances in health information technology, expanded data collection systems, and the use of computer-based treatments. Adoption of these new technology-based systems and therapies are necessary as an effective and cost-efficient means to directly support the systemic change goals promoted by health care reform. When addiction treatment is driven by fully integrated electronic medical records; automated utilizing computer-based or internet-based screening, treatment, or continuing care monitoring; and measured with comprehensive population-based utilization and outcomes data, then overall quality, safety, and efficiency improves. Less well understood, however, are the indirect effects of new technology on systemic change, including its profound impact on the patient and provider interface—the "doctor–patient" relationship.

Impact of Connectivity

When persons in America with addiction do receive care, it is mostly in specialty clinics and treatment centers that are technologically ill equipped to adopt electronic health record (EHR) systems or e-prescribing, or integrate into larger EHR networks alongside general medical care.[98] This disparity is exacerbated by the Health Information Technology for Economic and Clinical Health Act of 2009 (HITECH), which incentivized the expansion EHR systems through specific Medicare and Medicaid payments upon demonstration of "meaningful use of certified EHR technology"[99] but specifically excluded "meaningful use" incentives for providers of mental health and addiction treatment, many of whom are small, independent, nonprofit agencies.[100,101] Additionally, federal regulations intended to support the ACA, promote a national health information technology infrastructure more suitable for traditional medical or surgical delivery than for clinics that provide care to persons with addiction.[102] It remains to be seen whether recently introduced federal legislation or the newly formed state Health Information Exchanges—which are established coincident with state Health Insurance Exchanges to provide the framework through which health information from one health information system platform can be shared with another health information system—can facilitate the incorporation of behavioral health information into general medical care.

The practical aspects of providing integrated behavioral health information are obvious: emergency departments, primary care physicians, and other physicians can access health information regardless of the location where health care services are obtained. Dramatic improvements in health care quality will result from improved medical decision making and medical cost savings through reductions in duplicate diagnostic and laboratory tests and reduced medical errors.[100] Applied to substance use disorders treatment, the sharing of integrated medical information sounds promising. Patients with substance use disorders, who appear in emergency departments or other crisis clinics requesting refills of opioid pain medications, can be quickly triaged to appropriate care. Similarly, patients on the alcoholism treatment medication, disulfiram, who present with elevated liver functions, may be appropriately assessed by primary care providers. Before these improvements in integration are realized, however, current barriers to health information sharing must be overcome.

Chapter 42 Part 2 of the Code of Federal Regulations (42CFR) contains statutory language that protects and prohibits the release of any information obtained in the course of treatment by substance abuse treatment programs. Without prior written authorization, exemption from this confidentiality standard is permitted only under specific circumstances: in response to a court order, in a bona fide medical emergency, or to a qualified service organization that provides contracted services (eg, billing, lab collection) to the treatment program. In 2011, the Substance Abuse and Mental Health Services Administration issued a clarifying FAQ (Frequently Asked Questions) memo to assist health providers in navigating 42CFR confidentiality regulations under health care reform.[102] Nonetheless, clinicians and consumer advocates remain divided on the best means to handle these confidentiality standards during the expansion of electronic medical record keeping and health information sharing. Where one group sees improved quality for addiction care, the other sees potential for inappropriate rerelease of medical and addiction treatment information, sometimes resulting in adverse outcomes associated with discrimination, including loss of insurability (eg, life insurance), referral to the criminal justice (for using illegal drugs or participating in illegal activities), or loss of employment.[103–105] These concerns may not abate until broader national electronic information systems and standards are established to protect not only health information, but also financial and personal data as well.

Utilizing New Technology-Based Treatments

In 2012, 70 million persons utilized internet-based social media including chat rooms, personal blogs, and social network sites, reflecting major changes in nationwide patterns of social interaction. Despite this move toward greater online connectivity, the addiction treatment industry has been historically slow to adopt new technologies.[106,107] Treatment programs typically utilize face-to-face interventions based on therapeutic techniques developed in the 1970s during the heyday of 28-day "Minnesota Model" programs.[108] Overlooked are opportunities to engage new generations of young people with alcohol or other drug addiction through online screening, social network–based peer recovery, and online continuing care or monitoring programs.[109] Even remote telepsychiatry, which has broad mainstream support under ACA provisions to bring behavioral health care to rural or underserved areas, has largely been limited to general psychiatry and not implemented for addiction psychiatry, even though remote video-based assessment, substance abuse counseling, and medication-assisted treatment are quite feasible. If reimbursement mechanisms or the business case for utilizing these new innovations becomes more accessible, then the addiction treatment system has the opportunity to lead general health care with the development of programs that promote online recovery and wellness as well as establish whole communities of peers and providers dedicated to internet-assisted sobriety and health.

Moving Toward Accountable Outcomes

Underpinning much of our national reforms to our health care system are global concerns that the American health care system is inefficient. There is the concern that our health system should pay for results more than for processes, and should pay for outcomes that are generated rather than services that are rendered.[110] As general health care pushes toward improving quality, developing definitions of and measurements of quality, evaluating of the performance of systems and individual practitioners, comparing performance to "best practices" or benchmarks of "community standards of practice," insisting that services be "evidence-based," and requiring that measurement and metrics become more central to the health care enterprise, addiction medicine as a field must also improve its definitions of performance and quality.

Efforts are now underway to define addiction treatment outcomes and performance measures for patients, systems, and providers, but the hurdles are challenging.[111] For persons with addiction who are undergoing treatment, clinical measures of improvement are still not standard. Although the Addiction Severity Index[112] has been adopted widely, it is cumbersome to administer, even in its computerized form. Promising new measures include the Brief Addiction Monitor, which is undergoing pilot testing nationally by the Veterans Health Administration but still awaiting validation.[113] Regardless of the tool, health plans, purchasers, and agencies like the National Committee for Quality Assurance are demanding standardized outcomes, not just with systemic measures that compare how one health care delivery system performs with all the patients with addiction with others, but also for individual clinicians to see how well they perform when they encounter patients with addiction. As health reform moves forward, addiction treatment will not be able to move into "mainstream medicine" without adhering to accountability processes that apply to the rest of medical care. Addiction professionals must collect data on their clinical performance and clinical outcomes and become comfortable having these data publicly reported through public domain Websites, just like hospital data, and individual physician data are now collected regarding surgical, cardiology, and oncology care.

SUMMARY

This article outlined ways in which persons with addiction are currently underserved by our current health care system. However, with the coming broad scale reforms to our health care system, the access to and availability of high-quality care for substance use disorders will increase.[18] Addiction treatments will continue to be offered through traditional substance abuse care systems, but these will be more integrated with primary care, and less separated as treatment facilities leverage opportunities to blend services, financing mechanisms, and health information

---

Box 5
Essential recommendations to improve care for substance use disorders under health care reform

Persons in America with substance use disorders are underserved: 20.9 million people in need of treatment for an illicit drug or alcohol use problem did not receive it.[1] The following are essential recommendations to improve the care for substance use disorders under health care reform:

Coverage: Required expansion and protections of coverage for substance use disorders must comply with the Mental Health Parity and Addiction Equity Act to redress decades-old imbalance resulting from reliance on public funding to pay for US addiction treatment.[17]

Enrollment: State insurance exchanges and health plans must actively enroll and repatriate individuals with substance use disorders to reduce the preventable disease burden related to medical disenfranchisement.[22,13]

Benefits: Essential health benefits must support medically necessary treatment to assure optimal initiation, engagement, stabilization, and recovery from substance use disorders across the lifespan (including adolescents and adults). These benefits must minimally include[40–42]:

- Substance use prevention and early intervention activities, including universal screening and brief intervention in all clinical settings.
- At least 3 months outpatient or residential treatment to achieve psychosocial stabilization per episode.
- At least 3 years of continuing care in primary care or specialty outpatient settings.
- Medical detoxification, hospitalization, and care for medical and psychiatric comorbidities as needed.
- Medication-assisted therapy, including anticraving, anti-addiction, or opioid maintenance medications.
- Random drug toxicology testing.
- Placement in care that is determined by industry-accepted tools such as the American Society of Addiction Medicine's Patient Placement Criteria.[43]

Integration: Health researchers and administrators must collaboratively strive to understand the complex systemic, provider, and cultural changes required to effectively adopt and achieve maximal benefits through behavioral health integration. Electronic privacy and confidentiality regulations must allow medically necessary sharing of health information.

Treatment: Practice guidelines and performance measures for Screening and Brief Intervention must be universally implemented across health systems[68]; Tobacco care management systems must include routine assessment of tobacco use; develop tobacco user registries; provide comprehensive treatment, "direct to smoker" outreach, and centrally coordinated care across networks and plans; and report tobacco outcomes.[94] Regulations impacting federal and state reimbursement for opioid treatment programs must permit flexible funding to integrate medical and OTP care. Medication assisted therapy for opioid dependence should be an essential health insurance benefit. Reimbursement strategies must encourage expansion of new technology to permit remote or online access to services for substance use disorders.

Performance: Addiction professionals must collect and report data on their clinical performance and clinical outcomes through public domain websites.

Adapted from California Society of Addiction Medicine, Expansion of Substance Use Disorder Treatment within Reach through Health Care Reform, April 2011. San Francisco, CA. Available at: http://www.csam-asam.org/pdf/misc/CSAM_HCR.pdf.

---

systems under federally driven incentive programs.[29] To further these reforms, vigilance will be needed by consumers, clinicians, and policy makers to assure that the unmet treatment needs of individuals with addiction are addressed. Embedded in this article are essential recommendations to facilitate the improvement of care for substance use disorders under health care reform (**Box 5**).

Ultimately, as addiction care acquires more of the "look and feel" of mainstream medicine, it is important to be mindful of preexisting trends in health care delivery overall that are reflected in recent health reform legislation. Within the world of addiction care, clinicians must move beyond their self-imposed "stigmatization" and sequestration of specialty addiction treatment. The problem for addiction care, as it becomes more "mainstream," is to not comfortably feel that general slogans like "Treatment Works," as promoted by Substance Abuse and Mental Health Services Administration's Center for Substance Abuse Treatment during its annual Recovery Month celebrations, will meet the expectations of stakeholders outside the specialty addiction treatment community.[114] Rather, the problem is to show exactly *how* addiction treatment works, and to what extent it works—there have to be metrics showing changes in symptom level or functional outcome, changes in health care utilization, improvements in workplace attendance and productivity, or other measures. At minimum, clinicians will be required to demonstrate that their new systems of care and future clinical activity are in conformance with overall standards of "best practice" in health care.

ACKNOWLEDGMENTS

The authors graciously acknowledge Constance Weisner, DrPH, MSW (Kaiser Permanente Division of Research) for her helpful comments and review of this paper.

FACULTY DISCLOSURE AND CONFLICT OF INTEREST

The following authors have identified no professional or financial affiliations for themselves or their spouse/partner: Eric Goplerud, PhD, MA, Judith Martin, MD
The following authors identified the following professional or financial affiliations for themselves or their spouse/partner:
David R. Pating, MD:
Appointee: California Mental Health Services Oversight and Accountability Commission (no compensation).
Michael M. Miller, MD:
Consultant/Advisor: National Academy of Sciences Committee on Science, Technology and the Law (no compensation); Wisconsin State Council on Alcohol and Other Drug Abuse (no compensation).
Douglas M. Ziedonis, MD:
Grants: National Institute Drug Abuse (NIDA), National Cancer Institute (NCI), Massachusetts Department of Mental Health, Connecticut Department of Public Health, Legacy Foundation, and National Institute of Health/ARRA.
Consultant/Advisor: Skyland Trail Advisory Board, Educational Service District 112 – Washington State, American Psychiatric Institute, Community Health Link Advisory Board (no compensation); Veterans Affairs Health Care CHEQR (no compensation); and Rutgers University Scientific Advisory Board (no compensation).

REFERENCES

1. Substance Abuse and Mental Health Services Administration. Results from the 2009 National Survey on Drug Use and Health: volume I. Summary of National Findings (Office of Applied Studies, (2010) NSDUH Series H-38A, HHS Publication No. SMA 10-4586 Findings). Rockville, MD.
2. US Department of Health and Human Services. Mental Health: A Report of the Surgeon General—Executive Summary. Rockville (MD): U.S. Department of Health and Human Services, Substance Abuse and Mental Health Services Administration, Center for Mental Health Services, National Institutes of Health, National Institute of Mental Health, 1999.

3. Fleming M, Barry KL, Manwell LB, et al. Brief physician advice for problem alcohol drinkers: a randomized controlled trial in community-based primary care practices. JAMA 1997;277(13):1039–45.

4. Mark TL, Kranzler HR, Poole VH. Barriers to the use of medications to treat alcoholism. Am J Addictions 2003;12(4):281–94.

5. Jacobus-Kantor L, Goplerud E. The current state of commercial behavioral healthcare services: results from the 2010 Evalu8 Request for Information, Mental Health Works 2011. Available at: http://www.nxtbook.com/nxtbooks/apf/mentalhealthworks_2011q3/#/16. Accessed November 30, 2011.

6. Institute of Medicine. Improving the quality of health care for mental and substance-use conditions: Quality Chasm series. Washington, DC: National Academies Press; 2005.

7. Solberg LI, Maciosek MV, Edwards NM. Primary care interventions to reduce alcohol misuse ranking its health impact and cost effectiveness. Am J Prev Med 2008;34(2): 143–52.

8. American Society of Addiction Medicine. Public Policy Statement: Definition of Addiction, adopted April 12, 2011. Available at: http://www.asam.org/Definitionof Addiction-LongVersion.html. Accessed November 20, 2011.

9. McLellan AT, Lewis DC, O'Brien CP, et al. Drug dependence, a chronic medical illness: implications for treatment, insurance, and outcomes evaluation. JAMA 2000; 284(13):1689–95.

10. Buck JA. The looming expansion and transformation of public substance abuse treatment under the affordable care act. Health Affairs 2011;30(8):1402–10.

11. Mark TL, Levit KR, Vandivort-Warren R, et al. Changes in US spending on mental health and substance abuse treatment, 1986–2005, and implications for policy. Health Affairs 2011;30(2):284–92.

12. Berwick DM, Nolan TW, Whittington J. The triple aim: care, health and cost. Health Aff (Millwood) 2008;27(3):759–69.

13. The President's New Freedom Commission on Mental Health. Achieving the promise: transforming mental health care in America. SAMHSA Pub id: SMA03–3831, Jan 2003.

14. The Henry J Kaiser Family Foundation. Focus on Health reform: summary of new health reform law. Updated April 15, 2011. Available at: http://www.kff.org/healthreform/upload/8061.pdf. Accessed December 18, 2011.

15. Garfield RL, Zuvekas SH, Lave JR, et al. The impact of national health care reform on adults with severe mental disorders. Am J Psychiatry 2011;168:486–94.

16. US Department of Health and Human Services. The 2011 HHS Poverty Guidelines. Available at: http://aspe.hhs.gov/poverty/11poverty.shtml. Accessed November 20, 2011.

17. Barry CL, Huskamp HA. Moving beyond parity—mental health and addiction care under the ACA. N Engl J Med 2011;365:973–5.

18. Roy K, Miller M. Parity and the medicalization of addiction treatment, J Psychoactive Drug 2010; 42:115–20.

19. Goldman HH, Frank RG, Burnam MA, et al, Behavioral health insurance parity for federal employees. N Engl J Med 2006;354:1378–86

20. McConnell KJ, Gast SH, Ridgely MS, et al. Behavioral health insurance parity: does Oregon's experience presage the national experience with the Mental Health Parity and Addiction Equity Act? Am J Psychiatry 2012;169:31–8.

21. Mancuso D, Felver BE. Bending the health care cost curve by expanding alcohol/drug treatment. Department of Social and Health Services, RDA Report 4.81, Olympia, Washington. September 2010.

22. The National Association of State Alcohol and Drug Abuse Directors (NASADAD). The effects of health care reform on access to, and funding of, substance abuse services in Maine, Massachusetts, and Vermont. Washington, DC, 2010.
23. Institute of Medicine, Committee on Quality of Health Care in America. Crossing the quality chasm: a new health system for the 21st century. Washington, DC: National Academy Press; 2001.
24. Agency for Healthcare Research and Quality. Evidence report/technology assessment number 173: integration of mental health/substance abuse and primary care. AHRQ Publication No. 09–E003, Rockville, MD, 2008.
25. Treatment Improvement Protocol (TIP) Series 26. Substance Abuse Among Older Adults, Frederic C. Blow, Ph.D. Consensus Panel Chair, US Department of Health and Human Services, Rockville, MD, 1998.
26. Von Korf MR, Scott KM, Gureje O, editors. Global perspectives on mental-physical comorbidity in the WHO World Mental Health Surveys. Cambridge (UK): Cambridge University Press; 2009.
27. The National Center for Addiction and Substance Abuse at Columbia. Missed opportunity: national survey of primary care physicians and patients on substance abuse. New York; 2000.
28. American Academy of Family Physicians (AAFP), American Academy of Pediatrics (AAP), American College of Physicians (ACP), American Osteopathic Association (AOA). Joint Principles of the Patient-Centered Medical Home March 2007. Available at: http://www.aafp.org/online/en/home/media/releases/2007/20070305 pressrelease0.html. Accessed December 18, 2011.
29. Collins C, Hewson D, Munger R, et al. Evolving models of behavioral health integration in primary care. New York: Millbank Memorial Fund; 2010.
30. Integrated Behavioral Health Project (IBHP). Models of Behavioral Health Integration. Available at: http://www.ibhp.org/index.php?section=pages&cid=91. Accessed December 19, 2011.
31. (NASMHPD) Medical Directors Council, Parks J, Pollack D, editors. National Association of State Mental Health Program Directors. Integrating behavioral health and primary care services: opportunities and challenges for state mental health authorities. January 2005. Available at: http://www.nasmhpd.org/general_files/publications/med_directors_pubs/Final%20Technical%20Report%20on%20Primary%20Care%20-%20Behavioral%20Health%20Integration.final.pdf. Accessed December 18, 2011.
32. Weisner C, Mertens J, Parthasarathy S, et al, Integrating primary medical care with addiction treatment: a randomized controlled trial. JAMA 2001;286(14):1715–23.
33. Parthasarathy S, Mertens J, Moore C, et al. Utilization and cost impact of integrating substance abuse treatment and primary care. Med Care 2003;41(3):357–67.
34. Mertens JR, Flisher AJ, Satre DD, et al. The role of medical conditions and primary care services in 5-year substance use outcomes among chemical dependency treatment patients. Drug and Alcohol Dependence 2008;98(1–2):45–53.
35. Chi FW, Parthasarathy S, Mertens JR, et al. Continuing care and long-term substance use outcomes in managed care: initial evidence for a primary care based mode., Psychiatr Serv 2011;62(10):1194–2000.
36. Parthasarathy S, Chi FW, Mertens JR, et al. The role of continuing care on 9-year cost trajectories of patients with intakes into an outpatient alcohol and drug treatment program. Medical Care, In press.
37. U.S. Government Accountability Office. Report to congressional committees: mental health and substance use—employer's insurance coverage maintained or enhanced since MHPAEA, but effect of coverage on enrollees varied. GAO–12–63, 2011.

38. American Society of Addiction Medicine. Public policy statement of the relationship between treatment and self help: a joint statement of the American Society of Addiction Medicine, the American Academy of Addiction Psychiatry, and the American Psychiatric Association, adopted December 01, 1997. Available at: http://www.asam.org/RelationshipBetweenTreatmentAndSelfHelpAJointStatement.html. Accessed November 30, 2011.

39. Fortini A. Special treatment: the rise of luxury rehab. The New Yorker: 2008.

40. National Institute of Drug Abuse. Principles of Drug addiction treatment: a research-based guide, 2nd Edition. Rockville, MD: NIH Publication No. 09–4180, Revised April 2009.

41. California Society of Addiction Medicine, Expansion of Substance Use Disorder Treatment within Reach through Health Care Reform, April 2011. San Francisco, CA. Available at: http://www.csam-asam.org/pdf/misc/CSAM_HCR.pdf.

42. American Society of Addiction Medicine. Policy statement on core benefit for primary care and specialty treatment and prevention of alcohol, nicotine and other drug abuse and dependence. Adopted April 10 1993. Available at: http://www.asam.org/CoreBenefit.html. Accessed November 30, 2011.

43. Gastfriend DR, editor. Addiction treatment matching: research foundations of the American Society of Addiction Medicine (ASAM) Criteria. Binghampton (NY): Hayworth Press, 2004.

44. Gerstein DR, Harwood HJ, editors. Treating drug problems, Volume I. Washington, DC: National Academy Press, Institute of Medicine, 1990.

45. Institute of Medicine. Broadening the base of treatment for alcohol problems. Washington, DC: National Academies Press, 1990.

46. Mrazek PJ, Haggerty JR, editors, and Committee on Prevention of Mental Disorders, Institute of Medicine. Reducing risks for mental disorders: frontiers for prevention intervention research. Washington, DC: National Academy Press, 1994.

47. Fleming MF, Mundt MP, French MT, et al. Brief physician advice for problem alcohol drinkers: long-term efficacy and benefit-cost analysis. A randomized controlled trial in community-based primary care settings. Alcohol Clin Exp Res 2002;26:36–43.

48. Saitz R. Unhealthy alcohol use. N Engl J Med 2005;352:596–607.

49. Babor T, Higgins-Biddle J. AUDIT—The Alcohol Use Disorders Identification Test: Guidelines for Use in Primary Care (Second Edition), 2001. Available at: http://whqlibdoc.who.int/hq/2001/WHO_MSD_MSB_01.6a.pdf. Accessed November 30, 2011.

50. Babor T, Higgins-Biddle J. Brief intervention for hazardous and harmful drinking: a manual for use in primary care, 2001. Available at: http://whqlibdoc.who.int/hq/2001/WHO_MSD_MSB_01.6b.pdf. Accessed November 30, 2011.

51. Whitlock EP, Polen MR, Green CA, et al. Behavioral counseling interventions in primary care to reduce risky/harmful alcohol use by adults: a summary of the evidence for the U.S. Preventive Services Task Force. Ann Intern Med 2004;140: 557–68.

52. Miller WR, Wilbourne PL Mesa Grande: a methodological analysis of clinical trials of treatments for alcohol use disorders. Addiction 2002;97(3):265–77.

53. Cuijpers P, Riper H, Lemmers L, The effects on mortality of brief interventions for problem drinking: a meta-analysis, Addiction 2004;99:839–45.

54. Fleming M, Screening and brief intervention in primary care settings. Alcohol Research and Health 2003;28(5):57–62.

55. Gentilello LM, Donovan DM, Jurkovich GJ, et al. Alcohol interventions in a trauma center as a means of reducing the risk of injury recurrence. Ann Surg 1999;230(4): 473–83.

56. Storer RM, A simple cost-benefit analysis of brief interventions on substance abuse at Naval Medical Center Portsmouth. Military Medicine 2003;168(9):765–71.
57. Joint Commission. Hospital performance measure specification manual 2012, (2011). Available at: http://www.jointcommission.org/specifications_manual_for_national_hospital_inpatient_quality_measures/. Accessed November 30, 2011.
58. American Medical Association. Unhealthy alcohol use: screening & brief counseling. 2008. Available at: http://www.ama-assn.org/ama/pub/physician-resources/clinical-practice-improvement/clinical-quality/physician-consortium-performance-improvement/pcpi-measures.page? Accessed November 30, 2011.
59. Denny CH, Serdula MK, Holtzman D, et al. Physician advice about smoking and drinking: are U.S. adults being informed? Am J Prev Med 2003;24:1–4.
60. Coffield AB, Maciosek MV, McGinnis MJ, et al. Priorities among recommended clinical preventive services. Am J Prev Med 2001;21:1–9.
61. Saitz R, Mulvey KP, Plough A, et al. Physician unawareness of serious substance abuse. Am J Drug Alcohol Abuse 1997;23:343–54.
62. Millstein SG, Marcell AV. Screening and counseling for adolescent alcohol use among primary care physicians in the United States. Pediatrics 2003;111:114–22.
63. McGlynn EA, Asch SM, Adams J, et al. The Quality of Healthcare Delivered to Adults in the United States. N Engl J Med 2003;348:2635–45.
64. O'Rourke M, Richardson L, Wilets I, et al. Alcohol-related problems: emergency physicians' current practice and attitudes. J Emerg Med 2006;30(3):263–8.
65. Schermer CR, Gentilello LM, Hoyt DB, et al. National survey of trauma surgeons' use of alcohol screening and brief intervention. J Trauma 2003; 55(5):849–56.
66. Saitz R, Freedner N, Palfai T, et al. The severity of unhealthy alcohol use in hospitalized medical patients: the spectrum is narrow. J Gen Intern Med 2006;21:381–5.
67. Smothers BA, Yahr HT, Ruhl CE. Detection of alcohol use disorders in general hospital admissions in the United States. Arch Intern Med 2004;164:749–56.
68. Maciosek MV, Coffield AB, Edwards NM, et al. Priorities among effective clinical preventive services: results of a systematic review and analysis. Am J Prev Med 2006;31(1):52–61.
69. Okie S. A flood of opioids, a rising tide of death. N Engl J Med 2010;362(21):1981–84.
70. 2009 National Survey on Drug Use and Health (NSDUH): National Findings, SAMHSA (2010). Available at: http://www.oas.samhsa.gov/NSDUH/2k9NSDUH/2k9ResultsP.pdf. Accessed November 30, 2011.
71. Center for Disease Control and Prevention. Vital signs: overdoses of prescription opioid pain relievers United States, 1999 – 2008. MMWR Morb Mortal Wkly Rep 2011;60(43):1487–92.
72. Volkow ND, McLellan TA. Curtailing diversion and abuse of opioid analgesics without jeopardizing pain treatment. JAMA 2011;305(13):1346–7.
73. National Institutes of Health. Effective medical treatment of opiate addiction, consensus development conference statement,1997. Available at: http://consensus.nih.gov/1997/1998TreatOpiateAddiction108html.htm. Accessed November 30, 2011.
74. Strang J, Hall W, Hickman M, et al. Impact of supervision of methadone consumption on deaths related to methadone overdose (1993–2008): analyses using OD4 index in England and Scotland. BMJ 2010;341:c4851.
75. Mattick RP, Breen C, Kimber J, et al. Methadone maintenance therapy versus no opioid replacement therapy for opioid dependence. Cochrane Database Syst Rev 2009;3:CD002209.

76. Salsitz EA, Joseph H, Frank B, et al. Methadone medical maintenance (MMM): treating chronic opioid dependence in private medical practice—a summary report (1983 – 1998). The Mount Sinai Journal of Medicine 2000;67(5/6):388–97.

77. Novick DM, Joseph H, Salsita EA, et al. Outcomes of treatment of socially rehabilitated methadone maintenance patients in physicians' offices (medical maintenance): follow-up at three and a half to nine and a fourth years. J Gen Intern Med 1994;9(3): 127–30.

78. Kosten, TR, Fiellin DA, U.S. National Buprenorphine Implementation Program: Buprenorphine for office-based practice: Consensus conference overview. Am J Addictions 2004;13(Suppl 1):S1–S7.

79. Fiellin DA, O'Connor PG. Office-based treatment of opioid dependent patients. N Engl J Med 2002;347(11):818–23.

80. Cunningham CO, Giovanniello A, et al. A comparison of buprenorphine induction strategies: patient-centered home-based inductions versus standard-of-care office-based inductions. J Substance Abuse Treatment 2011;40:349–356.

81. Herman M, Gourevitch MN. Integrating primary care and methadone maintenance treatment: implementation issues. J Addict Dis 1997;16(1):91–102.

82. Neufeld K, Kidorf M, King V. Using enhanced and integrated services to improve response to standard methadone treatment: changing the clinical infrastructure of treatment networks. J Subst Abuse Treat 2010;38(2):170–7.

83. Harris KAJ, Arnsten JH, Litwain AH. Successful integration of hepatitis c evaluation and treatment services with methadone maintenance. J Addict Med 2010;4(1): 20–6.

84. World Health Organization. WHO report on the global tobacco epidemic. The MPOWER package. Geneva: World Health Organization; 2008.

85. Fiore MC, Jaen CR, Baker TB, et al. Treating tobacco use and dependence, 2008 update. Clinical practice guideline. Rockville, MD: U.S. Department of Health and Human Services. Public Health Service; 2008.

86. Work Group on Substance Use Disorders. Treatment of patients with substance use disorders, 2nd ed. American Psychiatric Association. Am J Psychiatry 2006;163(8 Suppl):5–82.

87. U.S. Preventive Services Task Force. Counseling and interventions to prevent tobacco use and tobacco-caused disease in adults and pregnant women: U.S. Preventive Services Task Force reaffirmation recommendation statement. Ann Intern Med 2009;21:150(8):551-5. Available at: http://www.ahrq.gov/clinic/uspstf/uspstbac2. htm. Accessed November 30, 2011.

88. Hughes JR, Fiester S, Goldstein M, et al. American Psychiatric Association's practice guidelines for the treatment of patients with nicotine dependence. Am J Psychiatry 1996;153:(10):S1–31.

89. Partnership for Prevention. Helping patients quit: implementing the Joint Commission tobacco measure set in your hospital. Washington, DC: Partnership for Prevention; 2011. Available at: www.actiontoquit.org. Accessed November 30, 2011.

90. Washington Health Foundation. Destination Tobacco-Free: a practical tool for hospitals and health systems. Seattle (WA): Washington Health Foundation; 2010. Available at: www.whf.org/DestinationTobaccoFree. Accessed November 30, 2011.

91. Stead LF, Perera R, Bullen C, et al. Nicotine replacement for smoking cessation. Cochrane Database Syst Rev 2008;1:CD000146.

92. Steinberg ML, Ziedonis DM, Krejci JA, et al. Motivational interviewing with personalized feedback: a brief intervention for motivating smokers with schizophrenia to seek treatment for tobacco dependence. J Consult Clin Psychol 2004;72(4):723–8.

93. Prochaska JJ, Delucchi K, Hall SM. A meta-analysis of smoking cessation interventions with individuals in substance abuse treatment or recovery. J Consult Clin Psychol 2004;72:1144–56.

94. Ziedonis DM, Zammarelli L, Seward G, et al. Addressing tobacco use through organizational change: a case study of an addiction treatment organization. J Psychoactive Drug 2007;39(4):451–9.

95. Maine Health. Becoming tobacco-free. A guide for healthcare organizations. Portland (ME): Maine Health; 2002. Available at: www.mainehealth.org/workfiles/mh_media/0Tobacco8-Final.pdf. Accessed November 30, 2011.

96. Rigotti N. Integrating comprehensive tobacco treatment into the evolving US health care system: It's time to act. Arch Intern Med 2011;17(1):53–5.

97. Institute of Medicine, Committee on Identifying Priority Areas for Quality Improvement. Priority areas for national action: transforming health care. Washington, DC: National Academies Press; 2003.

98. Clark W. Strategic Initiative #6: health information technology. In: Substance Abuse and Mental Health Services Administration. Leading change: a plan for SAMHSA's roles and actions 2011-2014. HHS Publication No. (SMA) 11–4629. Rockville (MD): Substance Abuse and Mental Health Services Administration; 2011.

99. Center for Medicaid and Medicare Services. The official web site for the Medicare and Medicaid electronic health records (EHR) incentive programs: overview. Available at: https://www.cms.gov/ehrincentiveprograms/. Accessed November 30, 2011.

100. Ghitza UE, Sparenborg S, Tai B. Improving drug abuse treatment delivery through adoption of harmonized electronic health record systems. Substance Abuse Rehab 2011;2:125–31.

101. Ingoglia C. Perspectives: include mental health, addiction providers in meaningful use incentives, iHealthBeat, July 20, 2001. Available at: http://www.ihealthbeat.org/perspectives/2011/include-mental-health-addiction-providers-in-meaningful-use-incentives.aspx. Accessed November 30, 2011.

102. Substance Abuse and Mental Health Services Administration. US DHHS, Applying the Substance Abuse Confidentiality Regulations 42CFR Part 2, released 12/8/2011. Available at: http://tools.store.samhsa.gov/emarketing/downloads/SAMHSA_42CFRPART2FAQII.docx. Accessed November 30, 2011.

103. American Society of Addiction Medicine, Public Policy Statement. Confidentiality of Patient Records and Protections Against Discrimination, Adopted July 1, 2010. Available at: http://www.asam.org/ConfidentialityPatientRecords.html. Accessed November 30, 2011.

104. Popovits RM. Confidentiality law: time for change? Behav Healthc 2010;30:11–13.

105. Legal Action Center. Confidentiality of alcohol and drug records in the 21st century, January 2010. Available at: http://www.lac.org/doc_library/lac/publications/Confidentiality_of_Alcohol_and_Drug_Records_in_the_21st_Century-1-20-10.pdf. Accessed November 30, 2011.

106. Thomas CP, McCarty D. Adoption of drug abuse treatment technology in specialty and primary care settings. In: Harwood HJ, Myers TG, editors. New treatments for addiction: behavioral, ethical, legal, and social questions. National Research Council (US) and Institute of Medicine (US) Committee on Immunotherapies and Sustained-Release Formulations for Treating Drug Addiction;. Washington, DC: National Academies Press (US); 2004.

107. Miller WR, Sorensen JL, Selzer JA, et al. Disseminating evidence-based practices in substance abuse treatment: a review with suggestions. J Sub Abuse Treat 2006;31:25–3.

108. Miller MM. Traditional approaches to the treatment of addiction. In: Graham AW, Schultz TK, editors. Principles of addiction medicine. 2nd edition. Annapolis Junction (MD): American Society of Addiction Medicine; 1998.
109. Cunningham JA, Kypri K, McCambridge J. The use of emerging technologies in alcohol treatment. Alcohol Research & Health 2011;33(4):321–6.
110. The Institute of Medicine. Rewarding provider performance: aligning incentives in Medicare. Washington, DC: The National Academies Press; 2006.
111. McLellan AT, Carise D, Kleber HD. Can the national addiction treatment infrastructure support the public's demand for quality care? J Substance Abuse Treat 2003;25:117–21.
112. McLellan AT, Luborsky L, Cacciola J, et al. New data from the Addiction Severity Index: reliability and validity in three centers. J Nerv Mental Dis 1985:173(7):412–23.
113. Drapkin ML, Oslin DW. Brief addiction monitor (BAM) in the VA substance abuse treatment system: implementation and clinical applications. Paper presented at: VA National Mental Health Conference. Baltimore (MD), July 1, 2010.
114. White W. Treatment Works! Is it time for a new slogan? Available at: http://www.bhrm.org, 2004, http://www.bhrm.org/advocacy/TreatmentWorks.pdf. Accessed December 26, 2011.

Serotonergic Hallucinogens and Emerging Targets for Addiction Pharmacotherapies

Stephen Ross, MD

KEYWORDS

- Serotonergic hallucinogens • Addiction • Treatment • Pharmacotherapy

KEY POINTS

- Converging lines of evidence from pharmacologic, electrophysiologic, and behavioral research in animals strongly suggest that activation of cortical 5-hydroxytryptamine-2A receptors is the most critical step in initiating a cascade of biological events that accounts for serotonergic hallucinogen (SH) psychoactive properties.
- Psilocybin produces hyperfrontality with divergent prefrontal–subcortical activation in such a way as to increase cognitive and affective processing in the context of reduced gating and reduced focus on external stimulus processing.
- In contrast to all other drugs of abuse, SHs are not considered to be capable of producing sufficient reinforcing effects to cause dependence (addiction) syndromes.
- Given that SHs increase extracellular glutamate levels and activity in the prefrontal–limbic circuitry, it is possible that a normalization in functional connectivity in this network through a glutamate-dependent neuroplastic adaptation could produce an anti-addictive effect.

INTRODUCTION

Hallucinogens are a broad group of drugs that are narrowly defined in the DSM-IV[1] to include only:

1. Serotonergic hallucinogens (SHs), agents that activate the 5-hydroxytryptamine-2A (5-HT$_{2A}$) receptor (2AR) such as lysergic acid diethylamide (LSD) and psilocybin

---

The author has nothing to disclose.
Division of Alcoholism and Drug Abuse, Bellevue Hospital Center and the New York University School of Medicine, 462 First Avenue, NBV 20E7, New York, NY 10016, USA
E-mail address: Stephen.ross@nyumc.org

Psychiatr Clin N Am 35 (2012) 357–374
http://dx.doi.org/10.1016/j.psc.2012.04.002
0193-953X/12/$ – see front matter © 2012 Elsevier Inc. All rights reserved.

2. The mixed amphetamine hallucinogen 3,4-methylenedioxymethamphetamine (MDMA [Ecstasy]).

However, they more broadly can include:

1. Dissociative anesthetics or *N*-methyl-D-aspartate (NMDA) antagonist hallucinogens (agents that antagonize the NMDA glutamate receptor such as phencyclidine [PCP], ketamine, and dextromethorphan)
2. Cannabinoid agonists (agents that activate the CB1 receptor)
3. κ opioid agonists (ie, salvinorum A)
4. Antimuscarinic agents (ie, scopolamine, atropine).

Most hallucinogens are included in the schedule I category as originally defined by the Controlled Substances Act of 1970.[2] As such, by definition they are classified as having no currently accepted medical use in the United States, lacking in safety for use under medical supervision, and possessing high addictive liability. From an addiction perspective, it is worth examining the evidence base for this classification to understand the true addictive liability of this class of agents. Moreover, given the history of research suggesting a role for certain hallucinogen treatment models to treat addictive disorders, it is further worth exploring how some of these drugs may confer anti-addictive effects.

A BRIEF HISTORY OF RESEARCH ON SHs

In 1943, Albert Hoffman, a Swiss chemist at Sandoz, accidentally discovered LSD-25 while examining alkaloids from the rye ergot fungus in search of a vasconstricting agent to reduce blood loss during pregnancy. A small amount of the agent came into contact with his skin and he had the first LSD experience. Sandoz began to test this new agent on animals and other Sandoz employees. The testing for toxicity in animals revealed LSD to be safe with no known human toxic dose (LD_{50}). In 1947, the company began marketing LSD as Delysid for two general indications: as a tool to explore the biological basis of psychosis and as an adjunct to psychotherapy. In 1958, after Albert Hoffman isolated psilocybin as the active ingredient in psychedelic mushrooms, psilocybin was also produced and marketed by Sandoz. This began a quarter century of research into the therapeutic applicability of hallucinogen treatment models, with much of the research centered in Europe and the United States. Two treatment models emerged[3]:

1. Psycholytic
2. Psychedelic

The **psycholytic** model came to predominate in Europe where lower doses of SHs (mostly LSD and to a lesser degree psilocybin) were used as tools to activate and enhance the psychoanalytic process by allowing greater access to unconscious material to effect personality changes in disease states such as personality disorders, neurotic spectrum disorders, and psychosomatic illness.

The **psychedelic** model utilized higher doses of the SHs to access novel dimensions of consciousness remarkably similar to mystical states of consciousness, with oneness, illuminative insight, a sense of the sacred, and ecstatic joy as core parts of the experience. This was a new therapeutic model with no previous basis within the field of mental health research, with parallels more toward religion and mysticism. Treatment of substance-use disorders (SUDs) was predominantly studied within this new model.

By the end of the nearly three decades of research, more than 1000 articles were published in the literature and more than 40,000 subjects were included in basic or therapeutic clinical hallucinogen research.[4] SUDs, mostly alcoholism, were the most studied of any of the psychiatric disorders, followed by psychological and spiritual distress associated with terminal cancer.[5–7] A treatment model that established the parameters of set (psychological frame of mind, intention, excluding participants with major mental illness or family history of such illness), setting (environment/room on dosing days), dose, preparation with therapeutic dyad teams, and integration of the experience was established.

Unfortunately, and perhaps predictably, the use of hallucinogens, in particular LSD, escaped from the human research laboratory and started to be misused by the general public. The adverse psychological effects (ie, anxiety, panic, psychosis) of the substances became apparent with their large-scale use without proper attention given to their unique properties, set, and setting. Their use for sacred intentional purposes in spiritual settings was replaced by abuse in party-like settings. They also came to be linked to politics in the United States and were associated with the counterculture movement. This and the reports of their adverse psychological effects were the main driving forces leading to the passage by Congress of the Controlled Substances Act of 1970 that established the controlled substances schedule system from I to V.[1] All of the SHs were placed in the most restrictive schedule I category, defined as lacking in safety for use under medical supervision, and with a high addictive liability. This effectively ended all clinical research into the therapeutic applicability of hallucinogen treatment models within the mental health field for the next two decades.

LSD AND ALCOHOLISM TREATMENT STUDIES

Overall, the studies looking at the effect of LSD in alcoholism during the 1950s and 1960s varied widely from astonishingly positive results to worsening of the alcoholism, depending on the design of the study, set, and setting of the dosing sessions and the degree to which preparatory and integrative psychotherapy was used. In 1971, Abuzzahab and Anderson reviewed 31 studies from 1953 to 1969 on the effects of LSD on approximately 1100 alcoholics. They were unable to offer any definitive conclusions about the overall efficacy or lack thereof of LSD-assisted therapy for alcoholics because of the overall wide variability in study designs, definitions of alcoholism, outcome measures, and effect of treatment setting. Overall, the vast majority of these studies were poorly designed by strict standards of modern methodologic paradigms to assess clinical efficacy. However, they were able to report in their final tally of results that[8]:

- 75% of participants receiving a single dose of LSD in the controlled studies were "improved" at 10-month follow-up compared to 44% of the controls.
- 58% of the multiple dosing patient were "improved" at approximately 20-month follow-up compared to 54% of the controls.

In 2012, Krebs and Johansen[9] performed a meta-analysis of previous studies examining the efficacy of single-dose LSD treatments for alcoholism that included the best designed trials in terms of randomization and the presence of a control group. Of the 536 adults identified from the 6 trials, 59% of patients in the LSD group were improved (in terms of a reduction of alcohol misuse at the first follow-up meeting) compared to 38% in the control arm ($P = .0003$), and the pooled odds ratio with respect to improvement in alcohol misuse between the LSD and control groups at the first follow-up was 1.96 (95% confidence interval [CI], 1.36–2.84; $P = .0003$). The significant treatment effects between the LSD and control groups on drinking behavior were observed up to 6-month follow-up but were not significant at 12-month follow-up. This suggests that repeated dosing may be necessary to confer longer lasting antidipsotropic effects.

THE NATIVE AMERICAN CHURCH/PEYOTE, THE UNIAO DO VEGETAL/AYAHUASCA, AND ANTI-ADDICTION

Two religious groups are legally allowed to use SHs in the United States as sacraments central to their religious practices: use of peyote (mescaline) by the Native American Church (NAC) and use of ayahuasca by the Uniao do Vegetal (UDV).

The legal use of peyote by the NAC was established under the American Indian Religious Freedom Act enacted by Congress in 1993,[10] and similarly the legal use of ayahuasca by the UDV was established by the US Supreme Court (in a unanimous 8–0 ruling) in 2006. In both religious communities (NAC/peyote; UDV/hoasca) the abuse of alcohol and drugs (ie, cocaine, heroin) is **proscribed**, whereas ongoing use of the SH is **prescribed**.[11,12] For both, ceremonies are conducted specifically to treat SUDs. In both groups, ethnographic and cross-sectional reports suggest low rates of SUDs, sustained abstinence, and no evidence of adverse psychological or cognitive effects in long-term members in both NAC/peyote and the UDV/ayahuasca research populations, suggesting a link between sacramental SH use in religious settings and anti-addictive effects.[13–19]

To truly determine if the peyote- and ayahuasca-based US religions have lower rates of alcohol or drug use disorders, formal epidemiologic inquiry is indicated. If it is indeed found that the rates are lower compared to those in the general population, then the next line of inquiry would be to ascertain potential causal mechanisms. It would be important to consider possible anti-addictive effects of SH itself, either from its biological effects or those related to its psychospiritual or mysticomimetic properties. It is also entirely possible that the effects have nothing to do the SH and are related to other factors such as **proscription** of drugs and alcohol in the NAC or social and spiritual factors related to membership and practice in the religion. Another possibility is some mix of ongoing effects of SH use and the social, spiritual, and communal aspects of the religion that give meaning to the spiritual experiences.

In addition to its use in traditional ayahuasca-based religions, the use of ayahuasca to treat addictive spectrum disorders has spread outside of religious contexts, with a well-known example being **Takiwasi,** a therapeutic community in Peru established by a group of French and Peruvian psychiatrists, psychologists, and anthropologists to treat drug dependence, in particular, cocaine use disorders. In this center, 15 to 20 addicted individuals are treated at one time; both the patients and the healers ingest ayahuasca (syntonic with the shamanic tradition of ayahuasca administration) and the putative treatment mechanisms are related to psychospiritual effects.[11]

CLASSIFICATION OF HALLUCINOGENS

The serotonergic or classic hallucinogens (which exert their hallucinogenic properties by activating the 2AR) can broadly be broken down into two main categories[20]:

1. Indolealkylamines
2. Phenylalkylamines

The **indolealkylamines** have a core structure similar to serotonin and include **tryptamines**, such as dimethyltryptamine (DMT, ie, found in ayahuasca), psilocybin and its psychoactive metabolite psilocin, semisynthetic ergolines or lysergamides (ie, LSD), and iboga alkaloids (ie, ibogaine).

The **phenylalkylamines** have a core structure more similar to that of norepinephrine and include **phenylethylamines**, such as mescaline (from the peyote cactus *Lophophora williamsii*); and the **phenylisopropylamines**, which are amphetamine derivatives such as 2,5-dimethoxy-4-methylamphetamine (DOM) and MDMA. Note that MDMA is not a classic hallucinogen because it does not directly agonize the 2AR.

NEUROBIOLOGY AND MECHANISMS OF ACTION OF SHs

All of the classic hallucinogens have marked affinity as agonists for the 2AR but also interact to some degree with 5-HT1, -4,- 5,- 6, and -7 receptors. In addition, the semisynthetic ergolines (ie, LSD) display high intrinsic activity at D_2 and α-adrenergic receptors.[21] Ibogaine has the most complicated pharmacodynamic profile of the SHs and interacts with the following neurotransmitter systems[22]:

1. **Serotonergic** effects: 2AR agonist (SH action), presynaptic release, and inhibition of serotonin reuptake pump (MDMA-like properties), 5-HT3 agonism
2. **Glutamatergic**: Noncompetitive NMDA antagonist (similar to PCP and ketamine)
3. **Opioidergic**: μ agonism (opioid-like effects), κ agonism (similar to salvinorum A)
4. **Cholinergic**: Muscarinic agonist, $\alpha3\beta4$ nicotinic antagonist.

Converging lines of evidence from pharmacologic, electrophysiologic, and behavioral research in animals strongly suggests that activation of cortical 2AR receptors is the most critical step in initiating a cascade of biological events that accounts for their hallucinogenic properties.[23] In humans, preadministration of ketanserin (a 2AR antagonist) abolishes almost all of the psilocybin-induced psychoactive effects.[24]

2AR activation by SHs modulates prefrontal network activity by causing marked increases in extracellular glutamate levels that account for increased activity of pyramidal neurons, most pronounced in layer V of the prefrontal cortex (PFC).[25,26] Also, activation of 2AR receptors in the medial PFC affects subcortical transmission by increasing the activity of serotonin neurons in the dorsal raphe and dopamine (DA) neurons in the ventral tegmental area (VTA), the latter resulting in increased DA transmission in mesocortical and mesostriatal areas.[27–29] In a human study, psilocybin induced an increase in striatal DA that was correlated with euphoria and depersonalization.[30] This is interesting to note in light of the lack of psilocybin's ability to produce dependence syndromes (see section on Addictive Liability of Serotonergic Hallucinogens).

Imaging studies of SH use on the brain

Human brain imaging studies have demonstrated that psilocybin produces a particular pattern of prefrontal–limbic activation/de-activation[23,31]:

1. Marked prefrontal activation (hyperfrontality): frontomedial, dorsolateral cortices, anterior cingulate, insula, and temporal poles
2. Decreased activation of areas important for gating or integrating cortical information processing such as the bilateral thalamus, right globus pallidus, bilateral pons, and cerebellum
3. Decreased activity in the somatosensory cortical areas, occipital cortex, and visual pathways.

Taken together, psilocybin produces hyperfrontality with divergent prefrontal–subcortical activation in such a way as to increase cognitive and affective processing in the context of reduced gating and reduced focus on external stimulus processing.

Animal models of SH use

In animal models, SHs increase brain-derived neurotrophic factor (BDNF) levels in prefrontal and limbic brain areas. There is also evidence that 2AR agonists activate differing intracellular signaling pathways depending on whether they have hallucinogenic properties or not (ie, lisuride).[32] The 2A receptor is a Gq-coupled G protein–coupled receptor

(GPCR) that responds to the endogenous neurotransmitter, serotonin, whereas the mGluR2 is a Gi-coupled, pertussis toxin–sensitive GPCR that responds to glutamate. It has been demonstrated that 2AR and mGluR2 receptors form a functional heteromeric complex through which classic hallucinogens cross-signal to the Gi-coupled receptor.[33] Furthermore, it was recently demonstrated that the formation of the mGluR2/2AR complex establishes an optimal Gi–Gq balance in response to glutamate and serotonin (increase in Gi and decrease in Gq) and that the classic hallucinogens may produce their pro-psychotic states by effecting decreases in Gi and increases in Gq.[34]

ADDICTIVE LIABILITY OF SHs

A commonality among all drugs that are capable of producing dependence or addictive syndromes is their ability to substantially increase extracellular DA levels in the mesoaccumbens pathway, either directly by enhancing DA transmission through reuptake inhibition or facilitating presynaptic DA release (ie, cocaine, amphetamine, MDMA) or by indirect γ-aminobutyric acid-ergic (GABAergic), cholinergic, or gluta-matergic mechanisms that affect DA-cell firing (ie, alcohol, sedatives, opioids, cannabis, nicotine, NMDA antagonists [PCP, ketamine, dextromethorphan]).[35]

In contrast to all other drugs of abuse, SHs are not considered to be capable of producing sufficient reinforcing effects to cause dependence (addiction) syndromes.[36] Animal models (ie, self-administration, conditioned place preference) have failed to reliably demonstrate addictive liability of the SHs, suggesting that they do not possess sufficient pharmacologic properties to initiate or maintain dependence.[32] Almost all of the SHs, with the exception of LSD,[37,38] lack affinity for DA receptors or the DA transporter and do not directly affect dopaminergic transmission. Interestingly, despite evidence that SHs have been shown to increase DA transmission in striatal areas in humans, they fail to significantly activate the nucleus accumbens (NA) in positron emission tomography (PET) imaging studies consistent, with the lack of evidence linking classic hallucinogens with dependence syndromes.[24,30,31]

In fact, in animals, ibogaine (as well as nor-ibogaine and 18-methoxycoronaridine [18-MC]) has been shown to decrease DA efflux in the NA in response to opioids[39–42] and nicotine.[43–45] Furthermore, rapid tachyphylaxis occurs with repeated administration of the classic hallucinogens (with the exception of N,N-dimethyltryptamine [DMT]) and with repeated daily dosing, psychological effects disappear within several days, an effect that correlates with and likely is mediated by 5HT$_{2A}$ downregulation.[46] In addition to the lack of biological evidence, epidemiologic studies have also failed to reliably demonstrate a link between SHs and their ability to engender dependence syndromes, and the National Institute on Drug Abuse does not consider the SHs drugs of "addiction" because they do not produce compulsive drug-seeking behavior and because most recreational users decrease or stop their use over time.[47,48]

IBOGAINE AND OPIOID WITHDRAWAL; IBOGAINE AND ADDICTION

Ibogaine is a psychoactive indole alkaloid that is the most abundant alkaloid found in the root bark of the Apocynaceous shrub *Tabernathe iboga* in West Central Africa. It has been used for centuries by the Fang peoples as a religious sacrament by the Bwiti and Mbiri tribes (in Gabon, the Cameroons, and the Republic of Congo) as part of a syncretic ancestor-worship religion.[49,50]

Research on ibogaine in the United States began in the early 1960s when a group of lay drug experimenters, led by Howard Lotsof, became interested in the psychotherapeutic potential of ibogaine as an SH. Over the last 50 years, research on ibogaine in animals and humans has demonstrated the following:

- *Heroin withdrawal:* Surprisingly, a heroin-dependent group reported the complete elimination of heroin withdrawal symptoms with a one-time use of ibogaine.[51] Since then, other human anecdotal reports and several case series studies have strongly suggested that ibogaine diminishes or eliminates opioid withdrawal symptoms[52–55] and drug craving for multiple drugs of abuse including opiates, cocaine, and amphetamines.[52,54,56] Furthermore, animal studies have confirmed the anti-addictive properties of ibogaine, demonstrating that ibogaine effectively attenuates heroin, morphine, cocaine, amphetamine, methamphetamine, nicotine, and alcohol-seeking behaviors.[22,40,57]
- *Alcohol self-administration:* In addition, ibogaine has also been shown to inhibit operant alcohol self-administration in rats and to reduce alcohol intake in a reinstatement paradigm.[58]
- *Chronic ibogaine administration:* Despite there being no significant history of ibogaine misuse or abuse in the United States, it was classified as a schedule I agent as part of the Controlled Substances Act in 1970. In animal self-administration paradigms for drug abuse, iboga alkaloids have not been demonstrated to maintain reliable drug self-administration or to produce a withdrawal syndrome after chronic administration.[55,59] In fact, ibogaine has become noteworthy only in the last several decades, during which evidence has begun to accumulate that it may be an effective anti-addictive treatment for a variety of drugs of abuse.

In 1991, NIDA began an ibogaine research project based on case reports and preclinical evidence suggesting its utility. In 1993, the US Food and Drug Administration (FDA) approved a phase I clinical trial of ibogaine that was never completed. Before the research project ended in 1995, NIDA had committed several million dollars in support of its ibogaine research project, in which ibogaine was administered to human subjects in an FDA-approved phase I study.[52] It remains unavailable for use in the United States because of concerns regarding its safety, specifically neurotoxic and cardiotoxic issues. The neurotoxicity of greatest concern relates to possible cerebellar damage, observed in rats but not in mice or primates.[52,60] The cardiac toxicity includes bradycardia and possible other forms of arrhythmia, including possible QT prolongation. Consistent with anthropologic reports of fatalities during initiation rites of the Fang people of West Africa, at least a dozen deaths have been reported within 72 hours of ibogaine use since 1990.[22,61]

The **clinical use of ibogaine** to treat SUDs in a medicalized setting began when Dr. Deborah Mash, a professor of neurology at the University of Miami and ibogaine researcher, set up a medically oriented ibogaine treatment clinic in St. Kitts in the Caribbean in 1996 to treat patients with SUDs and opiate dependence/withdrawal in particular. The clinic administered ibogaine with close cardiac monitoring under the supervision of emergency medicine personnel. The clinic operated for approximately 10 years, but is no longer active.

Currently, despite ibogaine not being officially approved as a therapeutic agent in the United States, it continues to be used in alternative treatment settings, by both lay treatment providers in nonmedical settings and by practitioners in conventional medical settings outside of the United State.[62] A worldwide expansion of ibogaine use to treat SUDs has occurred within the past decade. In an ethnographic study into the ibogaine subculture, Alper and colleagues estimated that as of early 2006, approximately 3400 individuals had taken ibogaine (a fourfold increase relative to 2001) and approximately three-quarters used ibogaine to treat an SUD and about half specifically used it to treat opioid withdrawal.[22] One of the expanded uses of ibogaine (including in the United States) has been in an underground lay provider treatment setting where nonmedical personnel administer ibogaine illegally and without medical monitoring. Given ibogaine's potential toxicity and link to fatalities, it is of concern that it is being used in such uncontrolled settings.

ANTI-ADDICTIVE MECHANISMS OF CHANGE
Potential Biological Change Mechanisms

Iboga alkaloids and the treatment of acute opioid withdrawal: biological mechanisms

Animal studies have provided strong and consistent evidence for the ability of ibogaine and a synthetic congener, 18-MC, to attenuate opioid withdrawal in rats, mice, and primates,[22] although the evidence has been mixed on the ability of ibogaine to attenuate opioid withdrawal precipitated by naloxone in animals.[63] The ability of ibogaine and related congeners to attenuate or suppress opioid withdrawal is unique among the SHs, with no evidence of other similar agents (ie, LSD, psilocybin, DMT, mescaline) having any efficacy diminishing opioid withdrawal. Regarding the potential of ibogaine to treat acute opioid withdrawal, agonism at the μ opioid receptor has to be considered. The main metabolite of ibogaine, metabolized by cytochrome P4502D6, is noribogaine, which is a strong candidate to account for diminished acute opioid withdrawal symptoms[64] because of noribogaine's longer half-life, full μ agonist effects, and greater μ opioid binding affinity (relative to ibogaine).[63] However, it may be that ibogaine diminishes opioid withdrawal through neuroadaptations related to opioid tolerance or dependence and may do this through modulation of intracellular signaling at the μ opioid receptor.[22] For instance, prior exposure to morphine augments ibogaine's decrease of sensitized DA efflux in the NA in response to morphine administration[65] and ibogaine is known to enhance the antinociceptive effects of morphine.[66]

DA antagonism, the NA, anti-addiction, iboga alkaloids

Increased transmission of DA antagonism in the NA is one of the core hallmark neurobiological features of the addictive process signaling reward/pleasure/reinforcement and beginning the process of neuroplasticity and associative learning between previously neutral stimuli that come to predict drug-seeking behavior in individuals who develop addictive spectrum disorders.[67] Accordingly, based on this, a traditional anti-addictive approach involves blocking DA activity in brain reward pathways (ie, NA) by either preventing delivery of the addictive agent to the receptor site (ie, vaccines) that mediates the drug's addictive liability, using DA receptor antagonists, or using antagonists that block a particular addictive mediating receptor.

In animal models, ibogaine, noribogaine, and 18-MC are known to decrease DA efflux in the NA in response to opioids[39–42] and nicotine.[43–45] The ability of iboga alkaloids to diminish DA activity in the NA therefore strongly suggests an acute anti-addictive property, whatever may be the specific mechanism by which this effect occurs.

DA agonism, the NA, anti-addictive effects, SHs

Although blocking DA mesolimbic reward circuitry has been traditionally studied in the development of pharmacotherapeutic interventions for addictive syndromes, a new line of inquiry involves activation of this circuitry. Blum and colleagues have coined the term *reward deficiency syndrome* to describe a genetically related hypodopaminergic syndrome at the level of the NA caused by genetic polymorphisms in the 2AR, D2 (DA D2 receptor), and catechol-O-methyl-transferase (COMT) receptors associated with impulsive, compulsive, and addictive behaviors.[68] This may relate to the well known genetic contribution to addictive syndromes, estimated to account for at least 50% of the risk of developing an addictive syndrome.[69] Irrespective of whether this hypodopaminergic state in the mesolimbic pathway in individuals at risk for addiction exists as a risk factor for addiction, it certainly develops temporally with dependence syndromes. Two effects that likely contribute significantly to the addicted state are[70]:

1. Changes in midbrain DA
2. PFC DA and glutamate function.

Damage to the DA system is one of the changes that likely contributes to the transition from abuse to dependence syndromes and is associated with decreased DA receptor density and release in the NA and PFC, diminishing the ability of DA to signal novel salient events, leading to underexcitability to biologically relevant stimuli.[71] Preclinical and animal studies have suggested that persistent low-grade stimulation of DA D2 receptors (by D2 agonists) can induce a proliferation of these receptors rather than downregulation,[72–74] which is interesting in light of evidence that low DA D2 receptor levels are associated with addictive behaviors in humans.[75,76]

In addition to the aforementioned anti-addictive approach of DA antagonism at the NA, another traditional approach is that of **agonist substitution** or replacement therapy in which an addictive agent is replaced with one that has less addictive liability based on pharmacodynamic and pharmacokinetic characteristics such as:

- Receptor potency/affinity (ie, agonist, partial agonist, antagonist)
- Rate of central nervous system (CNS) absorption (ie, slower rates of absorption associated with less addictive liability)
- Half-life (ie, receptor, distribution, elimination with longer duration preferable).

Examples of this approach with a substantial evidence base for anti-addictive effects include methadone and buprenorphine for opiate use disorders and nicotine replacement and varenicline for nicotine use disorders.[77] Agonist substitution partially works in a similar way to the aforementioned antagonism approach. By occupying a particular addictive mediating receptor (ie, μ opioid, nicotinic acetylcholine receptor [NAR]), an agonist will functionally antagonize a more addictive drug of abuse (ie, heroin/μ opioid receptor; inhaled nicotine/NAR) and prevent it from binding and activating the receptor leading to surges in DA in the NA associated with the initial rewarding effects and long-term damage and downregulation of DA neurons. Alternatively, these agonist substitution approaches may work similarly to the aforementioned approach of persistent low-grade stimulation of D2 receptors leading to upregulation and restoring normal functioning of these receptors to re-respond normatively to biologically oriented rewards and novel stimuli.

In trying to now tie this to potential anti-addictive properties of the SHs, it is important to reiterate that the SHs increase DA transmission in mesolimbic reward areas (except ibogaine which, as mentioned previously, decreases DA transmission) without causing dependence syndromes. Is it possible that these agents could induce low-grade DA transmission that could lead to regeneration of D2 receptors and restore them to normative functioning? If this were to be possible, it is unlikely that an acute time-limited effect on the order of several hours would be enough to engender prolonged anti-addictive change. Either repeated dosing or a longer-term biological process would have to be invoked for this to be plausible.

Hallucinogens and Potential Long-Term Anti-Addictive Biological Processes

5-HT$_{2A}$ downregulation

One type of neuroplastic change caused by classic hallucinogens is their ability to produce rapid downregulation and desensitization of cortical 2ARs (especially anterior cingulate and frontomedial cortices) in rats in response to a variety of agents including LSD, 2,5-dimethoxy-4-bromoamphetamine (DOB), 2,5-dimethoxy-4-iodo-amphetamine (DOI), and DOM.[46,78–80] Furthermore, frontolimbic 2AR density correlates positively with increased anxiety and an exaggerated stress response in humans.[81] Given that anxiety and stress (mediated by increased activation of the stress response system (ie, corticotropin releasing factor, cortisol)} are significantly involved in the relapse process,[82] it is possible that 2AR downregulation by classic hallucinogens could alter and diminish stress-induced substance use relapse.

Neurotrophic factors altered by SH

Another interesting area of longer-lasting effects of SHs relates to their ability to alter the expression of neurotrophic factors. Both BDNF and glial cell line–derived neurotrophic factor (GDNF) expression can facilitate or inhibit addictive behaviors in rats based on the drug type, brain site (ie, cortical or subcortical), and phase of addiction (ie, initiation, maintenance, abstinence/relapse). In addition, SHs have been shown in animals to increase cortical and subcortical levels of BDNF.[83,84] In terms of BDNF's anti-addictive effects, activating BDNF signaling in the dorsal striatum consistently decreases alcohol intake and self-administration. Regarding cocaine, activating BDNF signaling in the medial PFC diminishes cocaine-seeking behaviors while activation of BDNF signaling in the NA has opposite effects.[85]

Drug-craving reduction An interesting aspect of ibogaine treatment seems to be its ability to reduce drug craving for extended periods of time even after a single treatment. Anecdotal reports in humans with a single treatment have suggested that drug craving can be reduced ranging from several weeks to up to 6 months.[64] Animal studies have confirmed this as well; single treatments with ibogaine were able to induce extended periods of reduced cocaine self-administration[40,57] and a diminution of ethanol intake for up to 48 hours.[58]

From a neurobiological perspective, it is known that long-lasting structural and molecular alterations in dopaminergic neurons in the mesolimbic pathway result from neuroadaptative changes related to chronic drug or alcohol exposure and that a subset of these alterations can be reversed by activation of the GDNF signal pathway.[86]

Upregulation of GDNF pathway It has recently been suggested that upregulation of the GDNF pathway in the midbrain may mediate the anti-addiction properties of ibogaine. He and Ron, using a dopaminergic-like SHSY5Y cell line, observed that short-term ibogaine exposure resulted in a sustained enhancement of GDNF expression, mediated by induction of the long-lasting autoregulatory cycle by which GDNF positively regulates its own expression.[87] These findings strongly suggest the need for further research into possible clinical applications of agents, such as ibogaine, that can enhance GDNF functioning as a way to harness a novel anti-addiction pharmacotherapeutic strategy.

Translating anecdotal findings into supervised clinical setting Further research into the potential use of ibogaine with addictive disorders should continue with the goal of translating the anecdotal and preclinical findings into the supervised clinical setting as well as further characterizing its anti-craving mechanisms. Moreover, it would be important to use iboga alkaloid compounds that confer the therapeutic effects while minimizing or eliminating the toxic side effects. One such potential agent to consider is 18-MC, a synthetic ibogaine congener designed specifically for this purpose and without any psychoactive properties.[88] The anti-addictive properties of 18-MC are currently being studied at NYU and NIDA (K.R. Alper, personal communication, 2011).

Glutamatergic homeostasis: neuroplasticity

As addiction progresses, the neurocircuitry of the reward pathway becomes corrupted, reorganized, and dysregulated whereby the behavioral system changes from a DA-oriented one in the NA (involved in the acute high-salience attribution of novel stimuli and the initiation of learning and conditioned responses) to a glutamate-based system in the PFC (especially the anterior cingulate and orbitofrontal cortex) marked by altered glutamatergic transmission in projections from the PFC to the NA.[89] Specifically, there is an increased glutamatergic modulation of accumbens DA cell reactivity in response to drug-related cues and a decreased response to biologically oriented natural rewards.[90] Moreover, impaired plasticity (ie, long-term potentiation and long-term depression) has been demonstrated in animals in communication between the PFC and the NA that is thought to limit the ability of dependent individuals to make behavioral and motivational changes (ie, attend to natural rewards, novel stimuli, learn new conditioned associations) to compete with drug-seeking stimuli and behaviors.[90] Based on this glutamate homeostatic dysfunction model in functional connectively between the PFC and the NA in the addicted state, a new line of pharmacotherapeutic interventions centered on glutamatergic modulation is emerging and there is evidence in animals for promising therapeutic targets of restoring synaptic plasticity such as restoring the activity of cysteine–glutamate exchangers, glutamate transporters, and enhancing the NMDA receptor function.[91]

Given that SHs increase extracellular glutamate levels and activity in the prefrontal–limbic circuitry, it is possible that a normalization in functional connectivity in this network though a glutamate-dependent neuroplastic adaptation could produce an anti-addictive effect. One possible mediating mechanism might be through increased signaling in BDNF because, as mentioned previously, SHs increase BDNF transmission, which is related to decreased alcohol self-administration in the dorsal striatum and diminished cocaine-seeking behaviors in the medial PFC in animals.

Gene transduction

Multiple studies have now confirmed that 2AR activation alters gene expression, in particular in PFC regions. Increases in gene expression of the following genes have been identified: c-*fos*, arc (activity-regulated, cytoskeletal-associated protein localized in neuronal dendrites), *ania3* (involved in glutamate signaling), *EGR-1* (early growth response protein 1 endogin, a zinc-finger transcription factor), *EGR-2*, period-1 (a circadian rhythm-related gene), and *Beta-arrestin 2*.[23,32] How this might related to conferring anti-addictive effects is unknown.

CURRENT STATE OF RESEARCH IN THE UNITED STATES ON SEROTONERGIC HALLUCINOGEN TREATMENT MODELS FOR SUBSTANCE ABUSE

If research were undertaken to examine the therapeutic utility of hallucinogen-assisted treatment models for SUDs, what would be the essential elements to consider in the study design? Charles O'Brien has outlined the essential ingredients: specific diagnoses and validated psychometric diagnostic instruments (ie, structured clinical interview for DSM-IV [SCID]), randomization, placebo control, use of specific diagnoses using validated measures, inclusion of severity measures, informed consent to clearly inform the participant of the unique psychological risks and benefits of these drugs, placebo control, random assignment, the use of objective blind raters, clearly defined substance outcomes (ie, abstinence vs use reduction), the need for adequate follow-up, and a standardized dose of manual guided psychotherapy with adequate supervision.[92]

In addition, it would see key to assess other factors such as stage of illness, typology of illness, motivation for change, social support, and psychiatric and medical comorbidity. Attention to therapist training, fidelity of dyad treatment teams, and the nature of the preparatory versus integrative psychotherapy would have to be considered carefully as well. The setting of dosing sessions would have to be carefully constructed so as to resemble more of a comfortable living room–like setting with flowers, fruit, music, and personal and meaningful items of the participants so as to create a safe, comfortable environment that is more likely to occasion a mystical experience as opposed to a cold clinical type typical hospital-based setting that would be less likely to occasion such an experience and might be more likely to produce negative and adverse psychological effects. Eyeshades and focusing internally might also be important to consider to more likely occasion a mystical experience. Single versus multiple dosing paradigms would need to be considered. Importantly, it would be key to consider the type of psychotherapeutic/behavioral platform or container that would be utilized in these studies. One could consider motivational techniques that are not intrinsically spiritually oriented such as motivational interviewing (MI) or employing those that are spiritually oriented in nature such as 12-step facilitation (TSF) or mindfulness-based relapse prevention (MBRP).[93,94]

Single Versus Multiple Dosing Paradigms: Electroconvulsive Therapy Model

It would be naïve to think that a one-time experience with a hallucinogen, however profound or mystical in nature, could affect long-term sobriety in addicted individuals, especially without linkage to aftercare and psychosocial treatment. In some addicted individuals, a spiritual conversion experience can last a lifetime. However, the vast majority of patients with dependence syndromes need multiple repeated treatment attempts including with 12-step modalities. So, it may be that repeated dosing is necessary, similar to an electroconvulsive therapy (ECT) type model. On a psychological level it may be that incremental changes in motivation initiated by a psycholytic experience can be combined with psychosocial motivational interventions to gradually increase motivation for abstinence or use reduction. In this model, repeated dosing sessions combined with added motivational psychotherapies may be needed to continue the momentum of the change process. Alternatively, it may that a mysticomimetic experience causes a pronounced and sudden quantum change toward abstinence that is maintained with relapse prevention but then relapse occurs within a short period of time (ie, within weeks to several months). In this model, repeated dosing sessions may be needed to reignite motivational changes once they regress or to maintain motivation for sobriety and recovery as part of relapse prevention.

From a biological perspective, it may be that repeated dosing is necessary to sustain long-term changes that can account for prolonged anti-addictive molecular or genetic processes. As mentioned previously, some possibilities have to do with alterations in signaling in BDNF and GDNF and through glutamate-dependent neuroplastic adaptations that may restore functional connectivity between prefrontal cortical and limbic reward structures.

As mentioned in the early LSD alcoholism research, there appeared to be a treatment effect in the better designed controlled studies but it tended to be short lived, on the order of several months, suggesting the utility of a multiple dosing paradigm study design.[9,95]

Active Hallucinogen Treatment Studies

Currently, in the United States, there are several active or near-active hallucinogen treatment studies for SUDs:

- Johns Hopkins has an active pilot study examining the efficacy of psilocybin-assisted CBT for smoking addiction. A small sample (N = 4) has been successfully treated so far with long-term abstinence in all, with biologic markers showing no signs of active smoking (Johnson M, personal communication, 2012).
- Columbia University and the New York State Psychiatric Institute have an active controlled trial of ketamine-assisted MBRP for cocaine dependence. Several subjects have completed the trial, also with early promising signs of increased abstinence (Dakwar E, personal communication, 2012).

There are two studies in the early phases of approval examining repeated dosing of psilocybin-assisted psychotherapy to treat alcohol use disorders.

- At the University of New Mexico, a study examining psilocybin-assisted motivational interviewing is in an active phase of approval (Bogenschutz, personal communication, 2012).
- At NYU, a controlled trial of psilocybin-assisted psychotherapy to treat alcohol dependence will utilize a combination of MI and 12-step facilitation therapies (Ross S, personal observation, 2012).

It is worth noting that although all of these studies undergo rigorous governmental (ie, FDA and Drug Enforcement Administration [DEA]) and local (ie, institutional review board [IRB], Clinical Translational Science Institute [CTSI]) review processes and schedule I licenses are being granted for clinical research in academic medical centers, the funding for these studies comes largely from private foundations. The exception to this is the aforementioned ketamine-MBRP study funded by the National Institute on Drug Abuse as part of a K award.

SUMMARY

Only time will tell if serotonergic hallucinogen-assisted psychotherapy treatment paradigms for SUDs will prove to be safe and effective in double-blind, placebo-controlled clinical trials. If they are, they would truly constitute a novel psychopharmacologic–psychosocial treatment paradigm to treat addictive disorders, although the risk of adverse psychological events would have to be controlled through a careful screening process and the risk of misuse of the substances or developing use syndromes would have to be considered, although the overall risk would be low because, as mentioned, SHs are unlike all other drugs of abuse in that they do not appear to produce dependence syndromes. There effects on the NA and DA range from inhibition to slight activation, all this without producing addiction. The ability of these medicinal tools to treat a range of addictive, psychiatric, and existential disorders is remarkable in scope and possibility. They truly represent a potential paradigmatic shift within the field of psychiatry, too interesting to not explore further.

REFERENCES

1. American Psychiatric Association. Diagnostic and statistical manual of mental disorders. Fourth edition, text revision (DSM-IV-TR). Arlington (VA): American Psychiatric Association; 2000.
2. Controlled Substances Act. Pub. L. 91–513, 84 Stat. 1236, enacted October 27, 1970, codified at 21 U.S.C. §801.
3. Leuner H. Hallucinogens as an aid in psychotherapy: basic principles and results. In: Pletscher A, Ladewig D, editors. 50 years of LSD: current status and perspectives of hallucinogen research. 1st edition. New York: Parthenon; 1994. p. 175–89.
4. Malleson N. Acute adverse reactions to LSD in clinical and experimental use in the United Kingdom. Br J Psychiatry 1971;118:229–30.
5. Kast E. LSD and the dying patients. Chic Med Sch Q 1966;26:80–7.
6. Grof S, Goodman LE, Richards WA, et al. LSD-assisted psychotherapy in patients with terminal cancer. Int Pharmacopsychiatry 1973;8(129):129–44.
7. Pahnke WN. The psychedelic mystical experience in the human encounter with death. Harvard Theol Rev 1969;62:1–21.
8. Abuzzahab FS, Anderson J. A review of LSD treatment in alcoholism. Int Pharmacopsychiatry 1971;6:223–35.
9. Krebs TS, Johansen PO. Lysergic acid diethylamide (LSD) for alcoholism: meta-analysis of randomized controlled trials. J Psychopharmacol 2012. [Epub ahead of print].
10. H.R. 4230, 103 D Cong., US Government Printing Office, Washington: 1994 Congressional Record 10 (1994) (enacted).
11. Dobkin de Rios MD, Grob CS, Baker JR. Hallucinogens and redemption. J Psychoactive Drugs 2002;34(3):239–48.
12. Garrity JF. Jesus, peyote, and the holy people: alcohol abuse and the ethos of power in Navajo healing. Med Anthropol Q 2000;14(4):521–42.
13. Fabregas JM, Gonzalez D, Fondevila S, et al. Assessment of addiction severity among ritual users of ayahuasca. Drug Alcohol Depend 2010;111(3):257–61.
14. Halpern JH, Sherwood AR, Passie T, et al. Evidence of health and safety in American members of a religion who use a hallucinogenic sacrament. Med Sci Monit 2008; 14(8):SR15–22.
15. Doering-Silveira E, Lopez E, Grob CS, et al. Report on psychoactive drug use among adolescents using ayahuasca within a religious context. J Psychoactive Drugs 2005; 37:141–4.
16. Grob CS, McKenna DJ, Callaway JE, et al. Human psychopharmacology of hoasca, a plant hallucinogen use din ritual context in Brazil. J Nerv Ment Dis 1996;184:86–94.
17. Miranda CT, Labigalini E, Tacla C. Alternative religion and outcome of alcohol dependence in Brazol. Addiction 1995;90:847.
18. Menninger K. Navajo peyote use: its apparent safety. Am J Psychiatry 1971;128: 695–9.
19. Halpern JH, Sherwood AR, Hudson JI, et al. Psychological and cognitive effects of long-term peyote use among Native Americans. Biol Psychiatry 2005;58:624–31.
20. Glennon RA. The Pharmacology of Classical Hallucinogens and Related Designer Drugs. In: Ries RK, Fiellin DA, Miller SC, et al, editors. Principles of addiction medicine. 4th edition. Philadelphia: Lippincott Williams & Wilkins; 2009. p. 215–40.
21. Marona-Lewicka D, Thisted RA, Nichols DE. Distinct temporal phases in the behavioral pharmacology of LSD: dopamine D2 receptor-mediated effects in the rat and implications for psychosis. Psychopharmacologia [Berl] 2005;180:427–35.

22. Alper KR, Lotsof HS, Kaplan CD. The ibogaine medical subculture. J Ethnopharmacol 2008;115:9–24.
23. Vollenweider FX, Kometer M. The neurobiology of psychedelic drugs: implications for the treatment of mood disorders. Nat Rev Neurosci 2010;11(9):642–51.
24. Vollenweider FX, Vollenweider-Scherpenhuyzen MF, Bäbler A, et al. Psilocybin induces schizophrenia-like psychosis in humans via a serotonin-2 agonist action. NeuroReport 1998;9:3897–902.
25. Aghajanian GK, Marek GJ. Serotonin, via 5HT2A receptors, increases EPSCs in layer V pyramidal cells of prefrontal cortex by an asynchronous mode of glutamate release. Brain Res 1999;825:161–71.
26. Beique JC, Imad M, Mladenovic L, et al. Mechanism of the 5-hydroxytryptamine 2A receptor-mediated facilitation of synaptic activity in prefrontal cortex. Proc Natl Acad Sci U S A 2007;104:9870–5.
27. Puig MV, Celada P, az-Mataix L, et al. In vivo modulation of the activity of pyramidal neurons in the rate medial prefrontal cortex by 5-HT2A receptors: relationship to thalamocortical afferents. Cereb Cortex 2003;13:870–82.
28. Celada P, Puig MV, Casanovas JM, et al. Control of dorsal raphe serotonergic neurons by the medial prefrontal cortex: involvement of serotonin-1A, GABA(A), and glutamate receptors. J Neurosci 2001;21:9917–29.
29. Vazquez-Borsetti P, Cortes R, Artigas F. Pyramidal neurons in rat prefrontal cortex projecting to ventral tegmental area and dorsal raphe nucleus express 5-HT2A receptors. Cereb Cortex 2009;19:1678–86.
30. Vollenweider FX, Vontobel P, Hell D, et al. 5-HT modulation of dopamine release in basal ganglia in psilocybin-induced psychosis in man: a PET study with [^{11}C]raclopride. Neuropsychopharmacology 1999;20:424–33.
31. Geyer MA, Vollenweider FX. Serotonin research: contributions to understanding psychoses. Trends Pharmacol Sci 2008;29(9):445–53.
32. Nichols DE. Hallucinogens. Pharmacol Ther 2004;101:131–81.
33. González-Maeso J, Ang RL, Yuen T, et al. Identification of a serotonin/glutamate receptor complex implicated in psychosis. Nature 2008;452:93–7.
34. Fribourg M, Moreno JL, Holloway T, et al. Decoding the signaling of a GPCR heteromeric complex reveals a unifying mechanism of action of antipsychotic drugs. Cell 2011;147(5):1011–23.
35. Baler RD, Volkow ND. Drug addiction: the neurobiology of disrupted self-control. Trends Mol Med 2006;12(12):559–66.
36. O'Brien CP. Drug addiction and drug abuse. In: Hardman JGLimbird LEMolinoff PB, et al, editors. Goodman and Gilman's the pharmacological basis of therapeutics. New York: McGraw-Hill; 2001. p. 574–639.
37. Watts VJ, Lawler CP, Fox DR, et al. LSD and structural analogs: pharmacological evaluation at D_1 dopamine receptors. Psychopharmacology [Berl] 1995;118:401–9.
38. Giacomelli S, Palmery M, Romanelli L, et al. Lysergic acid diethylamide (LSD) in a partial agonist of D_2 dopaminergic receptors and it potentiates dopamine-mediated prolactin secretion in lactotrophs in vitro. Life Sci 1998;63:215–22.
39. Maisonneuve IM, Keller RW, Glick SD. Interactions of ibogaine, a potential anti-addictive agent, and morphine: an in vivo microdialysis study. Eur J Pharmacol 1991;199(1):35–42.
40. Glick SD, Kuehne ME, Raucci J et al. Effects of iboga alkaloids on morphine and cocaine self-administration in rats: relationship to tremorigenic effects and to effects on dopamine release in nucleus accumbens and striatum. Brain Res 1994;657(1–2): 14–22.

41. Glick SD, Maisonneuve IM, Dickinson HA. 18-MC reduced methamphetamine and nicotine self-administration in rats. NeuroReport 2000;11(9):2013–5.
42. Taraschenko OD, Shulan JM, Maisonneuve IM, et al. 18-MC acts in the medial habenula and interpeduncular nucleus to attenuate dopamine sensitization to morphine in the nucleus accumbens. Synapse 2007;61(7):547–60.
43. Benwell ME, Holtom PE, Moran RJ, et al. Neurochemical and behavioural interactions between ibogaine and nicotine in the rat. Br J Pharmacol 1996;117(4):743–9.
44. Maisonneuve IM, Mann GL, Deibel CR, et al. Ibogaine and the dopaminergic response to nicotine. Psychopharmacology [Berl] 1997;129(3):249–56.
45. Glick SD, Maisonneuve IM, Visker KE, et al. 18-Methoxycoronardine attenuates nicotine-induced dopamine release and nicotine preferences in rats. Psychopharmacology [Berl] 1998;139(3):274–80.
46. Buckholtz NS, Zhou DF, Freedman DX, et al. Lysergic acid diethylamide (LSD) administration selectively downregulates serotonin$_2$ receptors in rat brain. Neuropsychopharmacology 1990;3:137–48.
47. NIDA. Hallucinogens and dissociative drugs. National Institute on Drug Abuse research report series, vol. 01–4209. Rockville (MD): National Institute on Drug Abuse; 2001.
48. NIDA. LSD NIDA info facts. Rockville (MD): National Institute on Drug Abuse; 2005.
49. Dobkin de Rios M. Hallucinogens: cross-cultural perspective. Prospect Heights (IL): Waveland Press; 1984.
50. Fernandez JW. Bwiti: an ethnography of religious imagination in Africa. Princeton (NJ): Princeton University Press; 1982.
51. Lotsof HS, Alexander NE. Case studies of ibogaine treatment: implications for patients' management strategies. Alkaloids Chem Biol 2001;56:293–313.
52. Mash DC, Kovera CA, Buck BE, et al. Medication development of ibogaine as a pharmacotherapy for drug dependence. Ann NY Acad Sci 1998;844:274–92.
53. Schechter MD, Gordon TL. Comparison of the behavioral effects of ibogaine from three sources: mediation of discriminative activity. Eur J Pharmacol 1993;249:79–84.
54. Alper KR, Lotsof HS, Frenken GM, et al. Treatment of acute opioid withdrawal with ibogaine. Am J Addict 1999;8:234–42.
55. Alper KR, Beal D, Kaplan CD. A contemporary history of ibogaine in the United States and Europe. Alkaloids Chem Biol 2001;56:249–81.
56. Sheppard SG. A preliminary investigation of ibogaine: case reports and recommendations for further study. J Subst Abuse Treat 1994;11:379–85.
57. Cappendijk SL, Dzoljic MR. Inhibitory effects of ibogaine on cocaine self-administration in rats. Eur J Pharmacol 1993;241:261–5.
58. He DY, McGough NN, Ravindranathan A, et al. Glial cell line-derived neurotrophic factor mediates the desirable actions of the anti-addiction drug ibogaine against alcohol consumption. J Neurosci 2005;25:619–28.
59. Aceto MD, Bowman ER, Harris LS, et al. Dependence studies of new compounds in the rhesus monkey and mouse. NIDA Res Monogr 1991;119:513–58.
60. Molinari HH, Maisonneuve IM, Glick SD. Ibogaine neurotoxicity: a re-evaluation. Brain Res 1996;737(1–2):255–62.
61. Maas U, Strubelt S. Fatalities after taking ibogaine in addiction treatment could be related to sudden cardiac death caused by autonomic dysfunction. Med Hypotheses 2006;67(4):960–4.
62. Alper K, Lotsof HS. The use of ibogaine in the treatment of addictions. In: Winkelman M, Roberts T, editors. Hallucinogens and healing. Westport (CT): Praeger, Greenwood Publishing Group; 2007.

63. Maciulaitis R, Kontrimaviciute V, Bressolle FMM, et al. Ibogaine, an anti-addictive drug: pharmacology and time to go further in development. A narrative review. Hum Exp Toxicol 2008;27:181–94.
64. Mash DC, Kovera CA, Pablo J, et al. Ibogaine: complex pharmacokinetics, concerns for safety, and preliminary efficacy measures. Ann N Y Acad Sci 2000;914:394–401.
65. Pearl SM, Maisonneuve IM, Glick SD. Prior morphine exposure enhances ibogaine antagonism of morphine-induced dopamine release in rats. Neuropharmacology 1996;35:1779–84.
66. Sunder Sharma S, Bhargava HN. Enhancement of morphine antinociception by ibogaine and noribogaine in morphine-tolerant mice. Pharmacology 1998;57(5):229–32.
67. Kalivas PW. The glutamate homeostasis hypothesis of addiction. Nat Rev Neurosci 2009;10:561–72.
68. Blum K, Chen AL, Chen TJH, et al. Activation instead of blocking mesolimbic dopaminergic reward circuitry is a preferred modality in the long term treatment of reward deficiency syndrome (RDS): a commentary. Theor Biol Med Model 2008;5:24–39.
69. Swendsen J, Le Moal M. Individual vulnerability to addiction. Ann N Y Acad Sci 2011;1216:73–85.
70. Kalivas PW, Volkow ND. The neural basis of addiction: a pathology of motivation and choice. Am J Psychiatry 2005;162:1403–13.
71. Volkow ND, Fowler JS, Wang GJ, et al. Dopamine in drug abuse and addiction: results from imaging studies and treatment implications. Mol Psychiatry 2004;9:557–69.
72. Boundy VA, Pacheco MA, Guan W, et al. Agonists and antagonists differentially regulate the high affinity state of the D2L receptor in human embryonic kidney 293 cells. Mol Pharmacol 1995;48:956–64.
73. Boundy VA, Lu L, Molinoff PB. Differential coupling of rat D2 dopamine receptor isoforms expressed in *Spodoptera frugiperda* insect cells. J Pharmacol Exp Ther 1996;276:784–94.
74. Noble EP, Noble RE, Ritchie T, et al. D2 dopamine receptor gene and obesity. Int J Eat Disord 1994;15:205–17.
75. Pohjalainen T, Rinne JO, Nagren K, et al. The A1 allele of the human D2 dopamine receptor gene predicts low D2 receptor availability in healthy volunteers. Mol Psychiatry 1998;3:256–60.
76. Noble EP, Blum K, Ritchie T, et al. Allelic association of the D2 dopamine receptor gene with receptor-binding characteristics in alcoholism. Arch Gen Psychiatry 1991;48:648–54.
77. Ross S, Peselow E. Pharmacotherapies for addictive disorders. Clin Neuropharmacol 2009;32(5):277–89.
78. Buckholtz NS, Freedman DX, Middaugh LD. Daily LSD administration selectively decreases serotonin$_2$ receptor binding in rat brain. Eur J Pharmacool 1985;109:421–5.
79. Buckholtz NS, Zhou DF, Freedman DX. Serotonin$_2$ agonist administration down-regulates rat brain serotonin$_2$ receptors. Life Sci 1988;42:2439–45.
80. Leysen JE, Janssen PF, Niemegeers CJ. Rapid desensitization and down-regulation of 5-HT$_2$ receptors by DOM treatment. Eur J Pharmacol 1989;163:145–9.
81. Frokjaer VG, Mortensen EL, Nielsen FA, et al. Frontolimbic serotonin 2A receptor binding in healthy subjects is associated with personality risk factors for affective disorder. Biol Psychiatry 2008;63(6):569–76.
82. Sinha R, Li CS. Imaging stress- and cue-induced drug and alcohol craving: association with relapse and clinical implications. Drug Alcohol Rev 2007;26(1):25–31.

83. Vaidya VA, Marek GJ, Aghajanian GK, et al. 5-HT2A receptor-mediated regulation of brain-derived neurotrophic factor mRNA in the hippocampus and the neocortex. J Neurosci 1997;17:2785–95.
84. Cavus I, Duman RS. Influence of estradiol, stress, and 5-HT2A agonist treatment on brain-derived neurotrophic factor expression in female rats. Biol Psychiatry 2003;54:59–69.
85. Ghitza UE, Zhai H, Wu P, et al. Role of BDNF and GDNF in drug reward and relapse: a review. Neurosci Biobehav Rev 2010;35:157–71.
86. Ron D, Janak PH. GDNF and addiction. Rev Neurosci 2005;16:277–85.
87. He DY, Ron D. Autoregulation of glial cell line-derived neurotrophic factor expression: implications for the long-lasting actions of the anti-addictive drug, Ibogaine. Faseb J 2006;20:E1–E8.
88. Maissoneuve IM, Glick SD. Anti-addictive actions of an iboga alkaloid congener: a novel mechanism for a novel treatment. Pharmacol Biochem Behav 2003;75(3):607–18.
89. Kalivas PW. Cocaine and amphetamine-like psychostimulants: neurocircuitry and glutamate neuroplasticity. Dialogues Clin Neurosci 2007;9:389–97.
90. Kalivas PW. The glutamate homeostasis hypothesis of addiction. Nature Rev Neurosci 2009;10:561–72.
91. Javitt DC, Schoepp D, Kalivas PW, et al. Translating glutamate: from pathophysiology to treatment. Neuroscience 2011;102(3):1–13.
92. O'Brien CP, Jones RT. Methodological issues in the evaluation of a medication for its potential benefits in enhancing psychotherapy. In: 50 years of LSD: current status and perspectives of hallucinogens, 1st edition. New York: Parthenon; 1994. p. 213–22.
93. Brewer JA, Bowen S, Smith JT, et al. Mindfulness-based treatments for co-occurring depression and substance use disorders: what can we learn from the brain? Addiction 2010;105(10):1698–706.
94. Marlatt GA, Gordon JR, editors. Relapse prevention: Maintenance strategies in the treatment of addictive behaviors. New York: Guilford Press; 1985.
95. Bowen WT, Soskin RA, Chotlos JW. Lysergic acid diethylamide as a variable in the hospital treatment of alcoholism. J Nerv Ment Dis 1970;150(2):111–8.

Drug Treatments in Criminal Justice Settings

Benjamin R. Nordstrom, MD, PhD[a],*, A.R. Williams, MD, MBE[b]

KEYWORDS

- Drug addiction • Addiction treatment • Coerced treatment • Drug crime

KEY POINTS

- Studies have found that the direct effect of drug-related crime (ie, not including the cost of arrest, prosecution, and incarceration) is the largest single cost related to addiction.
- It has been estimated that people on probation and parole consume up to half of the cocaine and heroin brought into the United States.
- National Institute on Drug Abuse principles of drug addiction treatment, principle #11: treatment does not need to be voluntary to be effective.
- The available evidence suggests that drug treatment can lead to modest reductions in criminal offending for drug-using criminal offenders; considering the scope of the problem and expense in dealing with drug-related crime, even marginal improvements can lead to important aggregate savings in both economic and humanitarian terms.

Currently 8% (19.9 million) of Americans aged 12 or older are current users of illicit drugs. In addition, 6.9 million Americans over the age of 12 were classified as having either abuse of or dependence on illicit substances. This figure has been essentially stable since 2002.[1] Further, it has been estimated that 3% of the US population will meet criteria for dependence on an illicit substance at some point in their lives.[2] The Office of National Drug Control Policy reported that the total cost of drug abuse on society in 2002 was $180.9 billion, and the majority of these costs were crime-related.[3] Other studies have found that the direct effect of drug-related crime (ie, not including the cost of arrest, prosecution, and incarceration) is the largest single cost related to addiction.[4]

In the United States in 2007, violations of drug laws accounted for approximately 13% of the 14 million arrests made that year. Of those drug arrests, nearly 83% were for possession of drugs, whereas the remaining 17% were for drug trafficking.[5] Nearly 80% of the money the United States spends on incarceration is spent incarcerating drug-using offenders.[6] As many as 400,000 people are in jails and prisons on

[a] Dartmouth Medical School, DHMC, 1 Medical Center Drive, Lebanon, NH 03756, USA; [b] New York University, New York, NY, USA
* Corresponding author.
E-mail address: benjamin.r.nordstrom@dartmouth.edu

Psychiatr Clin N Am 35 (2012) 375–391
doi:10.1016/j.psc.2012.03.005
0193-953X/12/$ – see front matter © 2012 Published by Elsevier Inc.

drug-related charges.[7] Currently 52.2% of the offenders in federal prisons are convicted of drug offenses.[8]

In 2004, 17% of state prisoners and 18% of federal inmates reported having committed their current offense in order to get money to purchase drugs.[9] During 2002, 68% of offenders in local jails were found to be dependent on or abusing illicit drugs. The same survey revealed that approximately one-quarter of convicted property and drug offenders serving time in local jails had committed their crimes to get money with which to purchase drugs. Only 5% of violent offenders in local jails had similarly committed their crimes in order to purchase drugs.[10] Although violent drug-related crimes are less common than nonviolent drug-related crimes, they pose a greater cost to society because of the effects that such crimes impose on their victims.[11]

Among state prisoners, 30% of property offenders, 26% of drug offenders, and 11% of violent offenders had committed their crimes to obtain money with which to buy drugs. In federal prisons, 25% of drug users (but only 11% of property offenders) reported they had committed their crimes to obtain drug money.[12] According to the Uniform Crime Report, approximately 4% of the total 14,831 homicides that occurred in 2007 were coded as drug-related.[5]

The first national survey of adults on probation, which was undertaken in 1995, revealed that approximately 70% of probationers had used drugs in the past, and 32% of them used illegal drugs in the month leading up to their offense.[13] A later survey found that 30% of probationers (and 40% of mentally ill probationers) used illicit drugs in the month before their arrest.[14] In 2007 there were approximately 1.6 million adults on parole. Nearly one-quarter of parolees were recent users (ie, within the past month) of illicit drugs compared with 7.4% of adults not on parole or supervised release.[1]

DRUG USE PERSISTS WHILE UNDER CORRECTIONAL SUPERVISION

It has been estimated that people on probation and parole consume up to half of the cocaine and heroin brought into the United States.[15] The consequences of being caught for using drugs while on probation or parole can involve extremely harsh sanctions for even trivial illicit drug use.[15,16] Although it is risky to continue to use drugs on probation or parole, the chance of being caught for doing so is low, because urine toxicology screens are rarely performed.[17] Regardless, this group constitutes a large source of domestic demand for drugs, and this group's continued drug use leads to high rates of reoffending.[18]

ONGOING DRUG USE IS ASSOCIATED WITH INCREASED CRIME IN THIS POPULATION

It has been repeatedly demonstrated that criminally offending drug users commit a large number of crimes, especially when their drug use is active.[19–24] In 2002, 16% of convicted jail inmates reported they committed their offense to get money for drugs, and 75% of inmates in jail for drug or property offenses met criteria for substance abuse or dependence.[25] Illicit drug users are also 16 times more likely than nonusers to report being arrested for larceny or theft, and nine times more likely to be arrested for an assault charge.[26]

Despite these considerations, drug treatments provided to probationers and parolees can decrease the amount of drugs used by this population, as well as decreasing all-cause reoffending.[27] If an intervention could decrease the amount of drugs consumed by this population, it might diminish reoffending and reincarceration, and parolees and probationers would spend less time separated from their families and communities as well as constitute less of a burden in terms of criminal justice expenditures. Further, it could have a significant effect on reducing demand for illegal drugs.

DRUG USE AS THE PRODUCT OF OPERANT CONDITIONING

Drug use has been described as the product of operant conditioning. Operant conditioning holds that a given behavior will increase in frequency if it is reinforced.[28] Drug use, like other behaviors, is sensitive to environmental manipulations (eg, the presence of reinforcers or punishers). Alternative reinforcement holds that if a subject is given a choice between drugs and an alternative nondrug reinforcer (eg, a desired food item or money), the choice to use drugs will decrease. That such an environmental manipulation can decrease the frequency of the choice to use drugs has been repeatedly demonstrated in laboratory settings using rats[29] and nonhuman primates.[30–32] This result has also been repeatedly demonstrated in the human literature in studies offering subjects the choice between a dose of their drug of choice and money. As the magnitude of the alternative reinforcer and/or the dose of drug decreases, the frequency of the choice to use drugs diminishes.[33–38]

Like reinforcement, punishment can affect the choice to use drugs as well. Punishment can be positive—the application of an aversive stimulus—or negative—the removal of a pleasant stimulus.[39] The application of positive punishment (eg, an electric shock) has been shown to decrease self-administration of drugs of abuse by rhesus monkeys.[40–44] Negative punishment (a forced "time-out") has also been shown to decrease cocaine self-administration by monkeys.[45]

OPERANT PRINCIPLES HAVE GIVEN RISE TO CONTINGENCY MANAGEMENT TREATMENTS

The idea that changing environmental context can affect the choice to use drugs has given rise to a treatment modality known as contingency management. Contingency management is based on operant principles including that drug use is maintained by environmental influences and can be changed by altering the consequences of use, thus providing a system of incentives and disincentives to make abstinence a more attractive choice than continued drug use.[46] Many contingency management studies have demonstrated the efficacy of providing financial incentives for drug-free urine toxicology screens in either the form of cash or vouchers.[47–50]

Another form of contingency management includes the application of punishment for continued drug use. In an observational study in a methadone clinic, the application of limit-setting with respect to the ongoing use of illicit drugs, with termination from the clinic as the punishment, decreased illicit drug use.[51] Other descriptive reports tell of the efficacy of using positive punishment in the form of "contingency contracts" in drug-using populations.[52,53] One study of 21 male methadone maintenance "treatment failures" showed that the threat of negative punishment (having one's treatment terminated at the clinic) significantly reduced illicit drug use among this group.[54] A randomized study demonstrated that including consequences (termination from the clinic) for continued drug use significantly increased abstinence and treatment retention among methadone maintenance patients.[55] Two studies have compared contingency management interventions based on positive reinforcement and negative punishment.[56,57] Both showed that negative punishment was as equally effective as positive reinforcement in producing abstinence. Studies of a therapeutic workplace for drug users have found that adding contingency management strategies, including negative contingencies, significantly improves attendance and performance.[58,59]

TRANSLATING CONTINGENCY MANAGEMENT TO A CRIMINAL JUSTICE CONTEXT

Contingency management interventions using positive reinforcement have been studied in the criminal justice population.[60] However, this study did not take place in a criminal justice setting and focused on how criminal justice system–involved participants used the vouchers they had earned. Additional studies using contingency management in the drug-offending criminal justice population have been called for.[61]

It has been observed that compulsory supervision by the criminal justice system facilitates abstinence from narcotics.[62] Establishing early periods of sustained abstinence has been shown to correlate with longer term abstinence.[63] Coerced abstinence[15] works on the principle that the deterrent effect of drug monitoring on probation and parole will be greater if violations are detected routinely and sanctions applied swiftly. For probationers and parolees, urine screens are checked twice weekly, with each missed screen counting as positive. This practice is supported by clinical evidence that inconsistent urine screening undermines contingency management.[64] Any positive screen results in the immediate application of a series of graduated sanctions.

Graduated sanctions in the context of probation and parole mean that intermediate sanctions are applied for violations of probation or parole before revocation of probation or parole is considered.[65] For example, for the first positive screen the participant is transported to jail for one day (24 hours). For the second positive screen he stays 2 days (48 hours), and so forth. This differs from the current regime wherein one reoffense results in violation and being compelled to serve the duration of one's sentence in incarceration. Graduated sanctions allow drug users to learn from their mistakes and to modify their behavior without the scale of disruption posed by reincarceration. Both the certainty of detection of drug use and promptness of the application of sanctions are enhanced. In a metaanalysis of contingency management studies, both certainty of detection and celerity of the delivery of contingences were found to be significant moderators of outcome.[46]

In 1997 the state of Maryland initiated the Maryland Break the Cycle (BTC) initiative under the guidance of then Lieutenant Governor Kathleen Kennedy. This initiative contained many core elements of Kleiman's coerced abstinence, including more frequent urine toxicology screening and increased applications of sanctions for using drugs while under criminal justice supervision. The Urban Institute, an independent think tank, assessed the impact of this policy in 2003.[66] They found that in areas where BTC had been used probationers and parolees had significantly lower likelihood of arrests for drug offenses and fewer drug arrests, and that results were better in locations with greater program fidelity. They also found that for each dollar invested in the program, between $2.30 and $5.70 was saved. These data suggest that increasing the frequency of drug testing paired with graduated sanctions can be effective in reducing drug use and its associated harms in criminally offending drug users.

THE USE OF COERCION IN CRIMINAL JUSTICE SETTINGS

The use of coercion in the treatment for substance use disorders has gained significant traction in the past few decades.[67] An expert panel comprising the Addiction Committee of the Group for the Advancement of Psychiatry reviewed the literature on coerced drug treatment from 1998 to 2005 and found that mandated or coerced treatment has increasingly been shown to be as, or more, effective than "non-coerced" treatment.[68] These aggregate findings are consistent with the National

Institute on Drug Abuse (NIDA) Principles of Drug Addiction Treatment, specifically NIDA Principle #11: Treatment does not need to be voluntary to be effective.[69]

Coerced or mandated addiction treatment is now particularly common in criminal justice settings, capitalizing on judicial power and oversight to enforce swift consequences for aberrant behaviors, especially in unlocked and/or outpatient settings. By the late 1990s, criminal justice referrals constituted almost half of the publicly funded drug treatment population.[70] A study by Anglin and Hser[71] determined the four most important considerations for coerced treatment:

(1) Sufficient duration (at least 3 to 9 months)
(2) High level of structure and monitoring
(3) Flexibility to maintain enrollment despite occasional drug use (slips)
(4) Regular program evaluation (preferably external).

Outcomes of successful programs in the criminal system have been so robust that there has been renewed interest in the use of commitment and coercion in the civil system.

ADDICTION TREATMENT AND REOFFENDING

There are many studies that analyze the relationship between participation in addiction treatment and criminal justice outcomes. One observational study of opiate addicts seeking treatment in outpatient methadone maintenance programs attempted to study the salutatory effects of treatment on criminal offending.[72] The sample consisted of 315 Australian opiate-addicted people who applied to enter two separate methadone maintenance clinics. Of this group, 231 people were enrolled in treatment while the remaining 84 were rejected for either not completing the assessment or having an insufficiently severe addiction to warrant methadone maintenance. Information regarding social and personal history as well as on a history of drug use and treatment and criminal convictions was culled from admission interviews. Official records of arrests and convictions were used to supplement the self-report data. The investigators classified official convictions into six categories:

(1) Drug offenses
(2) Property offenses
(3) Violent offenses
(4) Traffic offenses
(5) Technical offenses (eg, failure to appear, violation of parole)
(6) Solicitation.

The subjects were then followed for between roughly 1.5 to 2.5 years.

The sample was predominantly (72%) male, and the mean age was 26.4 years. Only 11% of the sample had worked full-time in the 6 months prior to the assessment. 75% of the sample reported that at least some of their income was produced illegally. The treatment group differed from the rejected group in that the latter group was significantly younger, had used heroin for shorter periods of time, and was less likely to be physically dependent on opioids.

The majority of crimes were property offenses (50%) and drug offenses (26%). There were so few crimes in the other categories that they were dropped from analysis. Preassessment conviction rates declined with increasing age at assessment, but neither the duration of addiction nor the age of first drug use were significant predictors of crime rates. The age of first conviction was, however, and analyses all adjusted for the effect of age, sex, and age of first conviction.

The results of the study showed that the rejected group had significantly greater reductions in conviction rates in both drug and property offenses in the postassessment period. In fact, convictions for property offenses rose in the treatment group. However, even controlling for the declining propensity to be convicted over time, there was a progressively reduced risk of conviction with increasing duration of treatment.

A secondary analysis of these data was undertaken to further elucidate the drug-crime relationship in this population.[73] These data showed that men were more likely to initiate opioid use after or during the initiation of their crime careers, whereas women were more likely to begin an addiction career and initiate crime later. They also found that the earlier a criminal career began, the higher the rate of convictions.

There are two major issues that limit the confidence one can have in the findings of these studies.

(1) There are profound implications to the significant differences between the treatment and rejected groups. That the rejected group was less criminally active and showed greater reductions in the post-assessment period compared to the treatment group may well be referable to the fact that their addictions are less severe, and that because they are not physically dependent on opioids that the impetus to generate income to buy drugs is relatively smaller.

(2) The emphasis on conviction data may well underestimate the crimes these people committed.

Another study by this group sought to extend on their previous findings.[74] In this study 304 people attending three different methadone maintenance clinics were interviewed on three occasions over 12 months. Interviewers gathered data about participants' social history, the number of days in the previous month in which they had been criminally active, and their involvement in these activities during the last period of addiction prior to presenting for treatment. Information about drug use and crime was gathered at the initial interview and the 12-month follow-up interview. Information about antisocial personality disorder (ASPD) was gathered at the second interview that was conducted 1 month after the initial assessment.

Of the 304 participants, 131 were female and 173 were male. The results of the study showed that for people who remained in treatment for at least 1 month, self-report of participation in acquisitive crime fell to one-eighth the of the level observed prior to treatment. No P values were presented here, but confirmatory analysis using official conviction records showed a statistically significant reduction in convictions in property crime in the posttreatment period. As heroin use and criminal activity fell on entry into treatment, linear regression showed that ongoing cannabis use was the strongest predictor of continued acquisitive crime.

Antisocial personality disorder was then added to the model for those 229 (of the original 304) who participated in the second interview, and linear regression was performed to identify correlates of continued criminal activity while in treatment. The three significant predictors of crime were

(1) ASPD symptom count
(2) Continued heroin use
(3) Treatment at one specific clinic (Clinic 1) of the three clinics studied.

Regarding this final point, the authors note "Clinic 1 stood out in having a prevailing atmosphere of chaos."

This study gave further evidence that entry into methadone maintenance treatment can reduce crime, but that continued involvement with drugs was correlated with ongoing criminal activity. Further, the more antisocial a person was, the more likely he or she was to remain involved in crime. This latter point may be somewhat spurious because the authors note that people with ASPD had been more criminally active prior to coming to treatment as well.

Another study also sought to understand how antisocial behavior interacts with treatment effect.[75] In this study, 89 13- to 19-year-old males admitted to an inpatient treatment program for delinquent, drug-involved youth were recruited to participate. The inclusion criteria were that they had to be admitted between May 1991 and May 1993, have a diagnosis of substance dependence, and have at least three symptoms of conduct disorder (the juvenile equivalent of antisocial personality disorder). The participants underwent thorough reviews of their mental health, substance use, and violence histories. They then were followed up with similar interviews at 6, 12, and 24 months.

Of 176 potential participants, only 8 did not meet criteria. Another 57 did not complete intake assessments ("usually" because the boys eloped from the treatment center). Of the 111 boys who met criteria and completed assessment, 89 were available for 2-year follow-up interviews. The researchers found that at the 2-year evaluation, there were significant reductions in criminal behavior, symptoms of conduct disorder, depression, and attention problems, whereas the prevalence of drug use was unchanged (there were reductions in the frequency of use, but these were not statistically significant). The researchers also found that early-onset conduct disorder and more severe conduct disorder (as measured by having more symptoms of conduct disorder) were significant predictors of worse outcomes in terms of continued conduct disorder and criminality.

The conclusions the authors can draw from this study are somewhat limited. Because there was no random assignment and no control condition, it not clear that the treatment caused the reduction in conduct disorder. This limitation is especially true given the fact that the team also found that treatment retention was not associated with a better outcome. But for this result, one could logically assume that the findings underestimate the effect of conduct disorder on outcomes, because the more severely conduct-disordered boys might have eloped immediately (and then presumably suffered worse outcomes). Regardless, despite these limitations, the study provides a converging line of evidence that more antisocial people do not enjoy the same benefits of treatment as nonantisocial people.

THE NATIONAL TREATMENT OUTCOME RESEARCH STUDY

One large study in Britain sought to investigate a variety of potential effects of substance abuse treatment. The National Treatment Outcome Research Study (NTORS) used a longitudinal prospective cohort design and recruited 1075 people seeking treatment for addictions from 54 treatment centers representing the main British treatment modalities. Inclusion criteria were: (1) starting a new treatment episode, (2) presenting with a drug-related problem, (3) providing a UK contact address for follow-up, and (4) not having previously been enrolled in NTORS. Follow-up data were acquired at 1 year. The researchers conducted structured interviews and gathered information about drug and alcohol use, health risk behavior, treatment history, physical health problems, psychological health problems, criminal behavior, and treatment history. Clients were recruited from a variety of inpatient drug treatment units, residential drug rehabilitation units, and methadone maintenance and methadone reduction outpatient programs. With respect to criminal behavior, the researchers found that in the 90-day period leading up to entry into treatment, 48%

of the clients had committed no crime (apart from drug dealing) whereas only 10% of the clients committed 76% of the reported criminal activity.[76,77]

One report from this study focused on the changes that occurred in crime after 1 year from entering treatment.[77] This study focused on the subset of 753 of the original 1075 participants who were available for interview at 1 year. At 1 year both the residential and community treatment groups had significantly reduced the number of incidents of acquisitive crime, shoplifting, burglary, and fraud. The residential treatment group also had significantly fewer reported robberies. There were reductions in the community group's robbery rate, but it fell short of statistical significance. The number of incidents of "other theft" was substantially lower for both groups but also did not reach threshold for statistical significance in either case.

The participation rate in all acquisitive crime, shoplifting, and burglary were significantly lower in both groups. The residential group also significantly reduced their participation rate robbery and fraud, whereas the reductions seen in the community group did not reach statistical significance. In all, the number of crimes was reduced to one-third of the pretreatment levels, and the participation rate was cut in half.

The researchers specifically looked at the 483 methadone-treated NTORS participants available for study at the 1-year outcome.[78] The investigators used cluster analysis using substance use outcomes and found that the methadone participants separated into four groups:

(1) Patients who dramatically reduced their use of opiates and benzodiazepines.
(2) Patients who dramatically reduced their opiate use but increased their illicit benzodiazepine use. (Of note, groups 1 and 2 were labeled "improved response" groups and accounted for 59% of the sample.)
(3) A "poor response" group (18% of the sample), that failed to show improvement over 1 year of treatment.
(4) A "low rate" group (22% of the sample), who used substances much less frequently than the other groups, and who significantly reduced their use of benzodiazepines at 1 year.

It was demonstrated that the levels of acquisitive crime and drug selling were significantly reduced at 1 year. The greatest reductions were found in group 1, and the smallest reductions were found in group 4. P values were not presented for specific within-group differences.

Although there was a 2-year follow-up analysis, crime data were not presented in the report.[79] Crime data were included in the 4- to 5-year follow-up data.[80] Of the original 1075 participants, 418 were available for follow-up at this interval. For the methadone clients, rates of acquisitive crime at 4- to 5-year follow-up were 23% of intake levels. Also, the methadone group's self-reported drug-selling was 17% of the intake level. Both findings were statistically significant. The residential group's level of acquisitive crimes was about 25% of their intake levels and their rate of drug selling was 36% of intake levels. Both of these findings were statistically significant. Participation rate data were not presented.

There are two main methodological limitations to the NTORS data:

(1) The design of the study does not allow for causal inference. There was no randomization to treatment groups and no control group. It is unclear if the reductions in crime are referable to receiving drug treatment, or if receiving drug treatment is indicative of a readiness to change a host of maladaptive behaviors.

(2) The high attrition in the study severely limits the conclusions that can be drawn. The researchers used logistic regression analysis to compare the characteristics of the drop-outs with those of the group available at 4 to 5 years and found them differing in only very few ways (none of which were crime-related). However, this result does not exclude the possibility that those who dropped out had more chaotic lifestyles, more ongoing drug use, or more criminal activity *after* receiving treatment. Given the large number of drop-outs (30% at 1 year and 61% at 4 to 5 years) it seems very possible that the findings regarding decreased crime could be nullified were these individuals available for study.

Last, although data on the frequency of crime commission was addressed, the team did not present the data regarding the rate of participation in crime at the 4- to 5-year follow-up. These data would be highly germane to the discussion of drug treatment as a turning point leading to desistance.

THE DRUG ABUSE TREATMENT OUTCOMES STUDY

In the United States a similar observational study to examine the effects of substance abuse treatment was undertaken.[81] The Drug Abuse Treatment Outcomes Study (DATOS) was a prospective cohort study of 10,010 clients entering treatment at 96 programs in 11 cities. The treatment modalities studied included

(1) Outpatient methadone maintenance
(2) Long-term residential
(3) Outpatient drug-free (ie, nonmethadone) clinics
(4) Short-term inpatient chemical dependence programs.

At study entry and at follow-up participants were interviewed regarding their drug use, mental health, physical heath, psychosocial difficulties, and criminal behavior.

A subset of 708 DATOS participants who were dependent on cocaine were followed up at 1 and 5 years after study entry.[82] The results showed that, compared with rates at study entry, significant reductions persisted in arrest rates and rates of illegal activity at the 5-year follow-up.

There was also an arm of DATOS that studied adolescents.[81] Participants were drawn from 30 programs in six cities and received treatment from long-term residential, short-term inpatient, or outpatient drug-free programs. An analysis was performed on the effects of drug treatment on criminal offending in this group.[83] In all, 1167 adolescents were enrolled into the program. Fifty-eight percent of participants were under criminal justice supervision (defined as being on probation, on parole, awaiting trial, or having been referred to treatment by the criminal justice system) at study entry whereas the remaining 42% were not. Of the 1167 subjects, 1004 (86%) participated in a follow-up interview at 12 months.

Differences between the criminal justice and noncriminal justice groups in terms of participation rates in the follow-up interview were not presented. However, the investigators used logistic regression to investigate differences between the criminal justice and noncriminal justice groups at study entry. They found that there were no differences between the two groups in terms of self-reported illegal activity or most measures of drug use prior to study entry. However, the criminal justice group was more likely than the noncriminal justice group to be young, male, nonwhite, from a single-parent or foster home, or conduct-disordered or to have had a history of suicidal thoughts or behavior.

Both groups showed significant reductions in any drug-related illegal activity at 1 year compared with study entry. However, the criminal justice group also showed significant reductions in drug-dealing arrests, property crime arrests, violent crime arrests, and any arrests, whereas the noncriminal justice group did not. Further analysis revealed that reductions in the use of alcohol and marijuana were independently associated with reductions in the likelihood of committing a crime.

There are three main limitations to this study:

(1) There is no random assignment, limiting any causal inferences from being made.
(2) There is no comparison group.
(3) The reliance on self-report data with respect to criminal activity may lead to underreporting of crime, especially by adolescents already in the kind of legal trouble that characterizes the "criminal justice" group.

DRUG COURTS

Drug courts have been in use in the United States since the late 1980s when they arose as a problem-solving measure to cope with the large number of drug-involved criminal offenders in the court system. Drug courts are specialized courts that offer drug-using offenders drug treatment and monitor their progress by regular appearances before a judge. Compliance and progress are facilitated by the application of sanctions and rewards. Sanctions are typically applied in a graduated fashion (ie, they become progressively more severe) and can include mandatory time spent watching court hearings, mandatory attendance at drug treatment for incarcerated offenders, and brief incarcerations. The rewards include avoiding incarceration, public praise and encouragement, and having one's current charge expunged from the record upon successful completion of the program.[61,84] Drug courts have become enormously popular. Out of the 3155 counties in the United States, 1416 have drug courts activity. In total, there are 2038 total drug courts in operation and another 226 are being planned.[85]

Four randomized, controlled studies of drug courts have been performed. The earliest of these was performed at the Maricopa County, Arizona, drug court.[86] In this study, 630 drug offenders were randomly assigned to either the drug court condition or to probation-as-usual and then followed for 1 year. There was no statistically significant difference between the rates of substance use or rearrest between the two groups.

Compared with those in the probation-as-usual condition, however, the drug court participants were significantly less likely to be sentenced to prison for new arrests (23% vs 9%, $P<.05$). Proponents of the drug court noted that the drug court did reduce workload, in that the probation-as-usual ran for 36 months whereas the drug court condition ran for 12 months. Even though the outcomes were no better, they were also no worse and achieved the same result in one-third of the time. This result taken with the evidence that drug court participants were significantly less likely to return to prison allowed proponents of the drug court to claim a qualified success.

A second early experiment evaluated the efficacy of the Superior Court Drug Intervention Program, a drug court program in Washington, DC.[87] In this study 1022 felony defendants were randomly assigned to one of three conditions: (1) weekly drug testing with judicial monitoring and the application of graduated sanctions, (2) intensive court-based drug treatment with weekly drug testing, (3) a standard docket.

Compared with the standard docket, both of the experimental conditions had significantly less drug use during pretrial release and were significantly more likely to test drug-free prior to sentencing. There were no differences in arrest rates between the three groups during the study. In the year following sentencing, the group assigned to graduated sanctions had a significantly lower arrest rate compared with the group assigned to the standard docket (19 vs 27%). This difference was largely accounted for by lower rates of drug-related offenses.

Another program evaluation that used an experimental methodology was the Baltimore City Drug Treatment Court.[88–91] In the Baltimore program, 235 participants were randomly assigned to a drug court condition that included intensive supervision, drug testing, drug treatment judicial monitoring, or a treatment-as-usual control group. At follow-up at 2 years, the drug court group had significantly less arrests (66.2% vs 81.3%, $P<.05$), fewer number of new arrests (1.6 vs 2.3, $P<.01$) and fewer new charges brought against them (3.1 vs 4.6, $P<.05$).[90]

More recently, a group published an experimental evaluation of the New South Wales Adult Drug Court.[92] In this study, 468 participants were randomized to either a drug court or to treatment as usual. This drug court included judicial monitoring and sanctions, random drug testing, and drug treatment (including pharmacotherapy when applicable).

Follow-up at 23 months showed that the drug court participants had significantly longer times to first shoplifting ($P = .016$) and drug offenses ($P = .005$). In addition, the drug court group had a lower rate of commission of drug-related offenses. Rates of other crimes were also lower, but none reached statistical significance.

In addition to these randomized, controlled trials, there have been a number of less methodologically rigorous studies of drug courts as well. Two systematic reviews have been performed that evaluate this data as well.[93,94] The authors conclude that there is support for the general efficacy of drug courts to reduce recidivism. Another review of the data on drug courts showed that these institutions are cost-effective.[95]

OTHER STUDIES

Another study performed by Washington State used public records of substance abuse treatment participation and arrest to examine the effect on receiving substance abuse treatment on the risk for criminal conviction.[96] For inclusion in this analysis participants had to (1) be eligible for Social Security Insurance benefits, (2) be in need of substance abuse treatment, (3) be between 18 and 64 years old, (4) have a record of arrest or conviction in the 24 months prior to either entering substance abuse treatment or being identified as needing such treatment, and (5) have survived the 1-year follow-up period. Rates of rearrest and reconviction were then calculated for the 1-year follow-up period.

In all, 8343 people met criteria for inclusion in the analysis. A total of 4341 of these people entered treatment, whereas 4002 people did not enter treatment. The group that did not receive treatment was more likely to be young and male. The two groups did not differ with respect to rates of criminal conviction in the 2 years leading up to the index event (76.9% for the treated group and 78.7% of the untreated group). No P values were presented for any of these demographic between group differences.

The results showed that, compared with people who primarily abused alcohol, people who identified cocaine, heroin, or amphetamine/methamphetamine as their primary substance of abuse were significantly more likely to be rearrested or convicted of a felony. Primarily using marijuana (as opposed to alcohol) was related to a significant reduction in the chance or reconviction for any offense. It was also found that being young, African American, and male corresponded to significantly increased risk of rearrest and reconviction.

Further, it was demonstrated that completing substance abuse treatment (or remaining in treatment at least 90 days) significantly reduced the likelihood of arrests and convictions during the follow-up period. Remaining in treatment for more than 90 days was associated with a significant reduction in the hazard of rearrest by 30% and of conviction of any offense by 27%. However, no effect was found for felony convictions.

There are two main limitations to this study:

(1) There was no random assignment into the two groups. The group that declined treatment was more likely to be young and male, two factors that were found to increase the chances of rearrest and reconviction in the follow-up period. It is also possible that people entering into substance abuse treatment were more willing to make substantial changes in many aspects of their behavior compared with those who chose not to enter treatment.

(2) The reliance on official records of arrest and conviction may seriously underestimate the true level of criminal activity in a population.

Finally, a recent study performed trajectory analysis to study the relationship between drug use, crime, and treatment outcomes.[97] Here the researchers analyzed data obtained from 792 men from three separate studies of drug treatment. By applying growth mixture models to the number of days of drug use and the number of months of incarceration during the 5 years prior to the first treatment, the researchers identified four separate groups:

(1) High incarceration–high drug use
(2) High incarceration–low drug use
(3) Low incarceration–high drug use
(4) Low incarceration–low drug use.

They then used the 5-year follow-up data from the studies to investigate the effect of treatment on the trajectory of the drug use and criminal behavior of the four groups.

The researchers found that although the high drug–use groups maintained higher levels of drug use than the low-use groups, the overall drug use decreased over time. They also found that after treatment, incarceration decreased steadily for the high-incarceration groups, but not for the low-incarceration groups. Although they found that pretreatment drug use was not a significant predictor of posttreatment incarceration, they found "some indication that a high level of pretreatment drug use increases the risk of later incarceration, at least among those with a low incarceration history."

A significant limitation of this study is its reliance on "incarceration" as a proxy for criminal behavior. Although incarceration is a highly relevant end point, it depends on successful detection, apprehension, prosecution, and sentencing. As such, a huge volume of potential crime will be undetected in this sample. Also, the study did not measure other potential life changes in the 5 years after treatment (eg, marriage, military service). The researchers are appropriately mindful of these limitations when they conclude: "The results indicate a modest effect of treatment on subsequent behavior and suggest the need for research on criminal careers to include the influence of social interventions when accounting for long-term patterns of deviant behavior such as drug use and crime."

In total, there is a great deal of data supporting the contention that addiction treatment can be associated with meaningful reductions in criminal activity. Because of the lack of studies involving random assignment into drug treatment in the treatment services research, a solid case for a causal relationship existing between drug treatment and desistance cannot be made.

The Swedish National Council on Crime Prevention recently undertook a metaanalytic review of various studies of how drug treatment can reduce crime.[98] The main finding of the statistical review was that drug treatment resulted in a relative reduction in crime of around 26%. The program types with the largest reductions in crime were therapeutic communities and community supervision, which reduced crime 51% and 47%, respectively.

SUMMARY

The available evidence suggests that drug treatment can lead to modest, but real, reductions in criminal offending for drug-using criminal offenders. Considering the scope of the problem of drug-related crime and the expense of dealing with these issues, even marginal improvements can lead to important aggregate savings in both economic and humanitarian terms. More randomized, controlled trials of drug treatment in criminal justice programs will lead to a more sophisticated understanding of what kind of treatment works best for this group.

REFERENCES

1. Substance Abuse and Mental Health Services Administration. Results from the 2007 National Survey on Drug Use and Health: national findings [NSDUH Series H-34, DHHS Publication No. SMA 08-4343]. Rockville (MD): Department of Health and Human Services; 2008.
2. Grant BF. Prevalence and correlates of drug use and DSM-IV drug dependence in the United States: results of the National Longitudinal Alcohol Epidemiologic Survey. J Subst Abuse 1996;8:195–210.
3. Office of National Drug Control Policy. The economic costs of drug abuse in the United States 1992–2002. Washington, DC: Office of National Drug Control Policy Executive Office of the President; 2004.
4. Healey A, Knapp M, Astin J, et al. Economic burden of drug dependency. Social costs incurred by drug users at intake to the National Treatment Outcome Research Study. Br J Psychiatry 1998;173:160–5.
5. Federal Bureau of Investigation. Uniform Crime Report 2007. Washington, DC: Department of Justice; 2008.
6. National Center on Addiction and Substance Abuse. Behind bars: substance abuse and America's prison population, vol. 1. New York: Columbia University; 1998.
7. MacCoun RJ, Reuter P. Drug war heresies: learning from other vices, times and places. New York: Cambridge University Press; 2001.
8. Federal Bureau of Prisons. Quick facts about the Bureau of Prisons. Washington, DC: Department of Justice; 2009.
9. Bureau of Justice Statistics. Drug use and dependence, state and federal prisoners, 2004 [NCJ 213530]. Washington, DC: Department of Justice; 2006.
10. Bureau of Justice Statistics. Substance dependence, abuse, and treatment of jail inmates, 2002 [NCJ 209588]. Washington, DC: Department of Justice; 2005.
11. Miller TR, Levy DT, Cohen MA, et al. Costs of alcohol and drug-involved crime. Prev Sci 2006;7:333–42.
12. Bureau of Justice Statistics. Substance abuse and treatment, state and federal prisoners, 1997 [NCJ 172871]. Washington, DC: Department of Justice; 1999.
13. Bureau of Justice Statistics Substance abuse and treatment of adults on probation, 1995 [NCJ 166611]. Washington, DC: Department of Justice; 1998.
14. Bureau of Justice Statistics. Mental health and treatment of inmates and probationers [NCJ 174463]. Washington, DC: Department of Justice; 1999.
15. Kleiman Mark AR. Coerced abstinence: a neo-paternalist drug policy initiative. Washington, DC: Brookings Institute Press; 1997.

16. Kleiman Mark AR. Controlling drug use and crime among drug-involved offenders: testing, sanctions and treatment. In: Heymann PH, Brownsberger WN, editors. Drug addiction and drug policy. Cambridge (MA): Harvard University Press; 2001. p. 168–92.

17. Petersilia J, Turner S. Intensive probation and parole. Crime and Justice 1993;17: 281–335.

18. Harrison LD. The revolving prison door for drug-involved offenders: challenges and opportunities. Crime and Delinquency 2001;47(3):462–85.

19. Ball JC, Nurco DN. Criminality during the life course of heroin addiction. NIDA Res Monogr 1984;49:305–12.

20. Ball JC, Shaffer JW, Nurco DN. (1983). The day-to-day criminality of heroin addicts in Baltimore–a study in the continuity of offence rates. Drug Alcohol Depend 1983;12(2):119–42.

21. Nurco DN, Ball JC, Shaffer JW, et al. The criminality of narcotic addicts. J Nerv Ment Dis 1985;173(2):94–102.

22. Nurco DN, Cisin IH, Ball JC. Crime as a source of income for narcotic addicts. J Subst Abuse Treatment 1985;2(2):113–5.

23. Nurco DN, Shaffer JW, Ball JC, et al. Trends in the commission of crime among narcotic addicts over successive periods of addiction and nonaddiction. Am J Drug Alcohol Abuse 1984;10(4):481–9.

24. Nurco DN, Shaffer JW, Ball JC, et al. A comparison by ethnic group and city of the criminal activities of narcotic addicts. J Nerv Ment Dis 1986;174(2):112–6.

25. Bureau of Justice Statistics. Substance dependence, abuse, and treatment of jail inmates, 2002 [NCJ 209588]. Washington, DC: Department of Justice; 2005.

26. Office of National Drug Control Policy. Drug-related crime. Washington, DC: Office of National Drug Control Policy Executive Office of the President; 2000.

27. Cornish JW, Metzger D, Woody GE, et al. Naltrexone pharmacotherapy for opioid dependent federal probationers. J Subst Abuse Treatment 1997;14(6):529–34.

28. Goldberg SR, Stolerman IP. Drugs as reinforcers: studies in laboratory animals. In: Goldberg SR, Stolerman IP, editors. Behavioral analysis of drug dependence. New York: Academic Press, Inc; 1986. p. 1–9.

29. Carroll ME, Lac ST. Autoshaping i.v. cocaine self-administration in rats: effects of nondrug alternative reinforcers on acquisition. Psychopharmacology 1993;110(1–2):5–12.

30. Campbell UC, Thompson SS, Carroll ME. Acquisition of oral phencyclidine (PCP) self-administration in rhesus monkeys: effects of dose and an alternative non-drug reinforcer. Psychopharmacology 1998;137(2):132–8.

31. Evans SM, Nasser J, Comer SD, et al. Smoked heroin in rhesus monkeys: effects of heroin extinction and fluid availability on measures of heroin seeking. Pharmacol Biochem Behav 2003;74(3):723–37.

32. Foltin RW. Food and cocaine self-administration by baboons: effects of alternatives. J Exp Anal Behav 1999;72(2):215–34.

33. Comer SD, Collins ED, Fischman MW. Choice between money and intranasal heroin in morphine-maintained humans. Behav Pharmacol 1997;8(8):677–90.

34. Donny EC, Bigelow GE, Walsh SL. Choosing to take cocaine in the human laboratory: effects of cocaine dose, inter-choice interval, and magnitude of alternative reinforcement. Drug Alcohol Depend 2003;69(3):289–301.

35. Donny EC, Bigelow GE, Walsh SL. Assessing the initiation of cocaine self-administration in humans during abstinence: effects of dose, alternative reinforcement, and priming. Psychopharmacology 2004;172(3):316–23.

36. Hart CL, Haney M, Foltin RW, et al. Alternative reinforcers differentially modify cocaine self-administration by humans. Behav Pharmacol 2000;11(1):87–91.

37. Higgins ST. The influence of alternative reinforcers on cocaine use and abuse: a brief review. Pharmacol Biochem Behav 1997;57(3):419–27.
38. Higgins ST, Bickel WK, Hughes JR. Influence of an alternative reinforcer on human cocaine self-administration. Life Sciences 1994;55(3):179–87.
39. Schuster CR. Implications of laboratory research for the treatment of drug dependence. In: Goldberg SR, Stolerman IP, editors. Behavioral analysis of drug dependence. New York: Academic Press, Inc; 1986. p. 357–85.
40. Grove RN, Schuster CR. Suppression of cocaine self-administration by extinction and punishment. Pharmacol Biochem Behav 1974;2(2):199–208.
41. Johanson CE. The effects of electric shock on responding maintained by cocaine injections in a choice procedure in the rhesus monkey. Psychopharmacology 1977; 53(3):277–82.
42. Negus SS. Effects of punishment on choice between cocaine and food in rhesus monkeys. Psychopharmacology 2005;181(2):244–52.
43. Poling A, Thompson T. Attenuation of ethanol intake by contingent punishment of food-maintained responding. Pharmacol Biochem Behav 1977;7(4):393–9.
44. Poling A, Thompson T. Effects of delaying food availability contingent on ethanol-maintained lever pressing. Psychopharmacology 1977;51(3):289–91.
45. Nader MA, Morgan D. Effects of negative punishment contingencies on cocaine self-administration by rhesus monkeys. Behav Pharmacol 2001;12(2):91–9.
46. Griffith JD, Rowan-Szal GA, Roark RR, et al. Contingency management in outpatient methadone treatment: a meta-analysis. Drug Alcohol Depend 2000;58(1-2):55–66.
47. Budney AJ, Higgins ST, Delaney DD, et al. Contingent reinforcement of abstinence with individuals abusing cocaine and marijuana. J Appl Behav Anal 1991;24(4):657–65.
48. Budney AJ, Higgins ST, Radonovich KJ, et al. Adding voucher-based incentives to coping skills and motivational enhancement improves outcomes during treatment for marijuana dependence. J Consult Clin Psychol 2000;68(6):1051–61.
49. Higgins ST, Budney AJ, Bickel WK, et al. Incentives improve outcome in outpatient behavioral treatment of cocaine dependence. Arch Gen Psychiatry 1994;51(7):568–76.
50. Piotrowski NA, Tusel DJ, Sees KL, et al. Contingency contracting with monetary reinforcers for abstinence from multiple drugs in a methadone program. Exp Clin Psychopharmacol 1999;7(4):399–411.
51. Nightingale SL, Michaux WW, Platt PC. Clinical implications of urine surveillance in a methadone maintenance program. Int J Addict 1972;7(3):403–14.
52. Anker AL, Crowley TJ. Use of contingency contracts in specialty clinics for cocaine abuse. NIDA Res Monogr 1982;41:452–9.
53. Crowley TJ. Contingency contracting treatment of drug-abusing physicians, nurses, and dentists. NIDA Res Monogr 1984;46:68–83.
54. Dolan MP, Black JL, Penk WE, et al. Contracting for treatment termination to reduce illicit drug use among methadone maintenance treatment failures. J Consult Clin Psychol 1985;53(4):549–51.
55. McCarthy JJ, Borders OT. Limit setting on drug abuse in methadone maintenance patients. Am J Psychiatry 1985;142(12):1419–23.
56. Iguchi MY, Stitzer ML, Bigelow GE, et al. Contingency management in methadone maintenance: effects of reinforcing and aversive consequences on illicit polydrug use. Drug Alcohol Depend 1988;22(1–2):1–7.
57. Stitzer ML, Bickel WK, Bigelow GE, et al. Effect of methadone dose contingencies on urinalysis test results of polydrug-abusing methadone-maintenance patients. Drug Alcohol Depend 1986;18(4):341–8.

58. Wong CJ, Dillon EM, Sylvest CE, et al. Contingency management of reliable attendance of chronically unemployed substance abusers in a therapeutic workplace. Exp Clin Psychopharmacol 2004;12(1):39–46.

59. Wong CJ, Dillon EM, Sylvest C, et al. Evaluation of a modified contingency management intervention for consistent attendance in therapeutic workplace participants. Drug Alcohol Depend 2004;74(3):319–23.

60. Roll JM, Prendergast ML, Sorensen K, et al. A comparison of voucher exchanges between criminal justice involved and noninvolved participants enrolled in voucher-based contingency management drug abuse treatment programs. Am J Drug Alcohol Abuse 2005;31(3):393–401.

61. Burdon WM, Roll JM, Prendergast ML, et al. Drug courts and contingency management. J Drug Issues 2001;31(1):73–90.

62. Vaillant GE. A twelve-year follow-up of New York narcotic addicts: IV. Some characteristics and determinants of abstinence. Am J Psychiatry 1966;123(5):573–85.

63. Higgins ST, Badger GJ, Budney AJ. Initial abstinence and success in achieving longer term cocaine abstinence. Exp Clin Psychopharmacol 2000;8(3):377–86.

64. Petry NM, Simcic F Jr. Recent advances in the dissemination of contingency management techniques: clinical and research perspectives. J Subst Abuse Treatment 2002;23(2):81–6.

65. Taxman FS. Graduated sanctions: stepping into accountable systems and offenders. Prison Journal 1999;79(2):182–205.

66. Harrell A, Roman J, Bhati A, et al. The impact evaluation of the Maryland Break the Cycle initiative. Washington, DC: Urban Institute Justice Policy Center; 2003.

67. Nace EP, Birkmayer F, Sullivan MA, et al. Socially sanctioned coercion mechanisms for addiction treatment. Am J Addict 2007;16:15–23.

68. Sullivan MA, Birkmayer F, Boyarsky BK, et al. Uses of coercion in addiction treatment: clinical aspects. Am J Addict 2008;17(1):36–47.

69. National Institute on Drug Abuse. Principles of drug addiction treatment: a research-based guide. 2nd edition. Rockville (MD): National Institute on Drug Abuse; 2009.

70. Anglin MD, Prendergast M, Farabee D. The effectiveness of coerced treatment for drug-abusing offenders. Presented at the Office of National Drug Control Policy's Conference of Scholars and Policy Makers. Washington, DC, March 23–25, 1998.

71. Anglin MD, Hser YI. Criminal justice and the drug-abusing offender: policy issues of coerced treatment. Behav Sci Law 1991;9:243–67.

72. Bell J, Hall W, Byth K. Changes in criminal activity after entering methadone maintenance. Br J Addict 1992;87:251–8.

73. Hall W, Bell J, Carless J. Crime and drug use among applicants for methadone maintenance. Drug Alcohol Depend 1993;31:123–9.

74. Bell J, Mattick R, Hay A, et al. Methadone maintenance and drug-related crime. J Subst Abuse 1997;9:15–25.

75. Crowley TJ, Mikulich SK, MacDonald M, et al. Substance-dependent, conduct-disordered adolescent males: severity of diagnosis predicts 2-year outcome. Drug Alcohol Depend 1998;49:225–37.

76. Gossop M, Marsden J, Stewart D, et al. Substance use, health and social problems of service users at 54 treatment agencies. Intake data from the National Treatment Outcome Research Study. Br J Psychiatry 1998;173:166–71.

77. Gossop M, Marsden J, Stewart D, et al. Reductions in acquisitive crime and drug use after treatment of addiction problems: 1-year follow-up outcomes. Drug Alcohol Depend 2000;58(1–2):165–72.

78. Gossop M, Marsden J, Stewart D, et al. Patterns of improvement after methadone treatment: 1 year follow-up results from the National Treatment Outcome Research Study. Drug Alcohol Depend 2000;60(3):275–86.

79. Gossop M, Marsden J, Stewart D, et al. Change and stability of change after treatment of drug misuse: 2-year outcomes from the National Treatment Outcome Research Study (UK). Addict Behav 2002;27(2):155–66.

80. Gossop M, Marsden J, Stewart D, et al. The National Treatment Outcome Research Study (NTORS): 4-5 year follow-up results. Addiction 2003;98:291–303.

81. Flynn PM, Craddock G, Hubbard RL, et al. Methodological overview and research design for the Drug Abuse Treatment Outcome Study (DATOS). Psychol Addict Behav 1997;11(4):230–43.

82. Simpson DD, Joe GW, Broome KM. A national 5-year follow-up of treatment outcomes for cocaine dependence. Arch Gen Psychiatry 2002;59:538–44.

83. Farabee D, Shen H, Hser YI, et al. The effect of drug treatment on criminal behavior among adolescents in DATOS-A. J Adolesc Res 2001;16(6):679–96.

84. Ritvo JI, Kirk GL. Community-based treatment. In: Galanter M, Kleber HD, editors. Textbook of substance abuse treatment. 3rd edition. Washington, DC: American Psychiatric Press, Inc; 2004. p. 475–585.

85. Bureau of Justice Assistance, Office of Justice Programs, and US Department of Justice, editors. BJA Drug Court Clearinghouse Project: summary of drug court activity by state and county. Washington, DC: American University; 2009.

86. Deschenes EP, Turner S, Greenwood PW. Drug court or probation: an experimental evaluation of Maricopa County drug court. Justice System Journal 1995;18:55–73.

87. Harrell A, Cavanagh S, Roman J. Final report: findings from the evaluation of the Superior Court Drug Intervention Program. Washington, DC: Urban Institute; 1998.

88. Gottfredson DC, Exum M.L.The Baltimore City drug treatment court: one-year results from a randomized study. Journal of Research in Crime and Delinquency 2002;39(3):337–56.

89. Gottfredson DC, Kearley BW, Najaka SS, et al. The Baltimore City drug treatment court: 3-year self-report outcome study. Eval Rev 2005;29(1):42–64.

90. Gottfredson DC, Najaka SS, Kearley B. Effectiveness of drug treatment courts: evidence from a randomized trial. Criminology and Public Policy 2003;2(2):171–96.

91. Gottfredson DC, Najaka SS, Kearley BW, et al. Long-term effects of participation in the Baltimore City drug treatment court: results from an experimental study. Journal of Experimental Criminology 2006;2:67–98.

92. Shanahan M, Lanscar E, Haas M, et al. Cost-effectiveness of the New South Wales adult drug court program. Eval Rev 2004;28(1):3–27.

93. Belenko S. Research on drug courts: a critical review 2001 update. National Drug Court Institute Review 2001;4:1–60.

94. Wilson DB, Mitchell O, Mackenzie DL. A systematic review of drug court effects on recidivism. Journal of Experimental Criminology 2006;2:459–87.

95. United States General Accountability Office. Report to congressional committees. Adult drug courts: evidence indicates recidivism reductions and mixed effects for other outcomes [GAO-05-219]. Washington, DC: General Accountability Office; 2005.

96. Luchansky B, Nordlund D, Estee S, et al. Substance abuse treatment and criminal justice involvement for SSI recipients: results from Washington State. Am J Addict 2006;15:370–9.

97. Prendergast M, Huang D, Hser YI. Patterns of crime and drug use trajectories in relation to treatment initiation and 5-year outcomes. Eval Rev 2008;32(1):59–82.

98. Holloway K, Bennett TH, Farrington DP. Effectiveness of treatment in reducing drug-related crime. Stockholm (Sweden): Swedish National Council for Crime Prevention; 2008.

Managing Co-Occurring Substance Use and Pain Disorders

Karen Miotto, MD*, Aaron Kaufman, MD, Alexander Kong,
Grace Jun, Jeffrey Schwartz, MD

KEYWORDS

- Psychiatric assessment • Chronic pain • Opioid addiction

KEY POINTS

- Chronic pain is one of the most common complaints in psychiatric and primary care settings—lower back pain, headaches, and neck pain are the most common pain reports.
- Pain can impair social and occupational functioning.
- Increased use of opioids for pain has helped many people but has also promoted an increase in opioid misuse, addiction, overdose, and diversion of medication for illegitimate uses.
- Taking extra time in the initial psychiatric assessment and gathering collateral information will help determine the appropriate treatment setting and consultations required or comanagement from mental health, addiction, or pain specialists.

Over the past 2 decades, prescription drug emergencies and fatalities have reached an epidemic level. A confluence of medical, regulatory, economic, and pharmaceutical industry–driven factors contributed to the expansion of opioid treatment for nonmalignant pain, which parallels the increase of nonmedical use and opioid addiction. Opioid-based treatments were proved beneficial for acute and cancer pain, and health care providers were encouraged to apply these same principles to the treatment of chronic nonmalignant pain. However, chronic pain often has complex causes exacerbated by comorbid psychiatric conditions and stressful life events. The unfortunate lessons learned from the effort to improve pain treatment are that the potential for misuse and addiction with long-term opioid exposure is elevated in vulnerable individuals.

PAIN CLASSIFICATIONS

Chronic pain is one of the most common complaints in psychiatric and primary care settings. As of 2011, at least 116 million adult Americans reported common chronic

Department of Psychiatry and Biobehavioral Sciences, University of California, Los Angeles, 760 Westwood Plaza, Mail Code 175919, Los Angeles, CA 90095-1563, USA
* Corresponding author.
E-mail address: kmiotto@mednet.ucla.edu

Psychiatr Clin N Am 35 (2012) 393–409
http://dx.doi.org/10.1016/j.psc.2012.03.006
0193-953X/12/$ – see front matter © 2012 Elsevier Inc. All rights reserved.

psych.theclinics.com

pain conditions.[1] Pain impacts an individual's quality of life and often impairs social and occupational functioning. Lower back pain, followed by headaches and neck pain, seem to be the most common pain disorders.[2]

Pain classifications are based on several criteria. Two of the main categories are

1. Neuropathic pain
2. Nociceptive pain.

Neuropathic pain is caused by nerve damage, whereas nociceptive pain is caused by nonneural tissue damage. Pain is also commonly classified based on the type of tissue involved, such as musculoskeletal pain. Additionally, certain types of pain are classified by their associated syndromes, such as myofascial pain syndrome or fibromyalgia. These classifications are important in guiding treatment because certain types of pain respond better to a particular intervention. The definition of pain by the International Association for the Study of Pain is multifaceted and encompasses the complexity behind the condition. "Pain is an unpleasant sensory and emotional experience associated with actual or potential tissue damage, or described in terms of such damage."[3]

Another category of pain familiar to psychiatrists is psychogenic, or somatoform, pain. The term *somatoform disorder* is currently used by the Diagnostic and Statistical Manual of Mental Disorders (DSM-IV).[4] Medical schools historically taught that there is a difference between real and psychogenic pain. However, with the increasing recognition that psychological factors alter biological functions, it became apparent that the term *psychogenic* did not contribute to an understanding of the multidimensional nature of pain. A pain disorder is classified as a mental disorder when psychological factors play an important role in the onset, severity, exacerbation, or perpetuation of the pain. This perspective serves to improve the physician-patient relationship because patients often find the experience of having clinicians question the authenticity of their pain as devastating as the pain itself.[5] The fact that patients with somatoform disorders commonly attempt to treat their pain with alcohol or other drugs further complicates this issue.

PSYCHIATRIC EVALUATION OF PAIN AND ADDICTION

All types of chronic pain are multifactorial conditions with biopsychosocial components, and psychiatrists are well-suited to evaluate the interplay of the biological, psychological, and social factors. Because pain is pervasive, the settings in which a psychiatrist evaluates the patient are diverse and may include consultation-liaison services, specialized pain clinics, and inpatient or outpatient psychiatric settings. The American Board of Psychiatry and Neurology offers a subspecialty certification in pain management, which is intended for those who have an extensive pain practice. Psychiatric evaluation and management are often requested for individuals with complaints of pain that are greater than would be expected for the given condition and for patients with psychiatric or substance use–related comorbidity. Evaluations are also requested for patients who demand medication not deemed appropriate or who have a poor response to treatment. Patients who fit these descriptions raise concerns about the psychosocial factors contributing to pain, treatment compliance, and the potential for pain medication misuse, addiction, or malingering.[6]

Psychiatrists skilled in addiction evaluation and treatment are frequently referred pain patients who are believed to have aberrant medication use behaviors or frank addiction. There are several routes to acquiring these skills or gaining specialization in addiction, such as obtaining certification offered by the American Board of Psychiatry and Neurology[7] or by the American Board of Addiction Medicine.[7] Many psychiatrists who work in addiction treatment programs have acquired on-the-job training by caring for patients who are in pain and suffering from opioid addictions. They have also advanced their skills by participating in the growing number of continuing medical education courses in this critical area.

DIAGNOSIS OF PAIN AND ADDICTION

The main DSM-IV criteria for opioid dependence are directly related to the physiologic response to sustained opioid treatment, including[4]

- Tolerance
- Physical dependence
- Withdrawal.

This terminology has led to confusion when assessing addiction in patients maintained on opioid analgesics. The limitations of the DSM-IV criteria in this population have been recognized, and other proposed characteristics include

- Preoccupation with obtaining prescription opioids for other than analgesic use
- Loss of control over use
- Presence of adverse consequences related to use.

Typical indicators of aberrant medication use or addiction in this population are described as drug-seeking behaviors, which include

- Obtaining medication from multiple unsanctioned sources
- Repeated requests for early refills
- Frequent requests to have lost prescriptions replaced.

Behaviors more telling of addiction are using medication by alternative routes of administration such as injecting oral medication and engaging in prescription theft and forgery.

Physical dependence and withdrawal syndromes are not diagnostic for opioid addiction, and in fact, certain types of drug seeking behaviors in response to undertreated pain are frequently described in the pain literature as pseudoaddiction.[8] The possibility of pseudoaddiction has created a dilemma for the clinician, who must consider: "Is the observed behavior due to inadequate pain control or is it a manifestation of addiction?"[9] There are at least two problems with the concept of pseudoaddiction:

1. It assumes that a patient has either addiction or pain, but not both.
2. It suggests that clinicians will be able to reliably discern between addiction and undertreated pain by increasing the dose of opioid analgesics.

The medical, ethical, and legal questions in treating chronic pain with opioids are complex and create the central fear of health care providers: Can I safely treat this patient's pain with opioids?

THE EXPANSION OF PRESCRIPTION OPIOID USAGE

A public health campaign 2 decades ago to educate physicians and consumers about the undertreatment of pain led to the dramatic expansion of opioid use for chronic pain. There was an exponential increase in opioid sales between 1997 and 2008, with over 1 million providers (approximately 40% of whom were primary care providers, including osteopaths and internists) prescribing controlled substances for pain.[10] This expansion resulted from a confluence of medical, regulatory, economic, and pharmaceutical industry–driven factors.[11] Opioid-based treatments had been proved effective and beneficial for acute and cancer pain, and health care providers were encouraged to apply these same principles to the treatment of chronic noncancerous pain. These principles assumed the somatic origins of pain and the authenticity of the patient's report of pain.

Sustained opioid treatment was assumed to be relatively safe. The side effects including constipation, nausea and vomiting, urinary retention, pruritus, myoclonus, and respiratory depression were considered manageable by most clinicians. The long-term side effects that were less appreciated by nonpalliative care providers were analgesic tolerance, opioid-induced abnormal pain sensitivity or hyperalgesia, and hormonal imbalance.[12,13] Respiratory depression was well-known as a leading cause of opioid-related death, but the existing literature described its role mainly in compromised cancer patients and heroin users.

LESSONS IN THE MANAGEMENT OF CHRONIC PAIN WITH OPIOIDS

It has become clear in the treatment of chronic nonmalignant pain that comfort alone is not an acceptable treatment goal, because opioid use in some individuals can foster incapacity and a greater risk of accidents and injury. More recent trainings encourage physicians to think about the risk-benefit framework and assess for potential benefits: What is the person's current function? What can the person be expected to do with opioid treatment that he or she cannot do now? The pneumonic SMART is used in the Oregon Health and Science guidelines; set **S**pecific, **M**easurable, **A**ction-oriented, **R**ealistic, **T**ime-dependent goals for opioid treatment. Time-dependent goals allow for the use of opioids as a "test," not a commitment to indefinite opioid prescription refills.[14]

The increased use of opioids for the treatment of chronic pain occurred without adequate prospective studies concerning the long-term risks or optimal structure of treatment.[12] The unfortunate lesson learned from the effort to improve pain treatment is that the potential for opioid misuse and addiction is high in vulnerable individuals. Chronic pain has no discernable end point; therefore, long-term strategies are essential. However, lifestyle modifications such as weight loss and exercise may actually be hindered by opioid treatment in at-risk individuals. The experience of chronic pain is subjective and strongly influenced by personal and situational judgments and can be exacerbated by stress and psychological suffering. Chronic opioid use can alter a person's stress response system, and an individual with psychiatric comorbidities may become reliant on opioids to cope with negative affective states. The increased use of opioids for pain has helped many people but also promoted an increase in opioid misuse, addiction, overdose, and diversion of medication for illegitimate uses.

During the past 20 years, the pharmaceutical industry increased the treatment options from small doses of opioids compounded with acetaminophen or a nonsteroidal antiinflammatory drug (NSAID) to include a number of high-potency immediate-release and extended-release monoproduct formulations. The daily opioid doses of the new formulations such as extended-release oxycodone and fentanyl preparations were not limited by the acetaminophen toxicity warnings, which were to not to exceed 4 grams per day. In fact, there were guidelines suggesting that extremely high-dose opioids may be required for analgesic efficacy in some individuals.[15] In step with the new opioid formulations came recommendations for around-the-clock dosing, as opposed to as-needed dosing, because it was assumed that this strategy would reduce preoccupation with the medication. However, there is no evidence that around-the-clock dosing for noncancerous pain provides more consistent pain relief or decreases the risk of tolerance or addiction.[15]

Sustained opioid exposure can also lead to the development of analgesic tolerance and opioid-induced hyperalgesia, as mentioned. Tolerance and opioid-induced hyperalgesia may result in a similar call for dose escalation. However, with opioid-induced hyperalgesia, the abnormal pain sensitivity may occur even in regions unaffected by the initial pain complaint. This sensitivity can lead to cycles of dose escalation and increasing analgesic tolerance, both of which may unwittingly improve only after opioid taper or detoxification.[16]

With the expansion of long-term opioid treatment, heath care providers were not aware of the interaction of positive and negative reinforcement, in particular the power of opioid withdrawal discomfort in perpetuating medication use even if the pain diminishes.[14] Some patients request opioid dose escalations because of a lack of awareness of withdrawal discomfort. Aches and pain in the morning before a patient's opioid dose are misinterpreted as an exacerbation in the underlying painful condition, which leads to a request for an increase in medication. Some patients would achieve amelioration of their pain and attempt to stop their medication only to find that their withdrawal symptoms were incapacitating. In general, there was a misperception that the physical dependence could only develop after a long duration of high-dose use.[17,18] Many health care providers were unfamiliar with the phenomenon of therapeutic dose withdrawal, much less treatments for opioid withdrawal. Often, providers felt their only option was to refer the treatment of opioid withdrawal to detoxification centers. Advancements in chronic pain treatment guidelines recommend educating patients and providers about the signs, symptoms, and treatment of opioid withdrawal, as well as taking precautions by developing an exit strategy before treatment initiation.[15]

THE SCOPE OF THE PROBLEMS RELATED TO OPIOID USE

The scope of opioid use problems varies by age and the target population but has an impact on two groups:

1. Opioid-treated patients
2. Those who are at risk because of the increased acceptability and availability.

In terms of general population risk, the data from the 2010 National Survey on Drug Use and Health, released annually by the Substance Abuse and Mental Health Services Administration (SAMHSA), reported nonmedical use of opioid pain relievers in approximately 2.7% of the population, whereas 8.9% or 22.6 million Americans aged 12 or older reported current use of illicit drugs. Young adults reported the highest rate of usage of nonmedical prescription drugs at 5.9%. The rates of nonmedical opioid use have not significantly increased for the past decade, suggesting that the opioid epidemic is not a consequence of the expansion in the rate of use, but instead it is an epidemic of prescription drug emergencies and fatalities. For example, the number of emergency department (ED) visits for opioid-related problems has increased by 236%.[19] The number of drug-related unintentional overdoses has also rapidly increased; in fact, drug-related deaths exceeded motor vehicle accidents in 2009.[20] Along with the increase in the number of ED visits, unintentional overdoses, and treatment admissions, there has been significant elevation in the risk of traumatic injury, accidents in the work force, crime-related violence, and suicides related to prescription opioid use.

Prescription opioid dependence is a leading cause of admission to addiction treatment programs. A new SAMHSA report of the Treatment Episode Data Set shows that, whereas the overall rate of substance abuse treatment admissions among those aged 12 and older in the United States has remained nearly the same from 1999 to 2009, there has been a dramatic rise (430%) in the rate of treatment admissions for the abuse of prescription pain relievers. The rate of treatment admissions primarily linked to these drugs rose from 10 per 100,000 in the population in 1999 to 53 per 100,000 in the population in 2009.[21] Individuals in treatment describe multiple points in the supply chain as sources of medication, including doctor-shopping, supplies from family members or friends, nonmedical purchases, Internet purchases, unwitting or dishonest doctors, fraudulent pharmacists, or larger scale diversion from distributions centers.

In the chronic opioid-treated population, a recent metaanalysis by Martell and colleagues[22] on the opioid treatment for chronic back pain identified aberrant opioid use behaviors in 5% to 24% of the sample, whereas estimates of opioid addiction vary between 3% and 26% depending on the population studied.[23–26] Current literature suggests that the main risk factors for drug use disorders in the general population also apply to prescription drug use disorders, such as

- Lifetime history of substance use disorder[27]
- Family history of substance abuse
- History of legal problems[28]
- Heavy tobacco use[29]
- History of significant depression and anxiety.[30]

Analysis of large samples of insurance claims data by Edlund and colleagues[31] attempted to identify risk factors before initiation of opioid treatment, and they found an especially large risk for individuals under age 50 years. Pretreatment mental health and substance use disorders, as well as sedative-hypnotic use, were also identified as strong predictors of abuse.[31] Risk factors for addiction that were identified after opioid treatment was initiated include a larger number of days' medication supplied at once and a large daily dose of schedule II opioids, with large dose defined by the Washington State Opioid Dosing Guidelines as greater that 120 mg of morphine equivalents per day.[32]

PSYCHIATRIC ASSESSMENT

A comprehensive biopsychosocial assessment is essential, regardless of whether the role of the psychiatrist is to evaluate the patient prior to initiating or after initiating opioids or to manage a comorbid condition. The initial assessment can identify the extent of the pain and complex comorbid conditions. Taking extra time in the initial assessment and gathering collateral information will help determine the appropriate treatment setting, consultations required, or comanagement from mental health, addiction, or pain specialists. Essential questions to guide the interview are included in **Box 1**.[33–35] The domains of the interview include information about the painful condition, opioid and substance use patterns, social and family factors, and the psychiatric history.[36]

The biopsychosocial assessment includes questions about a history of childhood trauma or abuse. A patient's experience and definitions of pain are a function of childhood, familial, and historical influences. The sexual or physical violation of a child or adolescent has far-reaching effects. It is a well-known risk factor for both chronic pain syndromes and addiction. Addressing a history of childhood trauma with coordinated care from mental health and pain providers can improve the symptoms of pain and the outcome of opioid treatment.[37,38]

Box 1
Prescription drug use questionnaire 3

Yes/No Evaluation of the Pain Condition
1. Does the patient have more than one painful condition (ie, chronic back pain complicated by acute migraines or frequent dental work)?
2. Is the patient disabled by pain (ie, unable to complete social or vocational activities of daily living)?
3. Is the patient receiving disability (ie, SSI, worker' compensation)?
4. Is the patient involved in litigation around the pain-precipitating incident?
5. Has the patient explored and/or tried nonopioid or nonpharmacologic pain management techniques (ie, physical therapy, TENS unit, relaxation, biofeedback) to manage pain?
6. Does the patient believe that his/her pain has been adequately treated over the past 6 months?
7. Does the patient express anger/mistrust of past health care providers?
8. Does the patient believe that he/she is addicted to opioid analgesics?
9. Does the referring physician believe that the patient is addicted to opioid analgesics?

Opioid Use Patterns (in months)
9a. How long has the patient been on continuous opioids?
10. Does the patient have more than one prescription provider (including dentists, ER physicians)?
11. Is there a pattern of the patient increasing prescribed analgesic dose or frequency?
12. Is there a pattern of the patient calling in for early prescription refills?
13. Does the patient report using analgesics for symptoms other than those prescribed for (ie, insomnia, anxiety, depression)?
14. Does the patient save/hoard unused medication or have partially unused bottles of medication at home?
15. Does the patient report supplementing analgesics with alcohol or other psychoactive drugs (ie, Soma, benzodiazepines)?
15a. If yes, please list:
16. Has the patient ever forged a prescription?
17. Is there a pattern of the patient reporting losing his/her medication?
18. Does the patient have preferences for specific analgesics and/or routes of administration (ie, IV, IM routes over oral)?
18a. If so, please list preferred opioids with routes:
19. Is there a pattern of the patient making emergency room visits for analgesics?
20. Has the patient ever obtained analgesic from nonmedical (street) sources?
21. Has any MD/DDS limited care, expressed concern, or refused to prescribe opioid analgesics because of patient's opioid use patterns?

Social/Family Factors
22. Have family members expressed concern that the patient is addicted?
23. Are family members concerned about opioid analgesic side effects or tolerance?
24. Is there a pattern of family interaction that sustains the patient's opioid analgesic use (ie, family member overly concerned regarding pain or withdrawal)?
25. Is there a pattern of family interaction that sustains the patient's illness behavior or pain symptoms (ie, family member assuming caretaker role)?
26. Does the spouse/significant other have a history of alcoholism/drug abuse/drug misuse?
27. Has a family member or friend ever obtained analgesic for the patient?
28. Has the patient ever taken analgesics prescribed for a friend or family member?
29. Does a family member or friend have access (either legal or illegal) to opioid analgesics (ie, a family member in the medical profession)?

Family History
30. Is there a positive history of addiction (to any drug including alcohol) in the patient's mother, father, sibling or blood relative?
31. Is there a positive family history of chronic pain in the patient's mother, father, sibling or blood relative?

Patient History of Substance Abuse

32. Did intoxication play a role in pain-precipitating incident?
33. Has the patient ever been diagnosed with addiction to any drug or alcohol?
34. Does the patient have a drug or alcohol treatment history?
35. Has opioid analgesic detoxification been previously attempted?

Psychiatric History

36. Has the patient ever been diagnosed with a psychiatric disorder?
37. Did psychiatric symptoms precede onset of pain?
38. Is there a large psychological component to the pain condition, other than those related to addiction (ie, multiple psychological stressors)?
39. Is there evidence of a somatoform disorder?
40. Does the patient report a history of sexual or physical abuse?
41. Does the patient currently meet DSM-IV criteria for any Axis I, II, or III conditions?
41a. If so, please list diagnoses:
42. Please list all pain-producing medical conditions:

Abbreviations: ER, emergency room; IM, intramuscular; IV, intravenous; SSI, Supplemental Security Income; TENS, transcutaneous electrical nerve stimulation.

From Compton P, Darakjian J, Miotto K. Screening for addiction in patients with chronic pain and "problematic" substance use: evaluation of a pilot assessment tool. J Pain Symptom Manage 1998;16(6):355–63.

Some other psychological factors that are identified in the pain literature that are associated with persistent pain and poorer outcome in treatment are[39]

- High levels of psychological distress
- Patients who hold negative beliefs and expectations about their pain
- Pain-related fear and avoidance of daily activities leading to significant disability
- Sustained attitude of anger, hostility, and alienation
- Maladaptive coping strategies and cognitive distortions or catastrophic thinking.

The response of the spouse or other family members to the patient's expressions of pain and analgesic use can also influence the extent of impairment and disability. When observing the patient's family or social interactions, it is important to determine if patterns exist that encourage pain, opioid medication use, or disability. An increased sensitivity to pain has been reported in relationships in which there are more frequent negative spouse responses to pain, as well as in relationships in which there is spousal reinforcement often referred to as the "solicitous spouse."[40] The spouse or partner of a chronic pain patient may unintentionally foster disability and justify medication overuse in an attempt to be sympathetic or to perpetuate his or her role as the caregiver. For some individuals the role of caregiver began in childhood, in a household where there was a parent suffering with a disabling disorder. Family therapy and community mutual-help groups such as Al-Anon, Families Anonymous, and CoDA (Codependents Anonymous) can be important resources in this situation.[41]

The assessment of a patient's past or current addiction history requires skill in motivational interviewing.[42] It has been demonstrated that a psychiatrist's sympathetic interest and verbal as well as nonverbal expressions of empathy influence the extent of the information obtained related to substance use.[43] Individuals may fear disclosing a history of addiction, because they believe it will complicate the patient-physician relationship or trust and their reports of pain will be discredited.

Screening instruments gauge an individual's potential for problems with opioid treatment and are a topic of much discussion in the primary care and pain treatment literature.[44] These instruments are important tools not only because they help to identify patients at risk for opioid use disorders, but they also help to stratify risk and identify which patients can be managed in their practice settings. Ideally, these instruments also provide an opportunity for prescribers and patients to discuss a potentially difficult subject, the possibility of prescription opioid abuse, addiction, and diversion.[45] It is important for the psychiatrist to advocate the use of these screening instruments and to be aware of the resources. Two of the patient-administered instruments include the revised Screener and Opioid Assessment for Patient in Pain and the Opioid Risk Tool.[46,47] An example of a clinician-administered instrument is the Diagnosis, Intractability, Risk, Efficacy instrument.

Two important objective assessments for screening patients before and during opioid treatment are body fluid or urine toxicology tests and use of prescription drug monitoring programs (PDMPs). Drug tests are useful to detect the patient's medication use or lack of use or use of illicit drugs. Assays for reliable point-of-care testing, such as on oral fluid, are being developed to simplify the process and provide immediate in-office results. PDMPs provide an important source of collateral information on what controlled substances are prescribed to a patient. PDMPs are electronic databases, available in most states, documenting the number of prescriptions for controlled substances, the name of the prescriber, and the pharmacy for a given patient. The data are intended to serve as a tool for health care practitioners when prescribing controlled substances to reduce doctor-shopping and diversion.[48] Similarly, it can be useful for clinicians to review prescription profiles that may be sent on behalf of a patient's insurance provider. These profiles are generally sent when there are multiple physicians prescribing controlled substances.

UNIVERSAL PRECAUTIONS IN PAIN MEDICINE

The comprehensive screening and monitoring of opioid-treated patients has been incorporated into a universal precautions approach by Gourlay and Heit.[49] The universal precautions of opioid treatment are practice recommendations with the goals to improve patient education and care, decrease provider worry, and contain the overall risk. The adoption of universal precautions assumes a strong patient-practitioner relationship, adequate encounter time, and a system of care wherein opioid informed consent and agreements are developed in advance. The recommendations of Gourlay and Heit are summarized here:

- Evaluate and document the diagnosis of pain and the differential diagnoses. Comorbid conditions that impact the pain should be addressed early in treatment.
- Conduct an addiction assessment including a baseline drug of abuse screen and PDMP evaluation.
- Obtain written informed consent that describes the monitoring required and the risks of opioids including dependence, withdrawal, and addiction.
- Identify preopioid and postopioid treatment goals for pain reduction and functional restoration.
- Evaluate for 4 A's of pain medicine. These include
  1. **A**nalgesic response
  2. Increased **a**ctivity
  3. **A**dverse effects of opioids
  4. **A**berrant opioid use behaviors

- Review the evolution of the painful condition and any comorbid psychiatric disorders.
- Document the findings at each step of the way.

PHARMACOLOGIC CONSIDERATIONS AND STRATEGIES FOR PAIN

A variety of pharmacologic options are available to treat pain. Opioids should not be the first line treatment for chronic pain in most populations. Instead, the use of nonopioid medications should be maximized. Because of the complex pathophysiology of pain, combining various adjunctive medications and analgesics with different mechanisms of action can enhance effectiveness and decrease the likelihood of adverse events. The academic pain societies have recently developed excellent guidelines on treating chronic pain that describe pharmacologic and nonpharmacologic treatment options in great detail.[15,50] Ideally, all patients with significant chronic pain are treated in settings with multidisciplinary services that include physical and behavioral therapies as well as support for lifestyle modifications to prevent the physical deconditioning that afflicts so many patients with chronic pain. However, because of the limited availability of such services, the focus of this article is the care of opioid-treated patients and identification of some helpful pharmacologic strategies.

Many patients with chronic pain are treated with antidepressants. Pain and depression are the most common physical and psychological disorders with co-occurrence estimated as 30% to 50% of the time.[51] Antidepressants can serve several roles in providing relief from neuropathic pain and in treating psychological symptoms that exacerbate pain, such as anxiety, depression, and insomnia. The most commonly recommended adjuvant antidepressant medications used to treat pain include tricyclic antidepressants and serotonin-norepinephrine reuptake inhibitors (SNRIs) such as venlafaxine and duloxetine. There is more controversy concerning efficacy of selective serotonin reuptake inhibitors (SSRIs) in pain relief. Paroxetine and citalopram are somewhat useful in treating diabetic peripheral neuropathy, whereas escitalopram was comparable to duloxetine in a small trial for chronic low back pain.[52]

Anticonvulsants are often used in the management of neuropathic pain and for migraine prophylaxis. Antidepressants and anticonvulsants can be prescribed simultaneously when noradrenergic antidepressants alone prove to be ineffective or intolerable. Gabapentin and pregabalin are the most commonly prescribed, with the older anticonvulsants generally prescribed as second line options because of the need for laboratory monitoring and greater risk of adverse effects. Gabapentin has been described as an opioid-sparing agent because it has been found to be effective at reducing postoperative pain, opioid consumption, and opioid-related adverse effects based on a systematic review of several clinical trials.[53]

The safety of benzodiazepine use in the opioid-treated patient deserves special mention. Many patients receive benzodiazepines and opioids from different providers, and the concerns about the safety of this combination of medications may not be appreciated. Without a doubt, benzodiazepines have utility in the treatment of pain associated with anxiety, muscle spasticity, and insomnia. However, like opioids, benzodiazepines have the potential to cause central nervous system (CNS) depression, sedation, and decreased mental acuity. The 2010 Canadian Guideline for Safe and Effective Use of Opioids for Chronic Non-Cancer Pain states: "The use of opioids can result in respiratory depression and side effects include well known disturbances in the ventilation pattern."[50] The guideline recommends that for "patients taking benzodiazepines, tapering should be considered prior to opioid initiation. If tapering is not indicated or is unsuccessful, it is recommended that opioids be titrated more slowly and at lower doses." The rationale provided for this recommendation is that the combination increases the risk of sedation, overdose, and diminished function. The evidence referenced found serum concentration of opioids is lower in mixed over-doses than in pure overdoses, suggesting that other drugs significantly lower the lethal opioid dose.[54]

SOME TRANSDERMAL TREATMENT OPTIONS

Some of the topical and transdermal nonopioid and opioid formulations are important considerations in the treatment of pain when there is a concern about addiction, because they ameliorate the dosing interval dilemma and the questions of whether a particular dose of medication is being taken for physical pain, psychological pain, or craving.

- **Lidocaine-medicated patch.** Lidocaine-medicated patches (5%) have demonstrated analgesic effects in the treatment of neuropathic pain, lower back pain, and complex regional pain syndrome. One setting where transdermal preparations may be useful is in inpatient psychiatric settings for patients with musculoskeletal pain when the use of opioid medication is not indicated. Lidocaine patches are left in place for 12 hours and removed for 12 hours each day. A common nonopioid pain relief strategy is to alternate the lidocaine patch during the night and the diclofenac patch during the day.
- **Diclofenac epolamine patch.** The diclofenac epolamine patch is a topical NSAID. It consists of 1.3% diclofenac epolamine which, when applied to the skin over the painful area, provides analgesia for 4 to 5 hours. The typical oral NSAID gastrointestinal tract side effects do not occur with the topical treatments because hepatic first pass metabolism is bypassed and there is a slower rate of systemic circulation.[55–57]
- **Buprenorphine.** Buprenorphine is a schedule III controlled substance with partial agonist activity at the mu-opioid receptor and antagonist activity at the kappa-opioid receptor. Long before it was approved for the treatment of opioid dependence it was available as an analgesic intramuscular or intravenous injection. In 2010, the US Food and Drug Administration (FDA) approved a new formulation of buprenorphine; a once-weekly buprenorphine transdermal system for the management of moderate to severe chronic pain in patients requiring a continuous, around-the-clock opioid analgesic for an extended period.
- **Other transdermal medications.** A similar transdermal system has been marketed in Europe and Australia with indications for moderate chronic pain not responding to nonopioids. The prescribing information cautions that the medication is contraindicated in the management of acute or short-term pain or intermittent pain. This caution about treating intermittent pain with a continuous opioid medication was missing from the early campaign to end the undertreatment of pain.

DUAL MECHANISM OF ACTION MEDICATIONS

There are two drugs used in pain management that have an apparent dual mechanism of action:

1. Tramadol
2. Tapentadol.

The goal of these therapies is to provide a single medication with a dual mechanism of action without the potential risk of drug-drug interactions in multiple drug therapy.

Tramadol

The mode of action of tramadol is not completely understood, but it is mediated by CNS binding to mu-opioid receptors and reuptake inhibition of norepinephrine and serotonin. Psychiatrists need to appreciate the risk of serotonin syndrome, which may occur as a result of the combined use of tramadol with SSRIs or SNRIs. Although tramadol is generally believed to have a low addiction liability, it is notable that there are case reports describing an opioid withdrawal and an SSRI discontinuation syndrome after abrupt cessation of high-dose tramadol use. Other dangers of high-dose tramadol use are seizures in acute overdose and seizures in the context of withdrawal.[58] Finally, tramadol has been identified in the urologic literature as an on-demand for premature ejaculation, which has been associated with some clinical cases of abuse and diversion.

Tapentadol

Tapentadol is also a centrally acting analgesic useful in the treatment of chronic noncancer pain, and neuropathic pain. Tapentadol's dual mechanism of action includes mu-opioid receptor agonist activity and reuptake inhibition of norepinephrine. Tapentadol has an opioid-sparing property as a result of the dual mechanism of action. However, because it has an analgesic effect equivalent to morphine, there is a potential for abuse, although there are no case reports of addiction or withdrawal at this time. Nonetheless, it is important for clinicians to be vigilant of each new opioid preparation sold because the abuse liability may only be evident after several years of postmarketing surveillance. In an effort to improve the public health and safety of opioids, the FDA now requires pharmaceutical companies who market opioid drugs to submit a risk evaluation and mitigation strategy (REMS). The goals of the REMS programs are to increase patient and provider education and to ensure abuse-deterrent and tamper-resistant strategies are included in opioid drug development.[59]

MANAGING OPIOID TAPER OR WITHDRAWAL

Managing opioid withdrawal requires skill and sensitivity. Opioid withdrawal is not life-threatening. The signs and symptoms include

- Anxiety
- Insomnia
- Yawning
- Chills
- Anorexia
- Muscle cramps
- Nausea
- Diarrhea
- Miosis
- Elevated heart rate and blood pressure.

Although these signs and symptoms are generally not dangerous, unmanaged withdrawal can cause significant distress and trigger the resumption of opioid medication or relapse. The lack of recognition of opioid withdrawal discomfort may lead to cycles of dose escalation and increased tolerance. Patient education helps avoid the misinterpretation of the emergence of withdrawal as an exacerbation of the underlying painful condition. In addition, an important consideration is that in cases of opioid-induced hyperalgesia, medication discontinuation will diminish the pain. Nonopioid symptomatic management includes muscle relaxants, dicyclomine, loperamide, NSAIDs, and clonidine.

Methadone and buprenorphine are both options for the acute management of opioid withdrawal or maintenance treatment. Only federally licensed treatment facilities may dispense methadone treatment for opioid dependence as part of an addiction treatment program, but any physician may prescribe methadone for the treatment of pain. The safe use of methadone, whether for the treatment of pain, addiction, or both, requires an understanding of its unique pharmacologic properties and the regulatory issues; an extensive review of methadone safety and treatment can be found in *Lowinson and Ruiz's Substance Abuse: A Comprehensive Textbook.*[60]

Sublingual buprenorphine is available alone and in combination with naloxone. Buprenorphine can be used as an effective agent for opioid detoxification or maintenance or for the relief of pain. However, induction onto buprenorphine should begin 12 to 24 hours after cessation of short-acting opioid use and 24 to 48 hours after long-acting opioid use to minimize the risk of precipitating withdrawal. Unlike methadone, which is dispensed at a licensed clinic, buprenorphine can be prescribed for the treatment of addiction by physicians who have completed the required training and obtained a Drug Enforcement Agency waiver. Alternatively, the sublingual preparation can be prescribed off-label for the treatment of pain.[61,62]

SUMMARY

The safest pain treatment strategy for an individual at risk or recovering from addiction is a nonopioid and benzodiazepine-free approach. If an opioid treatment is necessary, the extent of the risk can be stratified by the use of a biopsychosocial assessment and opioid screening tools. Individuals at high risk should have the greatest amount of structure and monitoring. A written informed consent and treatment agreement can provide a framework for the patient and the patient's family, as well as the clinician. The structure of treatment should specify only that one prescribing physician will write a limited supply of opioids, without refills, until the analgesic efficacy, adverse events, and goals for functional restoration can be assessed. An additional recommendation is that prescriptions should be filled at the same pharmacy with no refill by phone or opportunity for replacement because of loss, damage, or stolen medications. Additionally, random urine drug screens and PDMP reports obtained will help determine if the patient is taking other substances, as well as monitor the patient's medication use patterns.

It is important to assess for risk factors in treating chronic pain with opioids; clinicians need to have a realistic appreciation of the resources available to them and the types of patients that can be managed in their practice. Chronic pain treatment with opioids should not be undertaken in patients who are currently addicted to illicit substances or alcohol. With the support of family and friends, ideally the patient can be motivated to participate in an intensive substance abuse treatment. In patients without an immediate risk, precautionary steps should be taken when prescribing opioids. Clinicians and patients need to review the risk factors for opioid-related problems including younger age, benzodiazepine use, and comorbid conditions such as depression, anxiety, and heavy smoking. Both the provider and the patient need a personal investment in the treatment plan and protocol to increase the safety of opioid treatment. New medications and treatment monitoring are being developed to provide maximal relief for the patient while protecting the public health. The optimal ingredients for safe opioid treatment include a strong provider-patient relationship and clinician training in the assessment and treatment of addiction and pain.

REFERENCES

1. Committee on Advancing Pain Research, Care and Education, Institute of Medicine of the National Academies. Relieving pain in America: a blueprint for transforming prevention, care, education, and research. Washington, DC: The National Academies Press; 2011.
2. Chartbook on trends in the health of Americans 2006, special feature: pain. Published 2006. Available at: http://www.cdc.gov/nchs/data/hus/hus06.pdf. Accessed January 10, 2012.
3. Classification of chronic pain. Descriptions of chronic pain syndromes and definitions of pain terms. Prepared by the International Association for the Study of Pain, Subcommittee on Taxonomy. Pain Suppl 1986;3:S1–S226.
4. American Psychiatric Association. Task Force on D-I. Diagnostic and statistical manual of mental disorders: DSM-IV-TR. Washington, DC: American Psychiatric Association; 2000.
5. Covington EC. Psychogenic pain—what it means, why it does not exist, and how to diagnose it. Pain Med 2000;1(4):287–94.
6. Eisendrath SJ. Psychiatric aspects of chronic pain. Neurology 1995;45(12 Suppl 9):S26–34.
7. Juul D, Scheiber SC, Kramer TA. Subspecialty certification by the American Board of Psychiatry and Neurology. Acad Psychiatry 2004;28(1):12–7.
8. Weissman DE, Haddox JD. Opioid pseudoaddiction--an iatrogenic syndrome. Pain 1989;36(3):363–6.
9. Bell K, Salmon A. Pain, physical dependence and pseudoaddiction: redefining addiction for 'nice' people? Int J Drug Policy 2009;20(2):170–8.
10. Okie S. A flood of opioids, a rising tide of deaths. N Engl J Med 2010;363(21):1981–5.
11. Horvath RJ, Romero-Sandoval EA, De Leo JA. Glial modulation in pain states: translation into humans. Boca Raton (FL): CRC Press; 2010.
12. Ballantyne JC. Chronic pain following treatment for cancer: the role of opioids. Oncologist 2003;8(6):567–75.
13. Lee M, Silverman SM, Hansen H, et al. A comprehensive review of opioid-induced hyperalgesia. Pain Physician 2011;14(2):145–61.
14. Nicolaidis C. Oregon Health & Science University. Society of General Internal Medicine 2008 Precourse; 2008.
15. Chou R. 2009 clinical guidelines from the American Pain Society and the American Academy of Pain Medicine on the use of chronic opioid therapy in chronic noncancer pain: what are the key messages for clinical practice? Pol Arch Med Wewn 2009; 119(7–8):469–77.
16. King T, Ossipov MH, Vanderah TW, et al. Is paradoxical pain induced by sustained opioid exposure an underlying mechanism of opioid antinociceptive tolerance? Neurosignals 2005;14(4):194–205.
17. Bailey CP, Connor M. Opioids: cellular mechanisms of tolerance and physical dependence. Curr Opin Pharmacol 2005;5(1):60–8.
18. Henry M. Opioids in pain management. Lancet 1999;353(9171):2229–32.
19. Substance Abuse and Mental Health Services Administration. Results from the 2010 National Survey on Drug Use and Health: summary of national findings [NSDUH Series H-41, HHS Publication No. (SMA) 11-4658]. Rockville (MD): Substance Abuse and Mental Health Services Administration; 2011.

20. Heron M. Deaths: leading causes for 2007. Natl Vital Stat Rep 2011;59(8):1–95.
21. Substance A, Mental Health Services A. Treatment episode data set (TEDS), 1999 – 2009: national admissions to substance abuse treatment services. Rockville (MD): Substance Abuse and Mental Health Services Administration; 2011.
22. Martell BA, O'Connor PG, Kerns RD, et al. Systematic review: opioid treatment for chronic back pain: prevalence, efficacy, and association with addiction. Ann Intern Med 2007;146(2):116–27.
23. Fleming MF, Balousek SL, Klessig CL, et al. Substance use disorders in a primary care sample receiving daily opioid therapy. J Pain 2007;8(7):573–82.
24. Banta-Green CJ, Merrill JO, Doyle SR, e tal. Measurement of opioid problems among chronic pain patients in a general medical population. Drug Alcohol Depend 2009; 104(1–2):43–9.
25. Becker WC, Fiellin DA, Gallagher RM, et al. The association between chronic pain and prescription drug abuse in veterans. Pain Med 2009;10(3):531–6.
26. Boscarino JA, Rukstalis M, Hoffman SN, et al. Risk factors for drug dependence among out-patients on opioid therapy in a large US health-care system. Addiction 2010;105(10):1776–82.
27. Reid MC, Engles-Horton LL, Weber MB, et al. Use of opioid medications for chronic noncancer pain syndromes in primary care. J Gen Intern Med 2002;17(3):173–9.
28. Michna E, Ross EL, Hynes WL, et al. Predicting aberrant drug behavior in patients treated for chronic pain: importance of abuse history. J Pain Symptom Manage 2004;28(3):250–8.
29. Skurtveit S, Furu K, Selmer R, et al. Nicotine dependence predicts repeated use of prescribed opioids. Prospective population-based cohort study. Ann Epidemiol 2010; 20(12):890–7.
30. Akbik H, Butler SF, Budman SH, et al. Validation and clinical application of the Screener and Opioid Assessment for Patients with Pain (SOAPP). J Pain Symptom Manage 2006;32(3):287–93.
31. Edlund MJ, Steffick D, Hudson T, et al. Risk factors for clinically recognized opioid abuse and dependence among veterans using opioids for chronic non-cancer pain. Pain 2007;129(3):355–62.
32. Edlund MJ, Martin BC, Fan M-Y, et al. Risks for opioid abuse and dependence among recipients of chronic opioid therapy: results from the TROUP Study. Drug Alcohol Depend 2010;112(1–2):90–8.
33. Portenoy RK. Opioid therapy for chronic nonmalignant pain: clinicians' perspective. J Law Med Ethics 1996;24(4):296–309.
34. Sees KL, Clark HW. Opioid use in the treatment of chronic pain: assessment of addiction. J Pain Symptom Manage 1993;8(5):257–64.
35. Miotto K, Compton P, Ling W, et al. Diagnosing addictive disease in chronic pain patients. Psychosomatics 1996;37(3):223–35.
36. Compton P, Darakjian J, Miotto K. Screening for addiction in patients with chronic pain and "problematic" substance use: evaluation of a pilot assessment tool. J Pain Symptom Manage 1998;16(6):355–63.
37. Davis DA, Luecken LJ, Zautra AJ. Are reports of childhood abuse related to the experience of chronic pain in adulthood?: A meta-analytic review of the literature. Clin J Pain 2005;21(5):398–405.
38. Wilsnack SC, Vogeltanz ND, Klassen AD, et al. Childhood sexual abuse and women's substance abuse: national survey findings. J Stud Alcohol 1997;58(3):264–71.
39. Turk DC, Okifuji A. Psychological aspects of pain. In: Warfield CA, Bajwa ZH, editors. Principles and practice of pain medicine. 2nd edition. New York: McGraw-Hill Professional; 2004. p. 139–47.

40. Weiss L, Kerns R. Patterns of pain-relevant social interactions. Int J Behav Med 1995;2(2):157–71.
41. Cano A, Weisberg JN, Gallagher RM. Marital satisfaction and pain severity mediate the association between negative spouse responses to pain and depressive symptoms in a chronic pain patient sample. Pain Med 2000;1(1):35–43.
42. Treasure J. Motivational interviewing. Advances in Psychiatric Treatment 2004;10(5): 331–7.
43. Chappel JN, Schnoll SH. Physician attitudes. Effect on the treatment of chemically dependent patients. JAMA 1977;237(21):2318–9.
44. Passik SD, Kirsh KL, Casper D. Addiction-related assessment tools and pain management: instruments for screening, treatment planning, and monitoring compliance. Pain Med 2008;9:S145–66.
45. Turk DC, Swanson KS, Gatchel RJ. Predicting opioid misuse by chronic pain patients: a systematic review and literature synthesis. Clin J Pain 2008;24(6):497–508.
46. Butler SF, Fernandez K, Benoit C, et al. Validation of the Revised Screener and Opioid Assessment for Patients With Pain (SOAPP-R). J Pain 2008;9(4):360–72.
47. Butler SF, Budman SH, Fernandez KC, et al. Development and validation of the Current Opioid Misuse Measure. Pain 2007;130(1–2):144–56.
48. Gugelmann HM, Perrone J. Can prescription drug monitoring programs help limit opioid abuse? JAMA 2011;306(20):2258–9.
49. Gourlay DL, Heit HA, Almahrezi A. Universal precautions in pain medicine: a rational approach to the treatment of chronic pain. Pain Med 2005;6(2):107–12.
50. Canadian guideline for safe and effective use of opioids for chronic non-cancer pain. Canada: National Opioid Use Guideline Group (NOUGG). Published 2010. Available at: http://nationalpaincentre.mcmaster.ca/opioid/. Accessed December 10, 2011.
51. Kroenke K, Wu J, Bair MJ, et al. Reciprocal relationship between pain and depression: a 12-month longitudinal analysis in primary care. J Pain 2011;12(9):964–73.
52. Saarto T, Wiffen PJ. Antidepressants for neuropathic pain. Cochrane Database Syst Rev 2007;4:CD005454.
53. Tiippana EM, Hamunen K, Kontinen VK, et al. Do surgical patients benefit from perioperative gabapentin/pregabalin? A systematic review of efficacy and safety. Anesth Analg 2007;104(6):1545–56.
54. Canadian Agency for Drugs and Technologies in Health (CADTH). Combination benzodiazepine-opioid use: a review of the evidence on safety [PDF]. Available at: cadth.ca/media/pdf/htis/sept.../RC0299_Benzodiazepines_final.pdf. Accessed January 10, 2012.
55. Gammaitoni AR, Alvarez NA, Galer BS. Safety and tolerability of the lidocaine patch 5%, a targeted peripheral analgesic: a review of the literature. J Clin Pharmacol 2003;43(2):111–7.
56. Wehrfritz A, Namer B, Ihmsen H, et al. Differential effects on sensory functions and measures of epidermal nerve fiber density after application of a lidocaine patch (5%) on healthy human skin. Eur J Pain 2011;15(9):907–12.
57. Bair MJ, Sanderson TR. Coanalgesics for chronic pain therapy: a narrative review. Postgrad Med 2011;123(6):140–50.
58. Nossaman VE, Ramadhyani U, Kadowitz PJ, et al. Advances in perioperative pain management: use of medications with dual analgesic mechanisms, tramadol & tapentadol. Anesthesiol Clin 2010;28(4):647–66.
59. Leiderman DB. Risk management of drug products and the U.S. Food and Drug Administration: evolution and context. Drug Alcohol Depend 2009;105(Suppl 1): S9–13.

60. Andrew J. Saxon KM. Methadone maintenance. In: Ruiz P, Strain E, editors. Lowinson and Ruiz's substance abuse: a comprehensive textbook. Philadelphia: Lippincott Williams and Wilkins; 2011. p. 419–36. Section 6, chapter 28.
61. McNicholas L. Clinical guidelines for the use of buprenorphine in the treatment of opioid addiction. Rockville (MD): US Department of Health and Human Services, Substance Abuse and Mental Health Services Administration, Center for Substance Abuse Treatment; 2004.
62. Center for Substance Abuse Treatment. Medication-assisted treatment for opioid addiction in Opioid Treatment Programs Inservice Training. HHS Publication No. (SMA) 09–4341. Rockville (MD): Substance Abuse and Mental Health Services Administration; 2008 [reprinted 2009].

Clinical Implications of Drug Abuse Epidemiology

Jeffrey D. Schulden, MD*, Marsha F. Lopez, PhD, MHS,
Wilson M. Compton, MD, MPE

KEYWORDS

- Drug abuse • Drug dependence • Drug use • Epidemiology

KEY POINTS

- Illicit drug use and drug use disorders are relatively common with initial use typically starting in mid to late adolescence and with marijuana as the most commonly used substance.
- Multiple studies have shown elevated prevalence of misuse of prescription drugs, such as hydrocodone and oxycodone, along with elevated rates for the problems associated with their misuse, including fatal and nonfatal opioid overdose.
- Large-scale epidemiologic studies have consistently shown a high degree of comorbidity of substance use disorders with other psychiatric disorders.
- Optimal treatment of either substance use or comorbid psychiatric disorders will not be achieved unless both are adequately treated.
- Genetic factors play an important role in the development of drug use disorders.
- Screening, Brief Intervention, and Referral to Treatment (SBIRT) programs for drug use should be an integral part of routine clinical care in a range of clinical settings, including primary care, psychiatric, and emergency department settings.

Findings from several large-scale, population-based surveys of drug use have indicated relatively high prevalence of illicit drug use and shifts in trends in illicit drug use, for example highlighting the elevated rates of prescription drug misuse and associated morbidity and mortality from their misuse. These studies have furthered understanding of the high comorbidity of drug use disorders with other psychiatric disorders and with the HIV epidemic. Building on an understanding of this research in substance abuse epidemiology, it is important for clinicians to learn to integrate

Disclaimer: The views and opinions expressed in this report are those of the authors and should not be construed to represent the views of NIDA or any of the sponsoring organizations, agencies, or the US government.

Division of Epidemiology, Services, and Prevention Research, National Institute on Drug Abuse (NIDA), 6001 Executive Boulevard, MSC 9589, Bethesda, MD 20892-9589, USA

* Corresponding author.

E-mail address: schuldenj@nida.nih.gov

Psychiatr Clin N Am 35 (2012) 411–423
http://dx.doi.org/10.1016/j.psc.2012.03.007
0193-953X/12/$ – see front matter Published by Elsevier Inc.

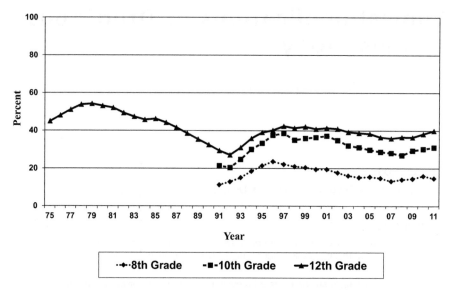

Source: The Monitoring the Future Study, 2011, University of Michigan[1]

Fig. 1. Trends in annual prevalence of illicit drug use, grades 8, 10, and 12. (*Data from* Johnston LD, O'Malley PM, Bachman JG, et al. Monitoring the future: National Survey Results on Drug Use, 1975–2011. Bethesda (MD): National Institute on Drug Abuse; 2011.)

strategies for prevention, screening, and linkage to substance abuse treatment programs available for the communities they serve. On-going research supports the important role of such Screening, Brief Intervention, and Referral to Treatment (SBIRT) programs in a range of settings, including primary care, mental health, and emergency departments.

TRENDS IN SUBSTANCE USE

Large, population-based, annual surveys, such as the National Survey on Drug Use and Health (NSDUH) and the Monitoring the Future study, provide a foundation for understanding patterns of illicit drug use over time.[1,2] After reaching a peak in the late 1970s, rates of illicit drug use among adolescents generally declined during the 1980s, increased somewhat during the 1990s, then have stayed relatively stable over the past several years, although with some indication of a possible slight upward trend in recent years (**Fig. 1**).[1] Nevertheless, multiple such epidemiologic studies suggest that illicit drug use is relatively common in the population, with initial use typically starting in mid to late adolescence. The 2010 NSDUH data, based on surveys conducted in a representative sample of US households, indicate that approximately 8.9% of persons ages 12 and older in the United States—an estimated 22.6 million individuals—have used any illicit drug at least once during the past month, 6.9% have used marijuana, and 2.7% have used prescription-type psychotherapeutic drugs nonmedically.[2] For comparison, the 2010 NSDUH data indicate that 51.8% of respondents age 12 and older reported having had alcohol in the past month.[2] The 2011 Monitoring the Future data, based on surveys conducted at a representative sample of US secondary schools, found that 20.1% of 8th grade students reported having ever tried an illicit drug, 37.7% of 10th graders, and 49.9% of 12th graders, showing a rising trend in use over the course of adolescence.[1] For comparison, 33.1% of 8th graders reported having ever tried alcohol, 56.0% of 10th graders, and 70.0% of 12th graders.[1] Thus, the prevalence of illicit drug use is generally closer to that of alcohol use among adolescents than among the United States population as a whole. Data from MTF also indicate that marijuana continues to be the most commonly used illicit drug, with 16.4% of 8th graders, 34.5% of 10th graders, and 45.5% of 12th graders reporting having ever tried marijuana.[1]

Such large-scale surveys have found that typically drug use increases from adolescence to young adulthood then gradually declines.[1-3] Given the high prevalence of illicit substance use, it is imperative that clinicians routinely screen for use among their patients, especially among adolescents and young adults.[4-6] Of note, the American Academy of Pediatrics has recently released a policy statement on substance use SBIRT for pediatricians, encouraging widespread adoption as a part of routine adolescent primary care screening and including recommended comprehensive algorithms for SBIRT in the pediatric setting.[7] Ideally, all clinicians would be able to offer patients integrated prevention, brief intervention, and referral to treatment services within well-coordinated health systems, although many communities still unfortunately face limited access to comprehensive drug abuse prevention and treatment services.[4-9]

PRESCRIPTION OPIOID MISUSE

These ongoing surveys have also found a high prevalence of misuse of prescription drugs, such as hydrocodone and oxycodone, along with elevated rates for the problems associated with their misuse, including fatal and nonfatal opioid overdose.[10-14] The heightened concern for the high prevalence of prescription drug misuse is due in part to evidence of elevated levels of abuse among adolescents.[12,15,16] In 2011, among 12th graders, past year use of prescription drugs was reported to be 15.2%.[1]

Clinicians must balance appropriately treating their patients while being alert for possible misuse of prescription opioids and other psychoactive medications such as stimulants and sedatives.[13,17-20] This balance can sometimes prove difficult, especially when treating chronic pain conditions. In general, clinicians treating persons with chronic analgesics or other psychoactive medications are advised to prescribe in limited, appropriate doses with regular follow-up appointments; to encourage the disposal of any unused medication; and to foster trusting relationships with patients in which personal and family history of substance abuse and risks of prescription medication misuse are openly discussed.[13,17-20] As possible, clinicians are advised to pursue analgesic treatment regimens that include nonopioid analgesics and include psychotherapeutic strategies for managing chronic pain, such as cognitive–behavioral therapy.[13,17-23]

DRUG ABUSE AND DEPENDENCE

A proportion of persons who use illicit substances develop ongoing dysfunctional patterns of use that may constitute drug abuse or dependence. Some large, population-based studies, such as the NSDUH and the National Epidemiologic Survey on Alcohol and Related Conditions (NESARC), have included actual diagnostic categories of drug abuse and dependence as defined in the *Diagnostic and Statistical Manual of Mental Disorders-IV* (DSM-IV). Recent data from the NESARC indicate that approximately 2.0% of adults living in US households had a DSM-IV drug use disorder in the prior 12 months (1.4% abuse, 0.6% dependence), and 10.3% reported a drug use disorder at any point in their lifetime (7.7% abuse, 2.6% dependence).[3] For comparison, data from the NESARC also indicate that approximately 8.5% of adults living in US households had an alcohol use disorder in the past 12 months (4.7% abuse, 3.8% dependence).[24]

Drug use disorders were also highly associated with measures of physical, social, and occupational disability, including missed work days and repeated hospitalizations.[3,25-27] The widespread nature of drug use disorders further highlights the substantial public health problem they represent and the need for integrated SBIRT programs in a range of clinical settings serving general patient populations, including primary care and emergency department settings.[4-9]

SPECIAL POPULATIONS

Although drug use disorders are found commonly throughout the population, several studies have suggested increased risk among some communities and demographic groups that may merit a heightened need for prevention and screening in clinical settings. For example, the NESARC and several other studies have shown drug use disorders to be much more common among men than among women.[2,3,28,29] Data from the NESARC have also suggested increased risk of drug use disorders among those who are younger; have less income; have less education; and have never married or are widowed, separated, or divorced.[3] Data from the NESARC further suggest an especially high prevalence of drug use disorders among Native Americans: 18.4% of Native Americans reporting a drug use disorder at some point in their lifetime (11.6% abuse, 6.9% dependence).[3]

These findings are similar to those found in regional studies among Native Americans and call attention to the tremendous need of this community for improved access to substance abuse prevention and treatment services.[3,30-33] Although younger age does continue to be generally associated with drug use disorders, recent data from the NESARC and other studies suggest that rates have also increased among older adults who came of age during the height of the drug epidemic of the 1970s.[2,3,29,34-36] These data suggest the possibility of rising rates of drug use disorders among future cohorts of older adults and highlight the need for geriatric clinicians to integrate drug abuse screening and referral into their assessments.[34-38]

Multiple studies have found that gay, lesbian, and bisexual individuals are at increased risk for drug use, drug use disorders, and a range of conditions that are commonly comorbid with drug use disorders, including depression and suicidality.[39-44] This disproportionate drug use among sexual minorities seems to emerge in adolescence and continue into adulthood, and has been found across multiple classes of substances.[39-43]

In addition, a high proportion of persons who enter into the criminal justice system in the United States have a history of substance abuse or dependence.[45,46] As such, criminal justice systems can serve as important settings for integrated drug abuse screening, brief intervention, and treatment.[45-47] Integrating such services in the criminal justice setting holds the promise not only to improve rates of drug use relapse among offenders, but also to reduce criminal recidivism related to illicit drug use.[45-47] It is important for clinicians to understand the unique epidemiologic risk profiles of the communities whom they serve and when appropriate to provided targeted screening and assessment for those at greatest risk.

COMORBID PSYCHIATRIC DISORDERS

Large-scale epidemiologic studies have also consistently shown a high degree of comorbidity of substance use disorders with other psychiatric disorders. Nationally representative studies such as the National Comorbidity Survey,[48] the Epidemiologic

Catchment Area Surveys,[49] the National Longitudinal Alcohol Epidemiologic Survey,[50] and the NESARC[3,51] have all indicated that a wide range of psychiatric disorders, including mood, anxiety, and some personality disorders, are highly associated with drug use disorders. Findings from several of these studies have further suggested that anxiety, mood, and antisocial personality disorders are more highly associated with substance dependence than substance abuse.[3,52,53] In addition, when these analyses controlled for the presence of multiple psychiatric disorders, the associations between individual psychiatric disorders and drug use disorders were reduced but overall remained substantial (**Table 1**).[3] This finding of the decreased magnitude of these associations suggests that common etiologies may underlie drug use disorders and other psychiatric disorders, findings consistent with twin and genetic studies.[54] Of note, numerous studies have found drug use disorders to be strongly associated with suicidal ideation and attempts, independent of other axis I and axis II disorders.[2,55-59] These findings also further highlight the importance of integrated drug abuse prevention, screening, and referral services in psychiatric treatment settings.[8,9,60-63] It is especially important for clinicians to recognize co-occurring substance use and psychiatric disorders and to treat them in an integrated and coordinated fashion.[8,9,61-64] Optimal treatment of either substance use or psychiatric disorders will not be achieved unless both are adequately treated.[8,9,60-63]

COMORBID HIV INFECTION WITH DRUG USE

Research on substance abuse epidemiology has also continued to examine the high degree of comorbidity of drug use with the ongoing HIV epidemic. Injection drug use remains an important risk factor for HIV infection, with an estimated 12% of persons with newly diagnosed HIV infections in the United States in 2009 reporting this as a contributing risk factor.[65] In addition, epidemiologic research has called increasing attention to the role that noninjection drug use has also played in fueling the epidemic.[66] Drugs such as methamphetamine are well-known to increase libido, reduce inhibitions, and cloud judgment, increasing the likelihood of high-risk behaviors that individuals might not have otherwise engaged in were it not for their drug use.[67,68]

A recent randomized, controlled trial among men who have sex with men who were methamphetamine dependent found that the addition of mirtazapine to substance use counseling significantly decreased not only methamphetamine use, but was also associated with decreases in a range of sexual risk behaviors.[69] Reductions in sexual risk behavior outcomes were associated with reductions in methamphetamine use among participants.[69] Larger scale replication trials are suggested, but the study findings highlight the importance of integrated prevention and treatment strategies for HIV and drug use disorders.

Multiple researchers now emphasize the importance of studying these comorbid epidemics of HIV and drug use disorders, along with other psychiatric disorders, as uniquely intertwined and fueled by a host of related social factors, referring to the combined phenomenon as a "syndemic."[70-72] Examining the multiplicity of factors related to these combined epidemics holds promise to shed new insights into the unique burden of these epidemics on some communities, in particular men who have sex with men and ethnic/racial minorities.[70,72,73] Multiple studies have suggested the value of combined, integrated approaches to the treatment of HIV, substance abuse, and mental health, with benefits including improved adherence to HIV treatment and improved HIV outcomes.[74-77] In particular, several studies have shown that combined opioid use disorder and HIV treatment is feasible and can be associated with improved initiation of antiretroviral therapy and improved CD4 counts.[74-76]

Table 1
Adjusted odds ratios (ORs) of 12-month DSM-IV drug use disorders and other psychiatric disorders controlling for demographic characteristics and comorbid psychiatric disorders in the NESARC study

Comorbid Disorder	ORs Adjusted for Demographic Characteristics[a]			ORs Adjusted for Demographic Characteristics and Other Psychiatric Disorders[b]		
	Drug Use Disorder OR (CI)[c]	Drug Abuse OR (CI)	Drug Dependence OR (CI)	Drug Use Disorder OR (CI)	Drug Abuse OR (CI)	Drug Dependence OR (CI)
Alcohol use disorder	9.0 (6.94–11.70)	6.4 (4.75–8.65)	15.0 (8.57–26.59)	5.6 (4.28–7.42)	4.5 (3.25–6.25)	7.0 (3.89–12.48)
Alcohol abuse	2.7 (1.98–3.71)	3.1 (2.18–4.50)	1.6 (0.88–3.01)	4.2 (3.03–5.85)	4.2 (2.87–6.13)	3.7 (1.79–7.58)
Alcohol dependence	9.7 (7.13–13.10)	5.7 (3.95–8.27)	18.7 (10.83–32.34)	6.8 (4.86–9.63)	4.8 (3.11–7.31)	9.0 (4.66–17.16)
Nicotine dependence	5.8 (4.41–7.63)	4.0 (2.86–5.69)	11.0 (6.89–17.56)	3.2 (2.38–4.38)	2.6 (1.76–3.79)	4.4 (2.63–7.42)
Any mood disorder	3.5 (2.66–4.53)	1.9 (1.34–2.70)	8.5 (5.27–13.64)	1.8 (1.33–2.41)	1.1 (0.73–1.67)	3.3 (1.92–5.56)
Major depressive disorder	2.2 (1.56–3.07)	1.4 (0.88–2.32)	3.8 (2.18–6.48)	1.4 (0.97–1.96)	1.0 (0.63–1.69)	2.2 (1.20–4.10)
Bipolar I	5.1 (3.35–7.80)	2.4 (1.38–4.21)	10.3 (5.75–18.62)	2.3 (1.49–3.67)	1.2 (0.61–2.24)	4.2 (2.14–8.35)
Bipolar II	2.4 (1.23–4.49)	2.1 (1.02–4.32)	2.6 (0.92–7.33)	1.2 (0.58–2.63)	1.2 (0.50–2.68)	1.4 (0.40–4.59)
Dysthymia	4.0 (2.17–7.20)	2.1 (0.85–5.25)	6.9 (3.28–14.67)	2.1 (1.15–3.84)	1.5 (0.62–3.76)	2.8 (1.16–6.67)
Any anxiety disorder	2.7 (2.05–3.67)	1.6 (1.15–2.25)	6.0 (3.74–9.55)	1.2 (0.88–1.73)	0.9 (0.62–1.34)	1.9 (1.07–3.24)
Any panic disorder	3.9 (2.58–5.87)	1.9 (1.02–3.62)	7.8 (4.31–14.05)	1.5 (0.91–2.39)	1.0 (0.49–2.10)	1.8 (0.85–3.81)
Panic with agoraphobia	5.6 (3.01–10.34)	3.2 (1.20–8.33)	9.2 (3.98–21.24)	1.7 (0.80–3.57)	1.4 (0.51–4.03)	1.5 (0.44–4.93)
Panic without agoraphobia	3.1 (1.87–5.14)	1.4 (0.62–3.32)	6.4 (3.21–12.58)	1.3 (0.75–2.28)	0.8 (0.32–2.13)	1.8 (0.85–3.94)
Social phobia	2.6 (1.69–4.15)	1.7 (0.94–3.00)	4.5 (2.53–8.16)	1.2 (0.71–1.93)	1.1 (0.58–2.04)	1.2 (0.58–2.48)
Specific phobia	2.3 (1.65–3.21)	1.6 (1.06–2.47)	3.8 (2.14–6.73)	1.0 (0.68–1.41)	0.9 (0.58–1.46)	1.0 (0.53–2.00)
Generalized anxiety	4.5 (2.80–7.09)	2.0 (0.98–4.00)	9.5 (4.82–18.83)	1.7 (0.97–2.92)	1.1 (0.51–2.28)	2.5 (1.02–5.88)

Any personality disorder	4.1 (3.27–5.15)	2.6 (1.94–3.49)	9.6 (6.44–14.43)	2.2 (1.71–2.91)	1.8 (1.26–2.48)	3.3 (2.00–5.33)
Avoidant	3.4 (2.25–5.12)	2.0 (1.05–3.69)	6.0 (3.19–11.34)	1.3 (0.85–2.05)	1.1 (0.56–2.30)	1.3 (0.63–2.60)
Dependent	7.3 (3.65–14.54)	2.4 (0.89–6.67)	14.9 (6.36–34.71)	2.2 (1.02–4.80)	1.1 (0.37–3.20)	2.4 (0.75–7.77)
Obsessive-compulsive	2.3 (1.65–3.15)	1.4 (0.87–2.17)	4.6 (2.91–7.34)	0.9 (0.57–1.33)	0.7 (0.40–1.23)	1.2 (0.69–2.10)
Paranoid	3.5 (2.49–4.86)	2.0 (1.28–3.00)	6.7 (4.09–11.07)	1.1 (0.66–1.68)	0.9 (0.48–1.50)	1.1 (0.59–2.22)
Schizoid	3.4 (2.33–5.03)	2.1 (1.26–3.56)	5.8 (3.35–10.11)	1.5 (0.88–2.44)	1.2 (0.66–2.32)	1.5 (0.74–3.21)
Histrionic	4.5 (2.98–6.77)	2.5 (1.45–4.21)	8.4 (4.69–14.92)	1.3 (0.79–2.20)	1.0 (0.58–1.86)	1.4 (0.63–3.03)
Antisocial	6.4 (4.77–8.56)	4.3 (2.84–6.50)	9.7 (6.29–15.10)	2.9 (2.08–4.12)	2.5 (1.57–3.99)	2.6 (1.45–4.53)

Note: Significant odds ratios are highlighted in boldface.

[a] Odds ratios adjusted for age, race-ethnicity, sex, education, income, marital status, urbanicity, and geographic region.

[b] Odds ratios adjusted for age, race-ethnicity, sex, education, income, marital status, urbanicity, geographic region, and other psychiatric disorders.

[c] CI = 99% confidence interval.

Data from Compton WM, Thomas YF, Stinson FS, et al. Prevalence, correlates, disability, and comorbidity of DSM-IV drug abuse and dependence in the United States: results from the National Epidemiologic Survey on Alcohol and Related Conditions. Arch Gen Psychiatry 2007;64:566–76.

GENETIC EPIDEMIOLOGY OF DRUG USE DISORDERS

Of the various risk factors for drug use disorders, family history has been identified as one of the most consistently and strongly associated factors. Large-scale family studies have consistently suggested the clustering of drug use disorders in families, and twin and adoption studies have provided support for the important role of genetic factors in this clustering.[54,78] Multiple such studies have shown significantly increased risk of substance use disorders in first-degree relatives and children of persons with a substance use disorder.[79–81] Moreover, genetic studies have provided substantial evidence for the combined role of genetic and environmental factors in drug use disorders.

Several studies have indicated that drug use disorders, but not drug use itself, are significantly associated with genetic factors.[54] This finding suggests the important role of developmental and environmental factors in determining who is exposed to and initiates illicit drug use, with genetic factors then contributing in determining an individual's risk of going on to develop a drug use disorder. For example, findings from several studies, including a large, longitudinal cohort study, suggest that childhood self-control—which itself is likely influenced by genetic, developmental, and other environmental factors—is strongly predictive of adult drug use disorders and a range of other outcomes, including adult physical health, income, and criminal involvement.[82–86] Such research suggests that interventions that target improved childhood self-control could have profound influence on a range of individual and societal outcomes, including rates of substance use, despite the role of other genetic and environmental factors in influencing these outcomes.[85,86] As with many common human disorders, it is likely that factors associated with drug use disorders include a large host of multiple possible genes, each exerting a small degree of influence, multiple developmental and environmental factors, and complex interactions among these factors.[54,81,86–88] Although still in its infancy, this research promises one day to improve clinicians understanding of the unique risk and protective factors affecting individual patients, for example, possibly allowing providers to assess which patients have unique opioid receptor polymorphisms that might place them at increased risk of prescription opioid misuse.[89–91]

SUMMARY

Research on the epidemiology of illicit drug use disorders provides continued critical insights into the distribution and determinants of drug use and drug use disorders in the United States. This research serves as a foundation for understanding the etiology of these disorders, helping to disentangle the complex interrelationship of developmental, genetic, and environmental risk and protective factors. Building on an understanding of this research in substance abuse epidemiology, it is important for clinicians to understand the unique trends in drug use in the overall communities that they serve and the unique risk factors for given individuals. The generally high prevalence of substance use disorders, along with their high comorbidity with other psychiatric disorders and with the HIV epidemic, make prevention, evaluation, and referral for treatment for drug abuse an important part of routine clinical practice in a range of clinical settings, including primary care, psychiatric, and emergency department settings. Ongoing efforts to ensure insurance coverage parity for the treatment of mental health and substance use disorders offer the promise of continued improvements in the integration and availability of such services in the broader US health care system.[92,93]

REFERENCES

1. Johnston LD, O'Malley PM, Bachman JG, et al. Monitoring the future: National Survey Results on Drug Use, 1975–2011. Bethesda (MD): National Institute on Drug Abuse; 2011.
2. Substance Abuse and Mental Health Services Administration. Results From the 2010 National Survey on Drug Use and Health: National Findings. Rockville (MD): DHHS; 2011.
3. Compton WM, Thomas YF, Stinson FS, et al. Prevalence, correlates, disability, and comorbidity of DSM-IV drug abuse and dependence in the United States: results from the National Epidemiologic Survey on Alcohol and Related Conditions. Arch Gen Psychiatry 2007;64:566–76.
4. Babor TF, McRee BG, Kassebaum PA, et al. Screening, Brief Intervention, and Referral to Treatment (SBIRT): toward a public health approach to the management of substance abuse. Subst Abus 2007;28:7–30.
5. Gryczynski J, Mitchell SG, Peterson TR, et al. The relationship between services delivered and substance use outcomes in New Mexico's Screening, Brief Intervention, Referral and Treatment (SBIRT) Initiative. Drug Alcohol Depend 2011;118:152–7.
6. Odgers CL, Caspi A, Nagin DS, et al. Is it important to prevent early exposure to drugs and alcohol among adolescents? Psychol Sci 2008;19:1037–44.
7. American Academy of Pediatrics Substance Use Screening, Brief Intervention, and Referral to Treatment for Pediatricians, 2011. Available at: http://aappolicy. aappublications.org/cgi/content/full/pediatrics;128/5/e1330. Accessed November 22, 2011.
8. Davoudi M, Rawson RA. Screening, brief intervention, and referral to treatment (SBIRT) initiatives in California: notable trends, challenges, and recommendations. J Psychoactive Drugs 2010;6(Suppl):239–48.
9. Madras BK, Compton WM, Avula D, et al. Screening, brief interventions, referral to treatment (SBIRT) for illicit drug and alcohol use at multiple healthcare sites: comparison at intake and 6 months later. Drug Alcohol Depend 2009;99:280–95.
10. Ballesteros MF, Budnitz DS, Sanford CP, et al. Increase in deaths due to methadone in North Carolina. JAMA 2003;290:40.
11. Hall AJ, Logan JE, Toblin RL, et al. Patterns of abuse among unintentional pharmaceutical overdose fatalities. JAMA 2008;300:2613–20.
12. Compton WM, Volkow ND. Major increases in opioid analgesic abuse: concerns and strategies. Drug Alcohol Depend 2006;81:103–7.
13. Ling W, Mooney L, Hillhouse M. Prescription opioid abuse, pain and addiction: clinical issues and implications. Drug Alcohol Rev 2011;30:300–5.
14. Paulozzi LJ, Jones CM, Mack KA, et al. Overdoses of prescription opioid pain relievers: United States, 1999–2008. Morbid Mortal Wkly Rep (MMWR) 2011;60:1487–92.
15. Boyd CJ, McCabe SE, Cranford JA, et al. Adolescents' motivations to abuse prescription medications. Pediatrics 2006;118:2472–80.
16. McCabe SE, Boyd CJ, Young A. Medical and nonmedical use of prescription drugs among secondary school students. J Adolesc Health 2007;40:76–83.
17. Lewis ET, Trafton JA. Opioid use in primary care: asking the right questions. Curr Pain Headache Rep 2011;15:137–43.
18. Meltzer EC, Rybin D, Saitz R, et al. Identifying prescription opioid use disorder in primary care: diagnostic characteristics of the Current Opioid Misuse Measure (COMM). Pain 2011;152:397–402.
19. Cheatle MD, O'Brien CP. Opioid therapy in patients with chronic noncancer pain: diagnostic and clinical challenges. Adv Psychosom Med 2011;30:61–91.

20. McCarberg BH. Pain management in primary care: strategies to mitigate opioid misuse, abuse, and diversion. Postgrad Med 2011;123:119–30.

21. Litt MD, Shafer DM, Kreutzer DL. Brief cognitive-behavioral treatment for TMD pain: long-term outcomes and moderators of treatment. Pain 2010;151:110–6.

22. Thorn BE, Day MA, Burns JW, et al. Randomized trial of group cognitive behavioral therapy compared with a pain education control for low-literacy rural people with chronic pain. Pain 2011;152:1–11.

23. Lamb SE, Hansen Z, Lall R, et al. Group cognitive behavioural treatment for low-back pain in primary care: a randomised controlled trial and cost-effectiveness analysis. Lancet 2010;375:916–23.

24. Grant BF, Dawson DA, Stinson FS, et al. The 12-month prevalence and trends in DSM-IV alcohol abuse and dependence: United States, 1991–1992 and 2001–2002. Drug Alcohol Depend 2004;74:223–34.

25. Mark TL, Coffey RM, King E, et al. Spending on mental health and substance abuse treatment, 1987–1997. Health Aff (Millwood) 2000;19:108–20.

26. Dilonardo J, Chalk M, Mark TL, et al; Team CCSE. Recent trends in the financing of substance abuse treatment: implications for the future. Health Serv Res 2000;35:60–71.

27. Office of National Drug Control Policy. The economic costs of drug abuse in the United States, 1992–1998. Washington, DC: Executive Office of the President; 2001.

28. Grant BF. Prevalence and correlates of drug use and DSM-IV drug dependence in the United States: results of the National Longitudinal Alcohol Epidemiologic Survey. J Subst Abuse 1996;8:195–210.

29. Teesson M, Baillie A, Lynskey M, et al. Substance use, dependence and treatment seeking in the United States and Australia: a cross-national comparison. Drug Alcohol Depend 2006;81:149–55.

30. Costello EJ, Farmer EM, Angold A, et al. Psychiatric disorders among American Indian and white youth in Appalachia: the Great Smoky Mountains Study. Am J Public Health 1997;87:827–32.

31. Wu L-T, Woody GE, Yang C, et al. Racial/ethnic variations in substance-related disorders among adolescents in the United States. Arch Gen Psychiatry 2011;68: 1176–85.

32. Gilder DA, Wall TL, Ehlers CL. Comorbidity of select anxiety and affective disorders with alcohol dependence in southwest California Indians. Alcohol Clin Exp Res 2004;28:1805–13.

33. Beals J, Novins DK, Whitesell NR, et al. Prevalence of mental disorders and utilization of mental health services in two American Indian reservation populations: mental health disparities in a national context. Am J Psychiatry 2005;162:1723–32.

34. Arndt S, Clayton R, Schultz SK. Trends in substance abuse treatment 1998–2008: increasing older adult first-time admissions for illicit drugs. Am J Geriatr Psychiatry 2011;19:704–11.

35. Arndt S, Gunter TD, Acion L. Older admissions to substance abuse treatment in 2001. Am J Geriatr Psychiatry 2005;13:385–92.

36. Lofwall MR, Schuster A, Strain EC. Changing profile of abused substances by older persons entering treatment. J Nerv Ment Dis 2008;196:898–905.

37. Gfroerer J, Penne M, Pemberton M, et al. Substance abuse treatment need among older adults in 2020: the impact of the aging baby-boom cohort. Drug Alcohol Depend 2003;69:127–35.

38. Colliver JD, Compton WM, Gfroerer JC, et al. Projecting drug use among aging baby boomers in 2020. Ann Epidemiol 2006;16:257–65.

39. Cochran SD, Ackerman D, Mays VM, et al. Prevalence of non-medical drug use and dependence among homosexually active men and women in the US population. Addiction (Abingdon, England) 2004;99:989–98.
40. Cochran SD, Mays VM. Burden of psychiatric morbidity among lesbian, gay, and bisexual individuals in the California Quality of Life Survey. J Abnorm Psychol 2009; 118:647–58.
41. Corliss HL, Grella CE, Mays VM, et al. Drug use, drug severity, and help-seeking behaviors of lesbian and bisexual women. J Womens Health (Larchmt) 2006;15: 556–68.
42. Corliss HL, Rosario M, Wypij D, et al. Sexual orientation and drug use in a longitudinal cohort study of U.S. adolescents. Addict Behav 2010;35:517–21.
43. Grella CE, Greenwell L, Mays VM, et al. Influence of gender, sexual orientation, and need on treatment utilization for substance use and mental disorders: findings from the California Quality of Life Survey. BMC Psychiatry 2009;9:52.
44. Almeida J, Johnson RM, Corliss HL, et al. Emotional distress among LGBT youth: the influence of perceived discrimination based on sexual orientation. J Youth Adolesc 2009;38:1001–14.
45. Zarkin GA, Cowell AJ, Hicks KA, et al. Benefits and costs of substance abuse treatment programs for state prison inmates: results from a lifetime simulation model. Health Econ 2011;14:1133–50.
46. French MT, Fang H, Fretz R. Economic evaluation of a prerelease substance abuse treatment program for repeat criminal offenders. J Subst Abuse Treat 2010;38:31–41.
47. Chandler RK, Fletcher BW, Volkow ND. Treating drug abuse and addiction in the criminal justice system: improving public health and safety. JAMA 2009;301:183–90.
48. Warner LA, Kessler RC, Hughes M, et al. Prevalence and correlates of drug use and dependence in the United States. Results from the National Comorbidity Survey. Arch Gen Psychiatry 1995;52:219–29.
49. Regier DA, Farmer ME, Rae DS, et al. Comorbidity of mental disorders with alcohol and other drug abuse: Results from the Epidemiologic Catchment Area (ECA) Study. JAMA 1990;264:2511–8.
50. Grant BF. Comorbidity between DSM-IV drug use disorders and major depression: results of a national survey of adults. J Substance Abuse 1995;7:481–97.
51. Grant BF, Stinson FS, Dawson DA, et al. Prevalence and co-occurrence of substance use disorders and independent mood and anxiety disorders: results from the National Epidemiologic Survey on Alcohol and Related Conditions. Arch Gen Psychiatry 2004;61:807–16.
52. Merikangas KR, Mehta RL, Molnar BE, et al. Comorbidity of substance use disorders with mood and anxiety disorders: results of the International Consortium in Psychiatric Epidemiology. Addict Behav 1998;23:893–907.
53. Swendsen JD, Merikangas KR. The comorbidity of depression and substance use disorders. Clin Psychol Rev 2000;20:173–89.
54. Kendler KS, Prescott CA, Myers J, et al. The structure of genetic and environmental risk factors for common psychiatric and substance use disorders in men and women. Arch Gen Psychiatry 2003;60:929–37.
55. Cheatle MD. Depression, chronic pain, and suicide by overdose: on the edge. Pain Med 2011;12(Suppl 2):S43–8.
56. Hakansson A, Schlyter F, Berglund M. Associations between polysubstance use and psychiatric problems in a criminal justice population in Sweden. Drug Alcohol Depend 2011;118:5–11.

57. Gao K, Tolliver BK, Kemp DE, et al. Correlates of historical suicide attempt in rapid-cycling bipolar disorder: a cross-sectional assessment. J Clin Psychiatry 2009; 70:1032–40.
58. Overholser JC, Braden A, Dieter L. Understanding suicide risk: Identification of high-risk groups during high-risk times. J Clin Psychol 2011;2:1–15.
59. Nordentoft M, Mortensen PB, Pedersen CB. Absolute risk of suicide after first hospital contact in mental disorder. Arch Gen Psychiatry 2011;68:1058–64.
60. Kessler RC, Nelson CB, McGonagle KA, et al. The epidemiology of co-occurring addictive and mental disorders: implications for prevention and service utilization. Am J Orthopsychiatry 1996;66:17–31.
61. RachBeisel J, Scott J, Dixon L. Co-occurring severe mental illness and substance use disorders: a review of recent research. Psychiatr Serv 1999;50:1427–34.
62. Havassy BE, Alvidrez J, Owen KK. Comparisons of patients with comorbid psychiatric and substance use disorders: implications for treatment and service delivery. Am J Psychiatry 2004;161:139–45.
63. Curran GM, Sullivan G, Williams K, et al. The association of psychiatric comorbidity and use of the emergency department among persons with substance use disorders: an observational cohort study. BMC Emerg Med 2008;8:17.
64. Durell J, Lechtenberg B, Corse S, et al. Intensive case management of persons with chronic mental illness who abuse substances. Hosp Community Psychiatry 1993;44: 415–6.
65. U.S. Centers for Disease Control and Prevention (CDC). HIV incidence. Available at: http://www.cdc.gov/hiv/topics/surveillance/incidence.htm. Accessed October 25, 2011.
66. Woody GE, Donnell D, Seage GR, et al. Non-injection substance use correlates with risky sex among men having sex with men: data from HIVNET. Drug Alcohol Depend 1999;53:197–205.
67. Mansergh G, Purcell DW, Stall R, et al. CDC consultation on methamphetamine use and sexual risk behavior for HIV/STD infection: summary and suggestions. Public Health Rep 2006;121:127–32.
68. Krawczyk CS, Molitor F, Ruiz J, et al. Methamphetamine use and HIV risk behaviors among heterosexual men: preliminary results from five northern California counties, December 2001–November 2003. MMWR 2006;55:273–7.
69. Colfax GN, Santos G-M, Das M, et al. Mirtazapine to reduce methamphetamine use: a randomized controlled trial. Arch Gen Psychiatry 2011;68:1168–75.
70. Walkup J, Blank MB, Gonzalez JS, et al. The impact of mental health and substance abuse factors on HIV prevention and treatment. J Acquir Immune Defic Syndr 2008;47(Suppl 1):S15–9.
71. Des Jarlais DC, Semaan S. HIV prevention for injecting drug users: the first 25 years and counting. Psychosom Med 2008;70:606–11.
72. Mustanski B, Garofalo R, Herrick A, et al. Psychosocial health problems increase risk for HIV among urban young men who have sex with men: preliminary evidence of a syndemic in need of attention. Ann Behav Med 2007;34:37–45.
73. Friedman SR, Tempalski B, Cooper H, et al. Metropolitan area characteristics, injection drug use and HIV among injectors. In: Thomas YF, Richardson D, Cheung I, editors. Geography and drug addiction. Washington, DC: Springer; 2008. p. 255–65.
74. Batkis MF, Treisman GJ, Angelino AF. Integrated opioid use disorder and HIV treatment: rationale, clinical guidelines for addiction treatment, and review of interactions of antiretroviral agents and opioid agonist therapies. AIDS Patient Care STDS 2010;24:15–22.

75. Altice FL, Bruce RD, Lucas GM, et al. HIV treatment outcomes among HIV-infected, opioid-dependent patients receiving buprenorphine/naloxone treatment within HIV clinical care settings: results from a multisite study. J Acquir Immune Defic Syndr 2011;56(Suppl 1):S22–32.
76. Uhlmann S, Milloy MJ, Kerr T, et al. Methadone maintenance therapy promotes initiation of antiretroviral therapy among injection drug users. Addiction (Abingdon, England) 2010;105:907–13.
77. Waldron PR, Angelino AF, Treisman GJ. Substance use disorders and HIV: common co-morbidities requiring co-ordinated management. European Infectious Disease 2009;24:44–51.
78. Bierut LJ, Dinwiddie SH, Begleiter H, et al. Familial transmission of substance dependence: alcohol, marijuana, cocaine, and habitual smoking: a report from the Collaborative Study on the Genetics of Alcoholism. Arch Gen Psychiatry 1998;55: 982–8.
79. Chassin L, Pitts SC, Prost J. Binge drinking trajectories from adolescence to emerging adulthood in a high-risk sample: predictors and substance abuse outcomes. J Consult Clin Psychol 2002;70:67–78.
80. Moss HB, Lynch KG, Hardie TL, et al. Family functioning and peer affiliation in children of fathers with antisocial personality disorder and substance dependence: associations with problem behaviors. Am J Psychiatry 2002;159:607–14.
81. Compton WM, Cottler LB, Ridenour T, et al. The specificity of family history of alcohol and drug abuse in cocaine abusers. Am J Addict 2002;11:85–94.
82. Bouchard TJ Jr, McGue M. Genetic and environmental influences on human psychological differences. J Neurobiol 2003;54:4–45.
83. Ebstein RP. The molecular genetic architecture of human personality: beyond self-report questionnaires. Mol Psychiatry 2006;11:427–45.
84. Kochanska G, Coy KC, Murray KT. The development of self-regulation in the first four years of life. Child Dev 2001;72:1091–111.
85. Caspi A, Moffitt TE, Newman DL, et al. Behavioral observations at age 3 years predict adult psychiatric disorders. Longitudinal evidence from a birth cohort. Arch Gen Psychiatry 1996;53:1033–9.
86. Moffitt TE, Arseneault L, Belsky D, et al. A gradient of childhood self-control predicts health, wealth, and public safety. Proc Natl Acad Sci U S A 2011;108:2693–8.
87. Caspi A, McClay J, Moffitt TE, et al. Role of genotype in the cycle of violence in maltreated children. Science 2002;297:851–4.
88. Foley DL, Eaves LJ, Wormley B, et al. Childhood adversity, monoamine oxidase a genotype, and risk for conduct disorder. Arch Gen Psychiatry 2004;61:738–44.
89. Nagashima M, Katoh R, Sato Y, et al. Is there genetic polymorphism evidence for individual human sensitivity to opiates? Curr Pain Headache Rep 2007;11:115–23.
90. Fukuda K-i, Hayashida M, Ikeda K, et al. Diversity of opioid requirements for postoperative pain control following oral surgery: is it affected by polymorphism of the mu-opioid receptor? Anesth Prog 2010;57:145–9.
91. Tremblay J, Hamet P. Genetics of pain, opioids, and opioid responsiveness. Metabolism 2010;59(Suppl 1):S5–8.
92. Barry CL, Huskamp HA. Moving beyond parity: mental health and addiction care under the ACA. N Engl J Med 2011;365:973–5.
93. Garfield RL, Zuvekas SH, Lave JR, et al. The impact of national health care reform on adults with severe mental disorders. Am J Psychiatry 2011;168:486–94.

Psychostimulant Treatment of Cocaine Dependence

John J. Mariani, MD[a,b,]*, Frances R. Levin, MD[a,b]

KEYWORDS

- Cocaine dependence • Psychostimulant • Substance abuse • Amphetamines
- Methylphenidate • Dopamine

KEY POINTS

- A reinforcer, in terms of mechanisms of addiction, can be defined operationally as any event that increases the probability of a response; psychostimulants increase extracellular dopamine in the brain, which is associated with both therapeutic and reinforcing effects.
- Substitution pharmacotherapy, which has been proven effective for opioid and nicotine dependence, is a promising strategy for cocaine dependence.
- Misuse, diversion, and addiction are inherent risks of prescribing controlled substances; all patients prescribed controlled substances should be assessed at each visit for signs of misuse, abuse, or addiction.

Cocaine dependence continues to be a substantial public health problem in the United States, yet no clearly effective pharmacotherapy has been identified. There are approximately 1.6 million current users of cocaine in the United States,[1] and the past-year prevalence of cocaine dependence is estimated to be 1.1%.[2] Controlled trials of behavioral treatments for cocaine dependence yield abstinence rates of up to 30%,[3] with the majority of patients continuing to use cocaine. Scores of double-blind, placebo-controlled pharmacotherapy clinical trials for cocaine dependence have been conducted[4-6] testing agents drawn from a wide variety of medication classes. Stimulants have shown promise as a treatment for cocaine dependence, despite resistance in the field to using controlled substances as therapeutic agents for addictive disorders.

Psychoactive drugs that cause addiction generally do so by increasing dopamine release within the nucleus accumbens.[7] Cocaine binds to the dopamine transporter and inhibits catecholamine reuptake,[8] directly increasing synaptic dopamine levels in

[a] Division of Substance Abuse, New York State Psychiatric Institute, 1051 Riverside Drive, New York, NY 10032, USA; [b] Department of Psychiatry, College of Physicians and Surgeons of Columbia University, 630 West 168th Street, New York, NY 10032, USA
* Corresponding author. Division of Substance Abuse, New York State Psychiatric Institute, 1051 Riverside Drive, New York, NY 10032.
E-mail address: jm2330@columbia.edu

Psychiatr Clin N Am 35 (2012) 425–439
http://dx.doi.org/10.1016/j.psc.2012.03.012
0193-953X/12/$ – see front matter © 2012 Elsevier Inc. All rights reserved.

the meso-cortico-limbic system. The increased levels of dopamine in the synaptic cleft result in increased activation of type 1 and type 2 dopamine receptors. Although the behavioral effects of cocaine are attributed primarily to the blockade of dopamine reuptake, cocaine also blocks the reuptake of the other major monoamines neurotransmitters, norepinephrine and serotonin.

Stimulant medications can be defined broadly as agents that produce behavioral arousal, typically acting, either directly or indirectly, through a sympathomimetic mechanism of action, stimulating α- and β-adrenergic receptors or increasing dopamine and norepinephrine in the synaptic cleft. Stimulant medications available in the United States for psychiatric treatment include amphetamine analogs, methamphetamine, methylphenidate, modafinil, and armodafinil. Other sympathomimetics that are available for short-term appetite suppression include benzphetamine, phentermine, diethylpropion, phenmetrazine, phendimetrazine, and mazindol. However, there are other medications, not usually classified as stimulants, that affect catecholamine reuptake and have some stimulantlike properties. Certain antidepressant medications, such as bupropion, which blocks the reuptake of dopamine and norepinephrine, have weak stimulant properties. Drugs such as levodopa increase dopamine release into the synaptic space in a manner similar to that of stimulant medications but do not cause behavioral activation and, for the purposes of this review, will be discussed as dopamine agonists. As a class of medications, classical psychostimulants, including the amphetamines and methylphenidate, have a rapid onset of action, immediate behavioral effects, and the propensity to induce tolerance, all of which present a risk of misuse and dependence in vulnerable individuals and have been classified as controlled drugs; their distribution and use are regulated by state and federal agencies.

Substitution pharmacotherapy, which has been proven effective for opioid[9] and nicotine[10] dependence, is a plausible strategy for treating cocaine dependence. Conceptually, the goal of substitution pharmacotherapy is to replace a drug of abuse with rapid onset and a brief half-life with an agent that has a more gradual onset of action and long half-life, resulting in less intoxication and withdrawal, reducing the cycle of compulsive use. Successful examples of this approach include the use of methadone or buprenorphine for the treatment of opioid dependence and the use of transdermal nicotine or varenicline for nicotine dependence. Long-acting replacement medications reduce craving and potentially blunt the effects of the primary substance by either receptor blockade (buprenorphine or varenicline) or inducing high levels of physiologic tolerance (methadone). Because cocaine is a short-acting psychostimulant with a rapid onset of action, a potential treatment strategy for cocaine dependence would be to substitute a longer-acting psychostimulant medication with a slower onset of action.

NEUROBIOLOGY OF STIMULANT TREATMENT FOR COCAINE DEPENDENCE

The concept of reinforcement is central to understanding the mechanism of addiction. A reinforcer can be defined operationally as any event that increases the probability of a response. When a drug is said to have reinforcing effects, exposure to the drug makes it likely that the animal or human will work to be re-exposed to the drug. For most substances that have addictive potential, the mechanism of reinforcement is thought to be via dopamine release in the nucleus accumbens.

The acute dosing of amphetamine has been associated with priming effects for rats previously trained to self-administer cocaine. Acute administration of dextroamphetamine into the basolateral amygdala, in combination with conditioned cue presentation, to rats trained to self-administer cocaine has been shown to potentiate reinstatement of cocaine-seeking behavior.[11] Amphetamine infusion in the absence of conditioned cues failed to reinstate the extinguished response. The facilitation of conditioned-cue reinstatement produced by amphetamine was apparent only during the initial half hour of the test session. These results suggest that while acute administration of amphetamine may potentiate cocaine reinforcement, more chronic exposure to amphetamine does not.

Animal laboratory studies have found that sustained dextroamphetamine administration can attenuate the reinforcing effects of cocaine. Dextroamphetamine has been shown to produce dose-dependent reductions in cocaine self-administration in rats.[12] In monkeys, oral dextroamphetamine pretreatment decreased responding for a sweetened cocaine fluid.[13] Dextroamphetamine administered by slow intravenous infusion has been shown to decrease cocaine self-administration in rhesus monkeys in a dose-dependent manner, possibly by attenuating the reinforcing effects of cocaine.[14,15] Further work with monkeys has suggested that continued treatment with dextroamphetamine may be necessary to produce a sustained reduction in the reinforcing effects of cocaine.[16] These preclinical data suggest that amphetamine administration must be of a sufficient dose and duration to affect cocaine reinforcement.

Human laboratory experiments have evaluated the effects of stimulant administration on models of cocaine self-administration. Initial studies investigated the possibility that stimulant treatment of cocaine-dependent patients would worsen cocaine craving and use. In a combination clinical trial and human laboratory study, Grabowski and colleagues[17] found that methylphenidate did not "prime" patients to use cocaine. Methylphenidate has been shown to be safe and not associated with increased cocaine craving or stimulant-related euphoria in the human laboratory.[18] Dextroamphetamine has been shown to be safe and well tolerated when co-administered with cocaine and attenuates some of the subjective effects of cocaine.[19] Dextroamphetamine has also been found to alter cocaine self-administration, most likely by altering the reinforcing effects of cocaine.[20] These human laboratory experiments support the potential utility of stimulant treatment of cocaine dependence.

In current medical practice, the most common clinical use of psychostimulant medication is to treat attention-deficit/hyperactivity disorder (ADHD). In patients with ADHD, stimulants have been found to be preferred to placebo using a laboratory choice procedure, although this preference is thought to be because of symptom relief rather than abuse potential.[21] In the human laboratory, methylphenidate administration has been found to reduce cocaine self-administration in individuals with and without ADHD.[22] These results suggest that stimulant pharmacotherapy is a potential approach for treating co-occurring ADHD and cocaine dependence.

Brain imaging studies of cocaine-dependent individuals have been used to examine the potential mechanism for psychostimulant pharmacotherapy of cocaine dependence. Functional magnetic resonance imaging has shown methylphenidate to be associated with robustly decreased stop signal reaction time, an index of improved control, in cocaine-dependent patients, a population in which inhibitory control is impaired.[23] Methylphenidate has also been shown using functional magnetic resonance imaging to increase responses to a salient cognitive task, and these improvements were correlated with attenuation of anterior cingulate cortex hypoactivation.[24] Using positron emission tomography and 2-fluoro-D-glucose to measure brain glucose metabolism as a marker of brain function, methylphenidate has been found to attenuate brain reactivity to cocaine cues.[25] Brain imaging using the positron emission tomography raclopride displacement procedure has shown that deficient dopamine transmission is associated with failure to respond to behavioral treatment.[26] Brain imaging of cocaine-dependent individuals receiving psychostimulants is at an early stage of development, but the initial results are quite promising in terms of both understanding the brain physiologic deficits associated with cocaine dependence as well as the potential therapeutic mechanisms of stimulant pharmacotherapy. If deficient dopamine transmission predicts poor response to behavioral interventions, then stimulant medication treatment could potentially reverse this deficit.

The association of deficient dopamine signaling with poor response to behavioral treatment[26] in particular highlights the proposed mechanism by which stimulant medications may be effective for treating cocaine dependence. Intact dopamine signaling is required for response to naturally occurring (eg, social or work relationships) or therapeutically manipulated (eg, vouchers) contingencies. In a dopamine-deficient state, noncocaine rewards are not as salient as the rewarding effects of cocaine. Stimulant medication may correct the deficits in dopaminergic signaling in cocaine-dependent individuals, thereby enhancing dopamine release in response to environmental contingencies, thereby improving the salience of competing reinforcers to cocaine.

STIMULANT PHARMACOTHERAPY FOR COCAINE DEPENDENCE

Double-blind, placebo-controlled trials of stimulant medications for cocaine dependence are listed in **Table 1**. The studies, arranged by therapeutic drug class, are discussed below.

Amphetamines

Amphetamines cause release of monoamines, in particular dopamine, and also block monoamine reuptake.[27] These actions are similar to those of cocaine (dopamine reuptake blockade), although the half-life of amphetamines, in particular long-acting formulations,[28] are much longer than cocaine.

Dextroamphetamine has been evaluated in outpatient clinical trials for cocaine dependence. Grabowski and colleagues[29] compared dextroamphetamine in 2 escalating dosing schedules (15 to 30 mg daily and 30 to 60 mg daily) with placebo for the treatment of cocaine dependence in 128 outpatients. Retention was best for the 15- to 30-mg group, and the proportion of positive urine toxicology samples was lowest for the 30- to 60-mg group, followed by the 15- to 30-mg group and then the placebo group. Grabowski and coworkers[30] also compared dextroamphetamine in 2 different escalating dose regimens with placebo for the treatment of cocaine- and opioid-dependent patients (n = 120) receiving methadone maintenance treatment. The higher-dose group of dextroamphetamine (30 to 60 mg/d) was superior to both the lower dose group (15 to 30 mg/d) and placebo. Shearer and colleagues[31] evaluated dextroamphetamine for the treatment of cocaine dependence in a sample of 30 patients. No between-group differences were detected, although the small sample size suggests lack of statistical power to do so. Participants in the active medication group experienced reductions in the proportion of cocaine-positive urines, craving scores, and other measures of cocaine dependence severity, whereas those in the placebo group did not improve on these measures.

Methamphetamine, an amphetamine analogue with a similar mechanism of action to cocaine, has been studied for the treatment of cocaine dependence. Mooney and coworkers[32] reported that in 82 cocaine-dependent outpatients, the sustained release preparation of methamphetamine was found to be associated with lower rates of cocaine-positive urine samples and greater reduction in craving than placebo, whereas the immediate-release formulation of methamphetamine was not superior to placebo for cocaine use outcomes. Despite these promising results, no other

Table 1
Psychostimulant and dopaminergic treatment of cocaine dependence: double-blind placebo-controlled clinical trials

Study	Publication Year	Population	Medication	N	Results
Anderson et al[36]	2009	Cocaine dependence	Modafinil	210	No significant effect on primary outcome of cocaine abstinence
Dackis et al[35]	2005	Cocaine dependence	Modafinil	62	Modafinil associated with more cocaine-negative urines and cocaine abstinence
Elkashef et al48	2006	Cocaine dependence	Selegiline	300	No differences between selegiline and placebo
Grabowski et al[17]	1997	Cocaine dependence	Methylphenidate	24	No differences between groups, limited statistical power
Grabowski et al[29]	2001	Cocaine dependence	Dextroamphetamine	128	Dextroamphetamine 30–60 mg superior to 15–30 mg and placebo for negative urine drug samples
Grabowski et al[30]	2004	Cocaine and opioid dependence receiving methadone	Dextroamphetamine	120	Reduction in cocaine use significant for 30–60 mg dosing of dextroamphetamine
Levin et al[42]	2007	Cocaine dependence and ADHD	Methylphenidate	106	Primary outcome not significant; secondary analysis showed lower probability of cocaine-positive urine samples for methylphenidate group; in methylphenidate group, ADHD responders more likely to have reduction in cocaine use
Margolin et al[33]	1995	Cocaine dependence	Bupropion	149	No differences between placebo and bupropion in primary analysis; depressed subgroup receiving bupropion with lower proportion positive urine toxicologies
Margolin et al[46]	1995b	Cocaine abuse and opioid dependence receiving methadone	Mazindol	37	No differences between placebo and mazindol, limited statistical power

(continued on next page)

Table 1
(Continued)

Study	Publication Year	Population	Medication	N	Results
Mooney et al[38]	2007	Cocaine dependence	Levodopa-carbidopa	189	No difference from placebo
Mooney et al[32]	2009	Cocaine dependence	Methamphetamine	82	Sustained-release formulation of methamphetamine associated with fewer cocaine-positive urines and less craving
Schubiner et al[41]	2002	Cocaine dependence and ADHD	Methylphenidate	48	ADHD symptoms improved on methylphenidate, no differences on cocaine use outcomes
Shearer et al[31]	2003	Cocaine dependence	Dextroamphetamine	30	No between-group differences, limited statistical power
Shoptaw	2008	Cocaine abuse or dependence	Bupropion	70	No differences between placebo and bupropion, no impact of depressive symptoms on outcome
Stine et al[34]	1995	Cocaine dependence	Mazindol	43	No difference between mazindol and placebo, possible limited statistical power

randomized, placebo-controlled clinical trials have tested the use of methamphetamine for cocaine dependence.

Mazindol, a sympathomimetic amine similar to amphetamine, is a catecholamine reuptake blocker, and was among the first stimulant medications studied for the treatment of cocaine dependence. Margolin and coworkers[33] conducted a small double-blind, placebo-controlled trial of mazindol in 37 opioid-dependent methadone maintenance patients with cocaine abuse and found no statistically significant difference between treatment groups. In a double-blind, placebo-controlled trial, Stine and colleagues[34] also evaluated mazindol in 43 cocaine-dependent outpatients and found no difference between treatment groups. These trials for testing mazindol did not yield significant results. However, given the relatively small sample sizes, these results are not likely to be definitive.

The results for dextroamphetamine and methamphetamine as potential treatments for cocaine dependence are promising, but there have been no large-scale, multisite trials confirming the results. A possible explanation for the lack of confirmatory studies despite promising initial results is that the field is resistant to investigating a controlled substance as a treatment for cocaine dependence. Other agents, with less or no abuse potential, including modafinil (discussed later)[35,36] and vigabatrin[37] proceeded relatively quickly to multisite trials based on the results of positive findings in single-site studies.

Dopamine Agonists

Medications that directly stimulate dopamine receptors or increase the levels of synaptic dopamine have a mechanism of action similar to stimulants, although they do not necessarily have the same activating effects on behavior. Mooney and coworkers[38] reported on 2 trials testing the combination of levodopa and carbidopa in 189 cocaine-dependent outpatients. Levodopa-carbidopa was well tolerated by cocaine-dependent patients but did not improve cocaine use outcomes compared with placebo. These results contrast the use of levodopa when combined with contingency management (discussed later).

Methylphenidate

Methylphenidate is structurally related to the amphetamines but differs in mechanism of action. The stimulant properties of methylphenidate are presumed to be mainly caused by inhibition of dopamine reuptake by binding to the dopamine transporter, whereas the primary action of amphetamine is to cause dopamine release into the synaptic cleft and secondarily block catecholamine reuptake.[39] Reuptake inhibition of norepinephrine by blockade for the norepinephrine transporter is presumed to be an important secondary mechanism of action of methylphenidate. The main clinical use of methylphenidate is, like for amphetamine, for the treatment of ADHD.

Methylphenidate has been investigated as a treatment for cocaine dependence. In a human laboratory study, methylphenidate has been found to be safe and well tolerated in doses up to 90 mg daily when co-administered with cocaine.[40] Grabowski and colleagues[17] compared methylphenidate with placebo for the treatment of cocaine dependence in 24 outpatients. Retention was equivalent between groups, with no significant differences in cocaine use outcomes, although statistical power was limited because of the small sample size. No significant adverse effects were reported. Larger, adequately powered studies examining the effect of methylphenidate on cocaine dependence have not been conducted.

Methylphenidate has also been studied as a treatment for cocaine dependence co-occurring with ADHD. Schubiner and colleagues[41] studied methylphenidate compared with placebo for the treatment of 48 cocaine-dependent adults with ADHD and found significantly greater ADHD symptom relief in the methylphenidate group but no group differences in cocaine use outcomes. Levin and coworkers[42] evaluated methylphenidate compared with placebo for the treatment of co-occurring ADHD and cocaine dependence in 106 outpatients. There were no significant between-group differences in ADHD symptom response or retention. Although the primary cocaine use outcome measure was negative, a secondary analysis using logistic regression found that methylphenidate was associated with a lower probability of cocaine-positive urine samples. Secondary analyses found that in the methylphenidate group, ADHD treatment responders were more likely to have a reduction in cocaine use compared with non-ADHD responders. These results suggest that methylphenidate has therapeutic effects on ADHD symptoms even in active cocaine users and that ADHD symptom response may be important for improving cocaine use outcomes in patients with co-occurring ADHD and cocaine dependence.

Modafinil and Armodafinil

Modafinil is a psychostimulant medication unrelated to the structure of amphetamine and has a differing profile of pharmacologic and behavioral effects.[43] Modafinil binds moderately to dopamine and norepinephrine transporters, increasing synaptic catecholamine levels. Elevations in other neurotransmitters appear to be secondary to changes in elevations in catecholamines.

Modafinil has been studied for the treatment of cocaine dependence and has been found to be safe and well tolerated when co-administered with cocaine.[44] Dackis and colleagues[35] conducted a pilot study of 62 cocaine-dependent participants and found that modafinil was superior to placebo in achieving abstinence and was associated with significantly more cocaine-negative urine samples. However, the follow-up multisite trial of 210 participants randomly assigned to placebo, modafinil 200 mg/d, or modafinil 400 mg/d, showed no advantage of modafinil on the primary outcome measure.[36] Secondary outcomes, including reduction of craving and the maximum number of consecutive nonuse days for cocaine, favored modafinil treatment, and a post hoc analysis showed a significant effect of modafinil on the weekly percentage of nonuse days in the subgroup of cocaine-dependent patients who did not have a history of alcohol dependence. Based on these data, modafinil does not appear to be effective for treating cocaine-dependent patients with a history of alcohol dependence but may be effective for cocaine-dependent patients without alcohol dependence. Future studies should exclude participants with alcohol dependence.

Stimulant Antidepressants

Bupropion is a novel antidepressant medication with a chemical structure dissimilar to existing antidepressant medications but slightly similar to the endogenous monoamine neurotransmitters, dopamine and norepinephrine. The presumed mechanism of action of bupropion has evolved over time and is now thought to be a result of reuptake inhibition of dopamine and norepinephrine by blocking the respective transporters.[45] The clinical profile of bupropion is that of mild stimulating effects.

Bupropion has been studied for the treatment of cocaine dependence. Margolin and coworkers[46] studied the bupropion for cocaine dependence in a multisite trial with 149 participants. No differences were observed between placebo and bupropion in cocaine use, depression, or psychosocial function. However, a secondary analysis found that among the subset of participants (n = 36) with baseline depression, there was a significant decrease in the proportion of urine toxicology samples positive for cocaine in the bupropion group. Shoptaw and colleagues[47] compared bupropion with placebo in a double-blind trail of 70 cocaine-dependent outpatients and found no differences between treatment groups. Secondary analyses found no significant differences by treatment group when controlling for baseline depression scores. The results of these 2 large clinical trials suggest that bupropion is not an effective treatment for cocaine dependence.

Selegiline is an irreversible selective inhibitor of monoamine oxidase type B. The inhibition of monoamine oxidase type B increases the concentration of dopamine and other neurotransmitters and is partially metabolized to *l*-methamphetamine and *l*-amphetamine. However, selegiline does not have consistent behavioral activation properties and should not be classified as a stimulant. Elkashef and colleagues[48] studied the use of a transdermal patch delivery system of selegiline for the treatment of 300 cocaine-dependent outpatients in a multisite, double-blind, placebo-controlled trial. No differences between selegiline and placebo were detected, suggesting that selegiline is not likely to have a role for treating cocaine dependence.

Table 2
Dopaminergic augmentation of contingency management treatment of cocaine dependence: double-blind, placebo-controlled trials

Study	Publication Year	Population	Medication	Behavioral Intervention	N	Results
Poling et al[51]	2006	Cocaine and opioid dependence receiving methadone	bupropion	Contingency management	106	Bupropion with contingency management more effective than bupropion alone
Schmitz et al[49]	2008	Cocaine dependence	Levodopa-carbidopa	Voucher incentives, CBT, and clinical management	161	Levodopa with vouchers associated with abstinence and negative urine tests
Schmitz et al[50]	2010	Cocaine	Levodopa-carbidopa	Contingency management of urine, attendance, or medication taking	136	Levodopa with CM-urine produced superior cocaine use outcomes, with effect moderated by medication compliance

DOPAMINERGIC AUGMENTATION OF CONTINGENCY MANAGEMENT

Dopaminergic medications have been tested in combination with contingency management behavioral interventions (**Table 2**). The theoretical framework for this approach is that cocaine-dependent individuals have difficulty responding to noncocaine rewards and that dopaminergic medications may normalize dopamine signaling and thereby increase the saliency of rewards offered as part of a behavioral treatment. In a clinical trial comparing levodopa-carbidopa to placebo combined with clinical management, cognitive behavioral therapy or voucher-based reinforcement therapy, levodopa combined with vouchers was associated with higher rates of abstinence and higher proportions of cocaine-free urine samples.[49] Levodopa-carbidopa was also evaluated in combination with 3 different contingency management (CM) targets (urine, medication, or attendance) and the combination of levodopa with CM-urine was associated with superior cocaine use outcomes, an effect moderated by medication compliance.[50] In a population of cocaine- and opioid-dependent methadone maintenance patients, bupropion was compared with placebo in combination with either CM or a voucher control condition, and the combination of CM with bupropion was associated with improved cocaine use outcomes compared with bupropion alone.[51]

However, studies of antidepressant medications that block reuptake of monoamines other than dopamine have also yielded positive results as augmenters of contingency management for cocaine dependence, including citalopram[52] and desipramine.[53] These results suggest that blocking the reuptake of monoamines in general may be responsible for the mechanism of augmentation of contingency management and not limited to dopaminergic effects per se. Further research is needed to elucidate the mechanism of the observed monoamine augmentation of contingency management treatment of cocaine dependence.

The strategy of augmenting contingency management interventions with drugs that enhance dopaminergic transmission is consistent with the hypothesis that cocaine-dependent individuals have deficient dopaminergic tone and that competing rewards to cocaine are less salient. A logical step in the development of this research would be to study more potent dopaminergic medications, such as amphetamines and methylphenidate, as augmenters of behavioral treatment.

CO-OCCURRING ADHD AND COCAINE DEPENDENCE

ADHD and cocaine dependence commonly occur. In clinical populations, the prevalence of ADHD in substance use disorder treatment settings ranges up to 24%.[54,55] In the general population, the prevalence of adult ADHD is 4.4%, whereas in individuals with a substance use disorder, ADHD co-occurs at a rate of 10.8%.[56] These data indicate that co-occurring ADHD and cocaine dependence will be routinely encountered in clinical settings.

Amphetamines[57] and methylphenidate[58] are effective treatments for treating adult ADHD. Because ADHD treatment is the main current clinical use of psychostimulant medications, concerns have been raised about the potential interaction between cocaine and psychostimulants. Stimulant therapy of ADHD in childhood is associated with a reduction in the risk for subsequent drug and alcohol use disorders.[59] However, psychostimulants increase extracellular dopamine in the brain, which is associated with both therapeutic and reinforcing effects. Volkow and Swanson[60] identified 4 variables that affected the therapeutic and reinforcing effects of methylphenidate, which included: (1) dose, (2) pharmacokinetics, (3) individual differences in sensitivity to methylphenidate, and (4) context. Large doses that penetrate the blood–brain barrier rapidly are associated with greater reinforcing effects, leading to the recommendation that the lowest possible dose that relieves symptoms be used and that sustained-release preparations are preferred for individuals with a predisposition to addiction.

ADDICTIVE POTENTIAL OF PSYCHOSTIMULANTS

Stimulant medications have the potential for misuse, diversion, and addiction.[61–63] Methylphenidate and dextroamphetamine have been shown to have reinforcing effects in individuals without histories of substance use disorders[64] and individuals with stimulant abuse histories.[65] The rate of onset of a drug's effect is an important determinant of its abuse potential. In a controlled laboratory evaluation, Kollins and colleagues[66] found that the sustained-release formulation of methylphenidate was associated with fewer ratings of "good effects" compared with the immediate-release formulation. These findings suggest that the abuse potential of the immediate-release preparation may be greater than that of the sustained-release preparation.

PRECAUTIONS IN PRESCRIBING STIMULANT MEDICATIONS

Misuse, diversion, and addiction are inherent risks of prescribing controlled substances, and a substantial minority of patients prescribed stimulants will divert their medications to others or misuse their own prescription.[61] An assessment of risk in a specific patient has to be determined at a specific point in time. All patients prescribed controlled substances should be assessed at each visit for signs of

---

Box 1
Red flags for diversion or misuse

- Symptoms of intoxication or withdrawal
- Demands for a particular, usually fast acting, medication (amphetamine IR)
- "Extended-release doesn't work for me"
- Repeated lost prescriptions
- Discordant pill count
- Excessive preoccupation with securing medication supply
- Multiple prescribers
- New development of cardiac symptoms
- New-onset psychosis

---

misuse, abuse, or addiction. Evaluations should be conducted using matter-of-fact and nonthreatening questioning (**Box 1**).

There are a number of strategies that can be used to minimize the risks presented when prescribing controlled substance psychostimulant treatment to patients with cocaine dependence. All patients with substance use disorders who are prescribed controlled substances should be advised of the risk of combining prescription medication with other substances. Patients should be warned about diversion and abuse liability of prescription stimulant medications. Delayed-release preparations are in general preferred over immediate-release preparations for behavioral safety. Small quantities of medication should be prescribed at a time, with pill count reconciled at each visit. Urine toxicology and breath alcohol testing can be useful in assessing a patient's overall clinical status. State prescribing databases can be consulted to check for multiple prescribers. Frequent patient visits may help detect problems or a change in clinical status sooner. In general, it should be emphasized to patients to take medications regularly, not on an as-needed basis, creating a structure of consistency and predictability around stimulant medication taking. Discussions with patients regarding safe storage and not advertising/sharing medications with others should occur regularly.

SUMMARY

The use of stimulant medications for the treatment of cocaine dependence is an evolving scientific line of research. To date, the most promising results are with the higher-potency medications, the amphetamine analogues, or a combination of a dopaminergic medication with a contingency management behavioral intervention. The development of effective pharmacotherapies for opioid and nicotine dependence using an agonist replacement approach suggests that these promising findings needs to continue to be vigorously investigated.

In clinical trial reports, there are very few instances of cardiovascular adverse events, which suggests that for well-selected patients with cocaine dependence, stimulant replacement therapy can be safe. However, clinical trial eligibility criteria excludes most high-risk patients from participating, and introducing stimulant substitution to the wider treatment community would likely expose more vulnerable patients to the medical risks associated with stimulant treatment while using cocaine. As treatment development research moves forward, attention must be paid to helping clinicians select patients who are most likely to benefit from stimulant substitution treatment and how to identify those at risk.

An additional concern with the use of stimulant medication treatment of cocaine dependence is prescribing controlled substances for patients with active substance use disorders. Again, within a clinical trial, medication supplies are monitored and distributed carefully in small quantities. In a community setting, misuse or diversion will be risks associated with prescribing controlled substances to patients with addictive disorders, but therapeutic strategies for monitoring and limiting that risk can be implemented.

Psychostimulant pharmacotherapy is a promising line of research for the treatment of cocaine dependence, a condition for which no effective pharmacotherapy has been identified. Further research is required to confirm positive results from single-site trials, in particular the study of amphetamines as a treatment for cocaine dependence. As this literature evolves, strategies to manage the risk of prescribing controlled substances to patients with addictive disorders need to be tested and refined. Biases against using controlled substances as a treatment for cocaine dependence should be challenged, much in the way the use of agonist treatment transformed the treatment of opioid dependence despite initial resistance from the field.

REFERENCES

1. SAMHSA. Results from the 2008 National Survey on Drug Use and Health: National Findings. Rockville (MD): Office of Applied Studies; 2009.
2. Compton WM, Thomas YF, Stinson FS, et al. Prevalence, correlates, disability, and comorbidity of DSM-IV drug abuse and dependence in the United States: results from the national epidemiologic survey on alcohol and related conditions. Arch Gen Psychiatry 2007;64(5):566–76.
3. Dutra L, Stathopoulou G, Basden SL, et al. A meta-analytic review of psychosocial interventions for substance use disorders. Am J Psychiatry 2008;165(2):179–87.
4. de Lima MS, de Oliveira Soares BG, Reisser AA, et al. Pharmacological treatment of cocaine dependence: a systematic review. Addiction 2002;97(8):931–49.
5. Elkashef A, Holmes TH, Bloch DA, et al. Retrospective analyses of pooled data from CREST I and CREST II trials for treatment of cocaine dependence. Addiction 2005; 100(Suppl 1):91–101.
6. Karila L, Gorelick D, Weinstein A, et al. New treatments for cocaine dependence: a focused review. Int J Neuropsychopharmacol 2008;11(3):425–38.
7. Cami J, Farre M. Drug addiction. N Engl J Med 2003;349(10):975–86.
8. White FJ, Kalivas PW. Neuroadaptations involved in amphetamine and cocaine addiction. Drug Alcohol Depend 1998;51(1–2):141–53.
9. Amato L, Davoli M, Perucci CA, et al. An overview of systematic reviews of the effectiveness of opiate maintenance therapies: available evidence to inform clinical practice and research. J Subst Abuse Treat 2005;28(4):321–9.
10. Berrettini WH, Lerman CE. Pharmacotherapy and pharmacogenetics of nicotine dependence. Am J Psychiatry 2005;162(8):1441–51.
11. Ledford CC, Fuchs RA, See RE. Potentiated reinstatement of cocaine-seeking behavior following D-amphetamine infusion into the basolateral amygdala. Neuropsychopharmacology 2003;28(10):1721–9.
12. Chiodo KA, Lack CM, Roberts DC. Cocaine self-administration reinforced on a progressive ratio schedule decreases with continuous D-amphetamine treatment in rats. Psychopharmacology (Berl) 2008;200(4):465–73.
13. Foltin RW, Evans SM. The effects of d-amphetamine on intake of food and a sweet fluid containing cocaine. Pharmacol Biochem Behav 1999;62(3):457–64.

14. Negus SS, Mello NK. Effects of chronic d-amphetamine treatment on cocaine- and food-maintained responding under a progressive-ratio schedule in rhesus monkeys. Psychopharmacology (Berl) 2003;167(3):324–32.

15. Negus SS, Mello NK. Effects of chronic d-amphetamine treatment on cocaine- and food-maintained responding under a second-order schedule in rhesus monkeys. Drug Alcohol Depend 2003;70(1):39–52.

16. Czoty PW, Martelle JL, Nader MA. Effects of chronic d-amphetamine administration on the reinforcing strength of cocaine in rhesus monkeys. Psychopharmacology (Berl) 2010;209(4):375–82.

17. Grabowski J, Roache JD, Schmitz JM, et al. Replacement medication for cocaine dependence: methylphenidate. J Clin Psychopharmacol 1997;17(6):485–8.

18. Roache JD, Grabowski J, Schmitz JM, et al. Laboratory measures of methylphenidate effects in cocaine-dependent patients receiving treatment. J Clin Psychopharmacol 2000;20(1):61–8.

19. Rush CR, Stoops WW, Hays LR. Cocaine effects during D-amphetamine maintenance: a human laboratory analysis of safety, tolerability and efficacy. Drug Alcohol Depend 2009;99(1–3):261–71.

20. Rush CR, Stoops WW, Sevak RJ, et al. Cocaine choice in humans during D-amphetamine maintenance. J Clin Psychopharmacol 2010;30(2):152–9.

21. Fredericks EM; Kollins SH. Assessing methylphenidate preference in ADHD patients using a choice procedure. Psychopharmacology (Berl) 2004;175(4):391–8.

22. Collins SL, Levin FR, Foltin RW, et al. Response to cocaine, alone and in combination with methylphenidate, in cocaine abusers with ADHD. Drug Alcohol Depend 2006; 82(2):158–67.

23. Li CS, Morgan PT, Matuskey D, et al. Biological markers of the effects of intravenous methylphenidate on improving inhibitory control in cocaine-dependent patients. Proc Natl Acad Sci U S A 2010;107(32):14455–9.

24. Goldstein RZ, Woicik PA, Maloney T, et al. Oral methylphenidate normalizes cingulate activity in cocaine addiction during a salient cognitive task. Proc Natl Acad Sci U S A 2010;107(38):16667–72.

25. Volkow ND, Wang GJ, Tomasi D, et al. Methylphenidate attenuates limbic brain inhibition after cocaine-cues exposure in cocaine abusers. PLoS One 2010;5(7): e11509.

26. Martinez D, Carpenter KM, Liu F, et al. Imaging dopamine transmission in cocaine dependence: link between neurochemistry and response to treatment. Am J Psychiatry 2011;168:634–41.

27. Fleckenstein AE, Volz TJ, Riddle EL, et al. New insights into the mechanism of action of amphetamines. Annu Rev Pharmacol Toxicol 2007;47:681–98.

28. Ermer JC, Adeyi BA, Pucci ML. Pharmacokinetic variability of long-acting stimulants in the treatment of children and adults with attention-deficit hyperactivity disorder. CNS Drugs 2010;24(12):1009–25.

29. Grabowski J, Rhoades H, Schmitz J, et al. Dextroamphetamine for cocaine-dependence treatment: a double-blind randomized clinical trial. J Clin Psychopharmacol 2001;21(5):522–6.

30. Grabowski J, Rhoades H, Stotts A, et al. Agonist-like or antagonist-like treatment for cocaine dependence with methadone for heroin dependence: two double-blind randomized clinical trials. Neuropsychopharmacology 2004;29(5):969–81.

31. Shearer J, Wodak A, van Beek I, et al. Pilot randomized double blind placebo-controlled study of dexamphetamine for cocaine dependence. Addiction 2003;98(8): 1137–41.

32. Mooney ME, Herin DV, Schmitz JM, et al. Effects of oral methamphetamine on cocaine use: a randomized, double-blind, placebo-controlled trial. Drug Alcohol Depend 2009;101(1–2):34–41.
33. Margolin A, Avants SK, Kosten TR. Mazindol for relapse prevention to cocaine abuse in methadone-maintained patients. Am J Drug Alcohol Abuse 1995;21(4):469–81.
34. Stine SM, Krystal JH, Kosten TR, et al. Mazindol treatment for cocaine dependence. Drug Alcohol Depend 1995;39(3):245–52.
35. Dackis CA, Kampman KM, Lynch KG, et al. A double-blind, placebo-controlled trial of modafinil for cocaine dependence. Neuropsychopharmacology 2005;30(1):205–11.
36. Anderson AL, Reid MS, Li SH, et al. Modafinil for the treatment of cocaine dependence. Drug Alcohol Depend 2009;104(1–2):133–9.
37. Brodie JD, Case BG, Figueroa E, et al. Randomized, double-blind, placebo-controlled trial of vigabatrin for the treatment of cocaine dependence in Mexican parolees. Am J Psychiatry 2009;166(11):1269–77.
38. Mooney ME, Schmitz JM, Moeller FG, et al. Safety, tolerability and efficacy of levodopa-carbidopa treatment for cocaine dependence: two double-blind, randomized, clinical trials. Drug Alcohol Depend 2007;88(2–3):214–23.
39. Leonard BE, McCartan D. White J, et al. Methylphenidate: a review of its neuropharmacological, neuropsychological and adverse clinical effects. Hum Psychopharmacol 2004;19(3):151–80.
40. Winhusen T, Somoza E. Singal BM, et al. Methylphenidate and cocaine: a placebo-controlled drug interaction study. Pharmacol Biochem Behav 2006;85(1):29–38.
41. Schubiner H, Saules KK, Arfken CL, et al. Double-blind placebo-controlled trial of methylphenidate in the treatment of adult ADHD patients with comorbid cocaine dependence. Exp Clin Psychopharmacol 2002;10(3):286–94.
42. Levin FR, Evans SM, Brooks DJ, et al. Treatment of cocaine dependent treatment seekers with adult ADHD: double-blind comparison of methylphenidate and placebo. Drug Alcohol Depend 2007;87(1):20–9.
43. Minzenberg MJ, Carter CS. Modafinil: a review of neurochemical actions and effects on cognition. Neuropsychopharmacology 2008;33(7):1477–502.
44. Dackis CA, Lynch KG, Yu E, et al. Modafinil and cocaine: a double-blind, placebo-controlled drug interaction study. Drug Alcohol Depend 2003;70(1):29–37.
45. Foley KF, DeSanty KP, Kast RE. Bupropion: pharmacology and therapeutic applications. Expert Rev Neurother 2006;6(9):1249–65.
46. Margolin A, Kosten TR, Avants SK, et al. A multicenter trial of bupropion for cocaine dependence in methadone-maintained patients. Drug Alcohol Depend 1995;40(2):125–31.
47. Shoptaw S, Heinzerling KG, Rotheram-Fuller E, et al. Bupropion hydrochloride versus placebo, in combination with cognitive behavioral therapy, for the treatment of cocaine abuse/dependence. J Addict Dis 2008;27(1):13–23.
48. Elkashef A, Fudala PJ, Gorgon L, et al. Double-blind, placebo-controlled trial of selegiline transdermal system (STS) for the treatment of cocaine dependence. Drug Alcohol Depend 2006;85(3):191–7.
49. Schmitz JM, Mooney ME, Moeller FG, et al. Levodopa pharmacotherapy for cocaine dependence: choosing the optimal behavioral therapy platform. Drug Alcohol Depend 2008;94(1–3):142–50.
50. Schmitz JM, Lindsay JA, Stotts AL, et al. Contingency management and levodopa-carbidopa for cocaine treatment: a comparison of three behavioral targets. Exp Clin Psychopharmacol 2010;18(3):238–44.

51. Poling J, Oliveto A, Petry N, et al. Six-month trial of bupropion with contingency management for cocaine dependence in a methadone-maintained population. Arch Gen Psychiatry 2006;63(2):219–28.

52. Moeller FG, Schmitz JM, Steinberg JL, et al. Citalopram combined with behavioral therapy reduces cocaine use: a double-blind, placebo-controlled trial. Am J Drug Alcohol Abuse 2007;33(3):367–78.

53. Kosten T, Oliveto A, Feingold A, et al. Desipramine and contingency management for cocaine and opiate dependence in buprenorphine maintained patients. Drug Alcohol Depend 2003;70(3):315–25.

54. Schubiner H, Tzelepis A, Milberger S, et al. Prevalence of attention-deficit/hyperactivity disorder and conduct disorder among substance abusers. J Clin Psychiatry 2000;61(4):244–51.

55. Levin FR, Evans SM, Kleber HD. Prevalence of adult attention-deficit hyperactivity disorder among cocaine abusers seeking treatment. Drug Alcohol Depend 1998; 52(1):15–25.

56. Kessler RC, Adler L, Barkley R, et al. The prevalence and correlates of adult ADHD in the United States: results from the National Comorbidity Survey Replication. Am J Psychiatry 2006;163(4):716–23.

57. Spencer T, Biederman J, Wilens T, et al. Efficacy of a mixed amphetamine salts compound in adults with attention-deficit/hyperactivity disorder. Arch Gen Psychiatry 2001;58(8):775–82.

58. Faraone SV, Spencer T, Aleardi M, et al. Meta-analysis of the efficacy of methylphenidate for treating adult attention-deficit/hyperactivity disorder. J Clin Psychopharmacol 2004;24(1):24–9.

59. Wilens TE, Faraone SV, Biederman J, et al. Does stimulant therapy of attention-deficit/hyperactivity disorder beget later substance abuse? A meta-analytic review of the literature. Pediatrics 2003;111(1):179–85.

60. Volkow ND, Swanson JM. Variables that affect the clinical use and abuse of methylphenidate in the treatment of ADHD. Am J Psychiatry 2003;160(11):1909–18.

61. Wilens TE, Adler LA, Adams J, et al. Misuse and diversion of stimulants prescribed for ADHD: a systematic review of the literature. J Am Acad Child Adolesc Psychiatry 2008;47(1):21–31.

62. Kollins SH, MacDonald EK, Rush CR. Assessing the abuse potential of methylphenidate in nonhuman and human subjects: a review. Pharmacol Biochem Behav 2001; 68(3):611–27.

63. Kollins SH. Abuse liability of medications used to treat attention-deficit/hyperactivity disorder (ADHD). Am J Addict 2007;16(Suppl 1):35–42 [quiz: 43–4].

64. Rush CR, Essman WD, Simpson CA, et al. Reinforcing and subject-rated effects of methylphenidate and d-amphetamine in non-drug-abusing humans. J Clin Psychopharmacol 2001;21(3):273–86.

65. Stoops WW, Glaser PE, Fillmore MT, et al. Reinforcing, subject-rated, performance and physiological effects of methylphenidate and d-amphetamine in stimulant abusing humans. J Psychopharmacol 2004;18(4):534–43.

66. Kollins SH, Rush CR, Pazzaglia PJ, et al. Comparison of acute behavioral effects of sustained-release and immediate-release methylphenidate. Exp Clin Psychopharmacol 1998;6(4):367–74.

Treatment of Opioid Dependence in the Setting of Pregnancy

Jessica L. Young, MD[a],*, Peter R. Martin, MD[b]

KEYWORDS

- Opioid dependence • Pregnancy • Addiction • Methadone • Buprenorphine

KEY POINTS

- Whereas 4% of pregnant women report current illicit drug use, a much higher rate of 16% is reported in teen pregnancies.
- In recent years, an increase in the abuse of prescription analgesics has been observed in the United States, as contrasted with observation of decrease in heroin use.
- Treatment plans for women using illicit drugs must take into consideration psychiatric and medical comorbidities while balancing risks and benefits for the maternal-fetal dyad.
- Treatment is best offered through a comprehensive treatment program designed to deliver opioid agonist maintenance treatment along with psychosocial and obstetric care.
- Buprenorphine as maintenance treatment of opioid dependence during pregnancy has promise and may offer some benefits, but more research is needed.
- Currently, methadone maintenance remains the standard of care for agonist treatment of opioid dependence in pregnancy against which other treatments must be compared.

Substance abuse in pregnancy is a major public health concern with risks for both mother and fetus. Four percent of pregnant women report current illicit drug use, with a much higher rate of 16% among teen pregnancies.[1] Illicit drugs that are commonly abused include cocaine, heroin, methamphetamine and related stimulants, and prescription analgesics, anxiolytics, and hypnotics. The prevalence of opioid use

The authors have no financial conflicts of interests to disclose.

[a] Vanderbilt University Medical Center, R-1217, Medical Center North, 1161 21st Avenue, Nashville, TN 37232, USA; [b] Division of Addiction Psychiatry and Vanderbilt Addiction Center, Vanderbilt Psychiatric Hospital, Suite 3068, 1601 23rd Avenue South, Nashville, TN 37212–8645, USA

* Corresponding author.

E-mail address: jessica.l.young@vanderbilt.edu

Psychiatr Clin N Am 35 (2012) 441–460
http://dx.doi.org/10.1016/j.psc.2012.03.008
0193-953X/12/$ – see front matter © 2012 Elsevier Inc. All rights reserved.

Box 1
Complications of opioid dependence in pregnancy

- Miscarriage
- Preterm labor
- Preterm premature rupture of membranes
- Malnutrition
- Intrauterine growth restriction
- Preeclampsia
- Stillbirth
- Neonatal abstinence syndrome
- Infectious disease exposure, ie, HIV, hepatitis C
- Concomitant substance use
- Co-occurring other psychiatric disorders

during pregnancy ranges from 1% to 21%.[2] In the past, this opioid use primarily consisted of heroin use. However, in recent years, an increase in the abuse of prescription analgesics has been observed in the United States. From 2002 to 2009 there was an increase in the rate of nonmedical use of prescription drugs by young adults (from 5.5% to 6.3%) that was fueled primarily by opioid analgesics.[3] Such a rise may be attributed to a change in physician prescribing habits. In 1997, the amount of opioid pain relievers prescribed was equivalent to 96 mg of morphine per individual. By 2007, rates had reached 700 mg of morphine per person, an increase of 600%.[4] Alarmingly, opioid pain relievers have recently surpassed heroin and cocaine in overdose deaths rivaling those from motor vehicle accidents, with a total of 73% of these deaths involving prescription analgesics.[5]

Of pregnant women who admitted to using illicit drugs, 27% reported use of heroin or prescription opioids.[6] It is estimated that over 54,000 pregnancies are affected annually by opioid dependence in the United States.[7] However, this figure is likely an underestimate because this prevalence rate is based on self-report, and the stigma of substance use in pregnancy may lead to significant underreporting. Additionally, the abuse of prescription opioids may be more difficult to identify and, as mentioned previously, these substances now account for the majority of opioid abuse/dependence. Accordingly, as opioid use and dependence rise among pregnant women, providers will increasingly be confronted with the challenges of identification and management of these patients.

COMPLICATIONS OF OPIOID DEPENDENCE DURING PREGNANCY
Inconsistent Prenatal Care

Opioid abuse during pregnancy leads to a substantial overutilization of healthcare resources and greatly influences management and outcome of the pregnancy. The complications associated with opioid dependence during pregnancy are shown in **Box 1**. Infants of opioid-dependent mothers are at risk for preterm delivery, low birth weight, and opioid withdrawal upon delivery (neonatal abstinence syndrome, NAS). In addition, women who are opioid-dependent tend to have less frequent and inconsistent prenatal care. Their living situations are often chaotic, with

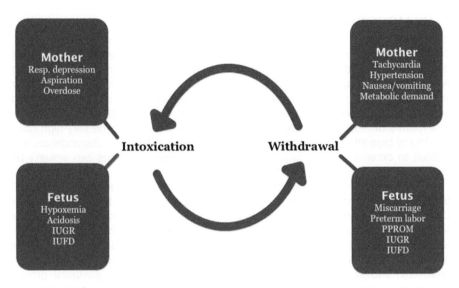

Legend: IUGR=Intrauterine growth restriction; IUFD=Intrauterine fetal demise;
PPROM=Premature preterm rupture of membranes

Fig. 1. Effects of opioid intoxication and withdrawal in pregnancy.

exposure to criminality and violence as well as inadequate food and housing. Maternal and fetal exposure to infectious diseases such as hepatitis B and C and human immunodeficiency virus (HIV) is also more likely as are other sexually transmitted diseases.[8,9] Consequently, these newborns have substantially increased neonatal intensive care unit stays and early childhood medical costs compared with healthy controls.[10] However, consequences of opioid dependence, co-occurring psychiatric disorders, and the associated lifestyle risk factors on the fetus may be difficult to disentangle from each other, but in combination they are synergistic and represent significant challenges for a healthy pregnancy outcome.

Cycles of Intoxication and Withdrawal

The pathophysiologic effects of repeated cycles of intoxication and withdrawal, so common in opioid dependence, represent a significant threat to the pregnancy **(Fig. 1)**. Intoxication with opioids suppresses respiratory drive in the mother and can be associated with hypoxemia in the fetus. Fetal hypoxemia can lead to fetal acidosis, a variety of metabolic and hematologic abnormalities, and intrauterine fetal demise (IUFD).[11] Opioid withdrawal causes maternal and fetal tachycardia and increased muscle activity and metabolism. Maternal hypertension and tachycardia cause decreased placental perfusion, reducing oxygen supply to the already stressed fetus. Severe withdrawal can stimulate uterine contractions, leading to preterm delivery with all of its subsequent risks including neonatal death. Thus, withdrawal can precipitate miscarriage in early pregnancy and preterm labor, preterm premature rupture of membranes, and stillbirth in later pregnancy.[12] Ultimately, repeated cycles of intoxication and withdrawal can lead to intrauterine growth restriction (IUGR) due to placental insufficiency.

Co-Use of Opioids with Other Drugs

Women who have opioid dependence are also more likely to use other drugs. Tobacco use during pregnancy is a particularly prevalent concern and compounds the risks of opioid dependence. The rate of cigarette smoking in this group is four times higher than that in the general population of pregnant women.[13] Tobacco use in pregnancy is associated with many of the same complications as have been noted with opioid dependence, namely miscarriage, IUGR, preterm labor, preterm premature rupture of membranes, and stillbirth. Therefore, because of the very high rates (>90%) of cigarette smoking among pregnant women with opioid dependence, it is difficult to determine how much of the associated poor outcomes can actually be attributed to opioids versus tobacco use.

Alcohol use is also highly prevalent in opioid users. In a study of 30,000 opioid-dependent people, 14% of women reported alcohol use to intoxication over the previous 30 days.[14] Fetuses exposed to alcohol during pregnancy are at risk for fetal alcohol spectrum disorders (FASDs), which include fetal alcohol syndrome (FAS), alcohol-related birth defects, and alcohol-related neurodevelopmental disorder (ARND). FAS may affect fetuses and infants exposed to high amounts of alcohol in utero with subsequent anomalies in three areas—prenatal and postnatal growth restriction, central nervous system dysfunction, and craniofacial abnormalities.[15] FASDs, particularly ARND, are far more common than FAS, with approximately 1% of pregnancies affected.[16] Consequences of milder forms of FASD include behavioral and neurocognitive disorders. A prospective cohort study of pregnant women showed that their offspring who were exposed to one or more drinks per day during the first trimester were three times more likely to develop conduct disorder in adolescence.[17] The outcomes of concomitant alcohol and opioid exposure in utero are yet to be elucidated but have the potential for long-term neurocognitive or behavioral effects.

Long-Term Risks to Children of Opioid-Dependent Mothers

Long-term risks for infants and children of opioid-dependent mothers may include sudden infant death syndrome and also various developmental delays with neurocognitive deficits, although once again, it may be difficult to distinguish the role of opioid use per se from other associated problems of these women. For example, a study of HIV-positive women showed an increased rate of sudden infant death syndrome for infants whose mothers chronically used opioids prenatally.[18] Children whose mothers were dependent on opioids during pregnancy have been shown to be at higher risk for neurocognitive delay and other behavioral disorders.[19] However, prematurity, which is more likely in these infants, is a major risk factor in its own right for cognitive delay. It is not clear how much of these complications are to be attributed to the unstable environment in which these children are often raised. Human and animal models have suggested that the brain functions underpinning addiction and parenting are closely related, because neural circuits subserving stress and reward converge in their representations in the brain. Theories posit that for a drug-addicted mother, caring for an infant may stimulate stress rather than reward pathways, which can result in continued drug use or relapse, poor mother-child bonding, and ultimately, ineffective mothering.[20]

Risks to Fetus of Opioid-Dependent Women

Finally, it is controversial and the subject of ongoing research whether exposure to opioids themselves during gestation may potentially represent a risk to the fetus.

> **Box 2**
> **Screening tools for substance abuse in pregnancy**
>
> - AUDIT-C (Alcohol Use Disorders Identification Test)
> - T-ACE (Tolerance, Annoyance, Cut down, Eye-opener)
> - TQDH (Ten Question Drinking History).
> - TWEAK (Tolerance, Worry about drinking, Eye-opener, Amnesia, K/Cut down)
> - 4Ps Plus (Parents, Partner, Past, Pregnancy)
> - Urine drug screen

Historically, opioids have been considered safe in pregnancy with no teratogenicity associated despite the fact that opioids readily cross the placenta. However, new data have emerged that raise concern that opioid use in the first trimester is associated with certain congenital anomalies. A 2011 report from The National Birth Defects Prevention Study showed an association between use of opioids early in pregnancy and cardiac defects, spina bifida, and gastroschisis.[21] However, this study did not take into account the degree of tobacco or alcohol use.[22] A study of the Tennessee Medicaid pregnant population from 2005 to 2009 showed that opioid use during the first trimester has increased from 8% in 2005 to 20% in 2009.[23] This increase illustrates the importance of answering the question of teratogenicity. At this time, it is difficult to make recommendations based on these data alone to women who are on opioid maintenance at the time of conception.

IDENTIFICATION OF OPIOID DEPENDENCE IN THE PREGNANT WOMAN

All pregnant women should be screened for substance use as part of routine prenatal care, regardless of perceived risk. The clinician should ask about the woman's use of alcohol, tobacco, illegal drugs, and nonmedical use of prescription drugs. Many pregnant women are reluctant to reveal drug use because of shame, guilt, or fear of rejection. Women also worry that disclosure will lead to legal action and loss of custody. An open-ended interview style may decrease the reluctance to admit to substance use.[24] **Box 2** lists the more common screening tools that can be used for screening.[25–32]

Tools that have been validated in pregnant women include[25]

- T-ACE (Tolerance, Annoyance, Cut down, Eye-opener)
- AUDIT-C (Alcohol Use Disorders Identification Test)
- 4Ps plus (Parents, Partner, Past, Pregnancy)
- TWEAK (Tolerance, Worry about drinking, Eye-opener, Amnesia, K/Cut down)
- TQDH (Ten Question Drinking History).

Common screening tools for alcohol and substance abuse have not been validated in a pregnant sample.[25]

- CAGE (Cut down, Annoyed, Guilty, Eye-opener)
- MAST (Michigan Alcohol Screening Test)
- DAST (Drug Abuse Screening Test).

Tools range from 4 to 28 questions in length. For initial screening, the clinician may opt for a tool that has been validated for pregnancy and that fits into the clinician's

Table 1		
Tools with highest sensitivity for use during pregnancy		
Tool	Sensitivity	Specificity
T-ACE	69%–88%	71%–89%
TWEAK	71%–91%	73%–83%
AUDIT-C	95%	85%

personal style and clinic flow. The tools with the highest sensitivity during pregnancy are shown in **Table 1**.[26]

Some experts advocate routine urine drug screening as part of prenatal labs for all pregnant women. If routine urine drug screening is implemented, informed consent should be obtained prior to the test. Women may be averse to covert attempts to discover drug use. By instilling a sense of mistrust, testing without consent could lead to disengagement or limited prenatal care. Conversely, sensitively obtaining the woman's consent for drug testing can help strengthen the physician-patient alliance.[33]

If prenatal screening is effectively conducted, pregnancy offers a unique opportunity for the addicted woman to enter addiction care services. Those found to have a positive screen result by their obstetrician can be referred to receive a comprehensive psychiatric diagnostic evaluation. This transition may sometimes be difficult and is highly dependent on the therapeutic alliance already established. However, it can be facilitated by using the principles of motivational interviewing.[34] The ensuing evaluation can be used to determine the extent of the problem and how best to care for the woman's addiction during pregnancy and beyond.

DIAGNOSTIC EVALUATION FOR ADDICTION IN PREGNANCY

The diagnostic evaluation for addiction in pregnancy (**Box 3**) should focus on the precursors and complications of drug use as they affect multiple domains of the addicted woman's life. The high rates of co-occurring substance use and other psychiatric disorders make evaluation for these conditions an essential part of the assessment. A tool such as the Addiction Severity Index that globally assesses the impact of drug use in seven domains (medical, legal, family/social, psychiatric, employment, drug, and alcohol) can be used in the intake process to assist with comprehensive assessment.[35] In addition, the evaluation must include careful consideration of medical co-morbidities such as infectious diseases, malnutrition, and anemia.

Assessment for Co-Occurring Drug Use and Other Psychiatric Disorders

Polysubstance abuse is common in the context of opioid dependence, and hence, once a diagnosis of opioid dependence is made or suspected, it is important to consider other substances of abuse as well. For example, analyses from the MOTHER trial showed that approximately 34% of participants had used cocaine in the 30 days prior to study entry.[36] Abuse of benzodiazepines and alcohol, in particular, must be recognized because detoxification from these substances presents its own set of problems that complicate management of opioid dependence. As mentioned previously, tobacco use is very common among pregnant opioid users, and many of the fetal complications of smoking confound those of opioid dependence.[37]

Women with opioid dependence are often socially disadvantaged and should be carefully evaluated for psychiatric comorbidities that often complicate the clinical

---

Box 3
Evaluation of the pregnant opioid-dependent woman

Screening for substance use

- Tobacco
- Alcohol
- Benzodiazepines
- Cocaine
- Marijuana
- Amphetamines
- Prescription drugs

Laboratory tests

- Routine prenatal labs
- Urine drug screening
- Serum blood alcohol
- HIV
- Rapid plasma reagin
- Hepatitis B surface antigen
- Hepatitis C antibody

Screening for psychiatric comorbidities

- Substance intoxication/withdrawal
- Mood disorders
- Anxiety disorders
- Eating disorders
- Adjustment disorder
- Personality traits/disorders
- Disorders due to general medical condition

Imaging

- Fetal ultrasound

---

course. In a recent study of opioid-dependent pregnant women, 64.6% endorsed symptoms potentially reflecting a co-occurring psychiatric illness.[38] Those who endorsed psychiatric symptoms had greater severity of drug dependence and were more likely to have impairments in social/family functioning, employment status, and medical status. Depressive symptoms affected approximately 34% of opioid-dependent pregnancies. Anxiety and related symptoms were reported by 40%, including posttraumatic stress disorder, panic disorder, agoraphobia, social phobia, and obsessive-compulsive disorder.[38]

Identifying co-occurring psychiatric illness is important because untreated disorders may affect both the success of addiction treatment as well as the outcome of the pregnancy.[39] Depression in the setting of opioid dependence has been shown to have a negative effect on treatment outcomes.[40] However, it should be emphasized that the treatments used for concurrent other psychiatric disorders may have significant adverse effects on the fetus, and hence one must balance risk and benefit in treatment planning. There are few studies that have examined the long-term effects of in utero exposure to selective serotonin reuptake inhibitors (SSRIs).[41] For example, neonates exposed to SSRIs during the third trimester are at risk for SSRI-induced symptoms that may resemble or exacerbate NAS. Therefore, the risk-benefit equation during pregnancy is modified compared with considerations in nonpregnant patients. If psychosocial treatments may suffice, one should carefully consider whether psychotropic medication exposure during pregnancy is warranted. Consequently, only the most severely symptomatic women with co-occurring psychiatric diagnoses should receive medications with recognized adverse effects on the fetus. Moderate psychiatric symptoms may often be effectively managed with behavioral strategies, especially if these strategies can be provided at sufficient frequencies in a more intensive manner.

Assessment for Infectious Diseases

Infectious disease co-morbidities are highly prevalent in this patient population and can significantly influence maternal health and neonatal outcomes. The lifestyle associated with opioid dependence, including injection drug use and high-risk sexual behaviors, puts these women at risk for HIV and hepatitis B and C. For injection drug users, the rate of infection with these diseases is as high as 33%.[42] Screening should be done at entry into prenatal care and then repeated in the third trimester. Antiretroviral therapy is standard of care for HIV-infected women in order to prevent vertical transmission. However, pharmacokinetic interactions of opioids and antiretrovirals may occur at the level of hepatic metabolism, and this fact must be considered along with metabolic effects of pregnancy per se in appropriate medication dosing. For example, protease inhibitors have been shown to decrease serum concentrations of methadone so that methadone doses may need to be raised to achieve the same therapeutic effect. The nonnucleoside reverse transcriptase inhibitors have also been shown to induce an opioid abstinence syndrome due to induction of methadone metabolism.[43] Buprenorphine seems to have fewer interactions than methadone and thus may be more easily used in women treated with antiretrovirals.[44]

COMPREHENSIVE TREATMENT OF OPIOID DEPENDENCE DURING PREGNANCY
Components of a Comprehensive Treatment Program

In order to provide optimal prenatal care for an opioid-dependent woman and her fetus, a collaborative team approach consisting of psychiatry and obstetrics in conjunction with nurses and social workers who can provide effective case management is beneficial (**Box 4**). The importance of creating a therapeutic alliance between the woman and her providers cannot be stressed enough. Better maternal and fetal outcomes have been reported for women who receive integrated prenatal care and substance abuse treatment.[45]

Increased frequency of medical visits

The schedule of prenatal care for the opioid-dependent woman is not different from the general pregnant population. However, as noted, the rate of coexisting psychiatric illness is quite high in these patients. Therefore, ongoing psychiatric care is required to complement agonist medication maintenance and obstetric management. Accordingly, the opioid-dependent woman will need to be seen more frequently, often weekly, for management of her drug dependence and pregnancy. These visits may alternate

> **Box 4**
> **Comprehensive treatment of opioid dependence in pregnancy**
>
> - Psychiatric management
> - Prenatal care
> - Social work and counseling
> - Group therapy
> - Case management
> - Mutual support groups (eg, Twelve-Step)
> - Anesthesia consultation

between the psychiatrist and the obstetrician, with judicious use of midlevel providers, especially case management provided by addiction counselors, social workers, or nurses, depending on clinic organization and structure.

Laboratory tests to screen for infectious disease
Initial prenatal labs for the opioid-dependent pregnant woman should include screening for hepatitis B and C, syphilis, and HIV. Tuberculosis skin testing should be done if risk factors are present, such as incarceration.[24] At each visit, urine drug screening should be performed and the results may be used to enhance the therapeutic process. For example, studies have shown that opioid-dependent women enrolled in contingency management that rewards patients for negative drug screens have greater retention in prenatal care as well as drug treatment.[46] Typically reinforcement is in the form of monetary vouchers, so cost can prohibit implementing this program on a large scale. More recently, models for contingency management that are less costly (involving tickets to win prizes) have been shown to also be effective.[47,48]

Ultrasound studies
An ultrasound should be performed at entry to pregnancy care for purposes of dating and determining viability of the fetus. A screening ultrasound to determine anatomic characteristics of the fetus is done at 19 to 21 weeks gestational age. Because of the risk for intrauterine growth restriction, monthly ultrasound examinations are recommended to assess fetal growth after the initial anatomic scan. Additional antenatal fetal surveillance is not necessary unless indicated for co-occurring obstetric complications.

Psychosocial interventions
Nonpharmacologic psychosocial interventions are an important part of the prenatal care for opioid-dependent pregnant women. Social workers, nurses, or addiction counselors should assess and assist the woman with housing, insurance, transportation, and other needs that may affect retention in a treatment program. Data supporting psychosocial interventions such as motivational interviewing are mixed.[46] Attendance at groups such as Narcotics Anonymous is highly recommended as part of treatment program and has shown to be beneficial in the nonpregnant population.[49] The mutual support offered in the Twelve Step context may be especially valuable because many of these women often face their pregnancies alone or in turbulent relationships.

Rationale for Opioid Maintenance

Treatment options for opioid dependence during pregnancy include maintenance, detoxification, and discontinuation by tapering and should be tailored to the individual patient. The clinician must weigh the risks and benefits of each treatment option while considering challenges of co-occurring medical and psychiatric disorders as well as those associated with the lifestyle of these women. Since the 1970s, detoxification from opioids has not been the recommended course of treatment during pregnancy. A chart review, conducted in 1998, of 34 pregnant women who underwent opioid detoxification with either methadone or clonidine showed a successful detoxification rate of only 59%. Twenty-nine percent of the women resumed use of street drugs and 12% opted to start methadone maintenance.[41] Twenty-five percent who opted for detoxification went into active labor triggered by opioid withdrawal. The risk of precipitating severe withdrawal and its consequences, in addition to a high probability that detoxified women will return to using opioids again during the pregnancy, do not support opioid detoxification as a viable recommendation to opioid-dependent women.

For decades, maintenance treatment with methadone has been the standard of care for pregnant women. Methadone maintenance has been shown to significantly increase adherence to prenatal care, improve neonatal outcomes, and decrease severity of NAS.[37] Within the context of a comprehensive treatment program (psychopharmacologic management, counseling and group therapy, prenatal care, and social work services), administration of a therapeutic daily dose of methadone reduces drug craving and eliminates the repeated cycles of intoxication and withdrawal experienced by the mother during active addiction.[50] In addition, methadone maintenance as compared with active heroin addiction has been shown to result in increased fetal growth, decreased risk of HIV infection, preeclampsia, and foster care placement of the neonate.[51] Nevertheless, NAS of significant severity to require treatment with morphine is still observed in over 50% of births despite the benefits of methadone maintenance.[52]

Initiation of Maintenance Dosing for Methadone

Women who are already in methadone maintenance programs can be safely continued on their current dose of methadone. Induction of methadone in the pregnant woman who is actively abusing opioids is most safely accomplished as an inpatient and requires careful obstetric oversight. The starting dose of methadone is typically 10 to 20 mg/d and dosage is adjusted based on response to treatment.[53] The goal is to suppress withdrawal without causing intoxication. Because of its slow elimination rate from the body, methadone plasma levels can cumulate, so it is advisable to only increase the dose very slowly (no more often than 3 to 5 days after withdrawal symptoms are suppressed). Many women will need increased dosage in the third trimester because physiologic changes of pregnancy augment the rate of clearance of methadone plasma levels; on rare occasions, it is necessary to split dosage twice daily.[51] A challenge of methadone maintenance is that this controlled drug can only be dispensed for the treatment of opioid dependence through licensed methadone maintenance clinics. Particularly for pregnant women, there is considerable stigma associated with frequenting methadone clinics. Additionally, this daily visit to a clinic can be a barrier for women without transportation or from rural areas.

Buprenorphine Versus Methadone

Buprenorphine, a partial mu opioid agonist and kappa opioid antagonist, is now available for office-based maintenance treatment of opioid dependence. Increasing numbers of women have become pregnant while prescribed buprenorphine and thus, there is considerable impetus to continue this medication during pregnancy. Recent studies have shown that buprenorphine can be used during pregnancy with little risk to the fetus, and neonatal outcomes are not significantly different from those obtained with methadone.[52]

Buprenorphine, as a partial mu opioid agonist, has been shown to cause less activation of, and have greater affinity for the mu-opioid receptor than the full mu agonist methadone. Additionally, placental experiments in vitro have shown buprenorphine to have less placental transfer than methadone. Both these considerations should theoretically lead to decreased physical dependence of the fetus and less severe associated NAS upon delivery than may occur with methadone maintenance.[54,55] For example, the recent MOTHER study, a randomized controlled trial comparing buprenorphine and methadone exposure during pregnancy, has provided support for these predictions.[52] Infants exposed to buprenorphine during gestation were found to spend fewer days in the hospital and to require lower morphine doses over a shorter treatment period for NAS than those exposed to methadone. However, the addiction treatment outcomes in this trial were consistent with previous studies that showed that methadone and buprenorphine equally decreased illicit drug use.[56]

A significant benefit of buprenorphine maintenance is that physicians who have requisite training and a waiver from the Center for Substance Abuse Treatment of the Substance Abuse and Mental Health Administration can prescribe it in a private clinic setting. This certification often can eliminate barriers associated with daily visits to a methadone clinic. Also, insurance may cover buprenorphine prescribed by a physician during pregnancy while not covering treatment at a methadone clinic. For women already taking buprenorphine when they become pregnant, the recommendation is now clearly to continue buprenorphine at the same dose with only minor adjustments in dosage needed throughout pregnancy. Typically, these individuals have been prescribed buprenorphine-naloxone (Suboxone) prior to pregnancy and should be switched to buprenorphine alone (Subutex) for the course of their pregnancy. (Naloxone is combined with buprenorphine for nonpregnant patients to discourage diversion because injection of naloxone causes a withdrawal reaction.) In pregnancy, naloxone should be avoided to decrease the number of substances to which the fetus is exposed.

Disadvantage of buprenorphine use

A disadvantage of buprenorphine use is the difficulty of initiating this medication during pregnancy. Induction of buprenorphine in an opioid-dependent pregnant woman is a vitally important issue about which there is currently no consensus, and further research is clearly required. Precipitated withdrawal due to administration of a partial mu opioid agonist to a woman who is actively using opioids may pose a risk to the developing fetus as well as increase relapse rates. For example, in the MOTHER trial, an apparently higher (though statistically nonsignificant) early dropout rate in the buprenorphine compared with the methadone group (33% vs 18%) underlined the potential difficulties associated with initiating buprenorphine maintenance in actively using opioid-dependent pregnant women.[52] Therefore, from a practical perspective, this threat to the fetus can only be completely avoided if the woman is initiated and subsequently maintained on a full agonist medication (methadone) throughout pregnancy rather than a partial agonist (buprenorphine).

Initiation of Buprenorphine Maintenance

As mentioned previously, initiation of buprenorphine in the setting of pregnancy is challenging. If heroin, methadone, or other opioids are present in the body, buprenorphine, because of its high affinity for the mu opioid receptor and partial mu agonist effect, can readily trigger a severe withdrawal syndrome.[57] There is no evidence-based consensus on how buprenorphine induction should be conducted, including appropriate gestational age, setting, and fetal monitoring. At this time, initiation of buprenorphine should be reserved for those women in whom the benefits clearly outweigh the risks.[58] Women must be counseled regarding potential harmful effects of withdrawal including miscarriage, preterm labor, and IUFD. As in nonpregnant patients, induction should begin only when the patient demonstrates moderate withdrawal symptoms.

For patients abusing short-acting opioids prior to induction, buprenorphine administration should not be initiated until at least 6 hours after the last opioid dose, but the best guide is to document the presence of at least moderate opioid withdrawal prior to beginning buprenorphine at the lowest (2 to 4 mg) dose. The presence of significant withdrawal signs prior to initiating buprenorphine is particularly important when the patient has been using long-acting opioids, because the duration of withdrawal under these circumstances can be protracted and the severity of mild withdrawal can be greatly accentuated by administration of buprenorphine. As diminution (rather than exacerbation) of withdrawal is demonstrated with low doses of buprenorphine, the initial buprenorphine dose can be increased to one that diminishes drug-seeking optimally. Typically, if withdrawal symptoms are not sufficiently relieved by the initial dose, an additional 2 to 4 mg of buprenorphine can be administered 1 to 2 hours later.

Concurrent Abuse of Central Nervous System Depressant Medications

Women with concomitant abuse of alcohol and benzodiazepines should be detoxified from these substances in parallel with beginning opioid agonist maintenance. There is considerable evidence of increased morbidity and mortality associated with combined use of central nervous system depressants with either methadone or buprenorphine.[59] Detoxification from central nervous system depressants and initiation of agonist maintenance during pregnancy typically requires inpatient admission. Alcohol detoxification can effectively be accomplished using a symptom-triggered approach to diazepam dosing as illustrated in **Fig. 2**.[60] Patients are assessed every 3 to 4 hours with the Clinical Institute Withdrawal Assessment for Alcohol scale (CIWA-A), which determines withdrawal severity. The CIWA score determines the dose of diazepam administered. For women dependent on benzodiazepines, the typical approach of symptom-triggered phenobarbital loading for benzodiazepine withdrawal is not recommended because of the potential for teratogenicity of phenobarbital. Because the risk of benzodiazepines to the fetus is relatively small, tapering and then discontinuing may accomplish detoxification. The diazepam dose needed to suppress withdrawal symptoms is determined, and then the daily dosage can be decreased at a rate that is symptomatically tolerated, typically by about 25% each week.

Opioids Prescribed for Chronic Pain

For pregnant women who are prescribed oral opioids for chronic pain and do not meet criteria for an opioid use disorder, outpatient tapering is sometimes considered during pregnancy because of the desire to diminish risk to the fetus. However, care must be exercised not to precipitate withdrawal. There are no studies to show that

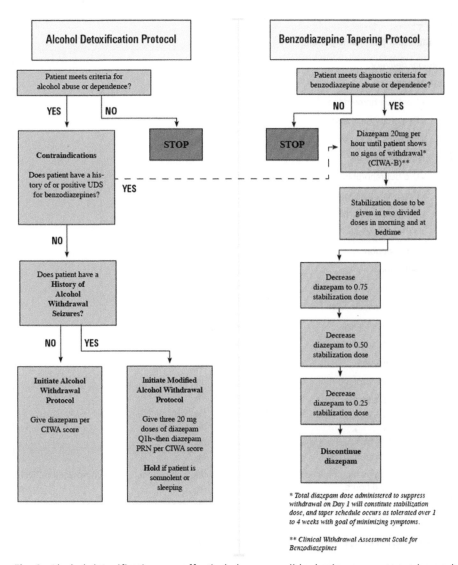

Fig. 2. Alcohol detoxification can effectively be accomplished using a symptom-triggered approach to diazepam dosing.

tapering opioids is reliably successful during pregnancy and results in prolonged discontinuation of use. The most common outcome is that opioids are used intermittently, which may be the most problematic for fetal health. In nonpregnant patients, switching form a short-acting to long-acting opioid and then gradually reducing the dose may effectively accomplish tapering and discontinuation. Regardless of the method of outpatient tapering, withdrawal may pose a significant risk and is not recommended for the majority of opioid-dependent pregnant women. Rather, the patient should be educated about maintaining consistent dosing with a long-acting opioid throughout the pregnancy so as to minimally stress the fetus.

Box 5
Intrapartum pain management

Vaginal delivery

○ **Methadone**

- Continue home dose
- Regional Anesthesia
- Comfort Measures

○ **Buprenorphinea**[a]

- D/c buprenorphine
- Regional anesthesia
- Comfort measures
- +/− methadone

Cesarean section

○ **Methadone**

- Continue home dose
- Regional anesthesia
- Local anesthetics
- Short-acting opioids

○ **Buprenorphine**[a]

- D/c buprenorphine
- Regional anesthesia
- Local anesthetics
- +/− methadone
- Short-acting opioids

[a] Alternative regimens: continue buprenorphine OR divide home dose of buprenorphine by 25% and give every 6 hours.

PAIN MANAGEMENT FOR LABOR AND DELIVERY

During the prenatal period, the strategy for delivery and postpartum care should be organized. The coordinated management of pain during labor or cesarean section may require input from psychiatry, obstetrics, and anesthesia providers on the care team (**Box 5**). Patients with addiction should not be deprived of pain control for fear of overdosing them. Because pain is a subjective symptom, the woman (not her physician) must be the final arbiter of how much pain she is willing to tolerate during this potentially exciting and rewarding time in her life. Opioid-dependent women may fear that their pain will not be adequately treated during labor, which leads to self-medication prior to admission. Formulating a plan prior to labor with the patient and care teams can assuage these fears. Chronic use of opioids causes tolerance as well as hyperalgesia.[61] This tolerance can make pain control difficult, and higher than normal doses of opioids are commonly required. For labor, the motivated patient may choose a delivery without pain medications and opt for management of pain using techniques such as showers, hot tubs, and position changes. Epidural and spinal analgesia can also be used safely in this population, and for cesarean delivery these approaches are preferred over general anesthesia. However, adequate levels of regional anesthesia may be more difficult to achieve. Nalbuphine (Nubain) and butorphanol (Stadol) should be avoided in the opioid-dependent patient, because these medications will precipitate withdrawal.[37]

Methadone-maintained pregnant women should be continued on routine dose of methadone, and short-acting opioids can be administered as needed.[62] For patients who are maintained on buprenorphine, there is less available data for the management of acute pain.

- For pain of short duration such as with a spontaneous vaginal delivery, patients may discontinue their buprenorphine prior to labor, and their pain can be managed with short-acting opioids as needed.[62] Subsequently, buprenorphine can easily be restarted.
- Alternatively, buprenorphine can be continued and pain can be managed with regional anesthesia. However, if buprenorphine is continued up until labor has begun, because buprenorphine has a high affinity for the mu-opioid receptor, higher doses of the short-acting opioids may be required, and patients should be monitored for signs of respiratory depression.
- Other strategies for the buprenorphine-maintained patient include dividing the daily buprenorphine dose by 25% and administering this dose every 6 hours and switching from buprenorphine to methadone with short-acting opioid supplementation.[63]

POSTPARTUM CONSIDERATIONS

Postpartum pain management should include use of nonsteroidal antiinflammatory drugs (NSAIDs) if the patient has no contraindication to such treatment. Scheduling NSAIDs while continuing maintenance dose of methadone or buprenorphine may be adequate for vaginal deliveries. However, the patient who has had a cesarean delivery or vaginal delivery complicated by significant laceration will require a short-acting opioid in addition to maintenance dose of methadone. For severe postoperative pain, buprenorphine will often need to be stopped so that short-acting opioids can effectively control pain. Infiltration of the incision site with a long-acting anesthetic can also help with the management of postpartum pain from cesarean delivery.[64]

Additional postpartum considerations include management of addiction, postpartum contraception, and breastfeeding.

A plan for **management of addiction postpartum**, including addressing other co-occurring psychiatric disorders, should be made prior to delivery. Opioid-dependent women are at increased risk for postpartum depression as well as exacerbation of other common coexisting psychiatric disorders. The stress of the early postpartum period can trigger relapse to active addiction. These factors make the postpartum period treacherous, and early follow-up with the treatment team should be facilitated.

Postpartum contraception should also be addressed prior to delivery because opioid-dependent women are at increased risk for unintended pregnancy. A 2011 study showed that 86% of pregnancies in a cohort of opioid-dependent women were unintended compared with 47% in the general population.[65] Pregnancy spacing has both maternal and fetal/infant health benefits in the general population and perhaps even more so for the opioid-dependent mother and her offspring.

Breastfeeding is safe for women who are maintained on either methadone or buprenorphine and should be supported as long as the woman is not abusing other substances and has no other contraindication to breastfeeding such as HIV infection.[66,67] Breastfeeding increases maternal-infant bonding, reduces severity of NAS symptoms, and increases maternal self-esteem.[68,69]

NEONATAL ABSTINENCE SYNDROME

Chronic exposure to opioids puts the fetus at risk for NAS, which is a group of symptoms associated with neonatal withdrawal. These symptoms include irritability, tremors, high-pitched cry, hypertonicity, difficulty feeding, vomiting, and diarrhea.[70] The treatment of NAS requires administration of opioids to diminish severity and is typically managed by pediatricians and neonatologists in a neonatal intensive care setting. Historically, paregoric and diazepam were used, but both agents have fallen out of favor. The former is no longer used because it contains potentially toxic compounds such as camphor and alcohol.[71] The latter has not been shown to be as effective as opioids and puts the infant at risk for late onset seizures, perhaps due to subsequent benzodiazepine dependence.[72] The preferred treatment for NAS in neonatal intensive care units is alcohol-free oral morphine sulfate solution (0.4 mg/mL) or morphine hydrochloride solution (0.2 mg/mL). Less commonly, methadone is used. Diluted tincture of opium is now rarely used because it contains small amounts of alcohol.[71] New data on buprenorphine treatment of NAS shows it to be safe and to reduce the length of hospital stay.[73] Phenobarbital and clonidine have been used as adjunctive therapy to oral morphine.[74–76] Neonates of opioid-dependent women must be monitored closely and assessed every 3 hours for signs of withdrawal. As mentioned, breastfeeding and bonding with the mother have been shown to decrease the severity of NAS symptoms and diminishes the need for treatment.[77]

SUMMARY

Opioid dependence in the setting of pregnancy provides a distinct set of challenges for providers. Treatment plans must take into consideration psychiatric and medical comorbidities while balancing risks and benefits for the maternal-fetal dyad. Treatment is best offered through a comprehensive treatment program designed to effectively deliver opioid agonist maintenance treatment along with psychosocial and obstetric care. As misuse of prescription analgesics increases in the United States, identification of the problem in pregnancy will become more important because this misuse is expected to lead to an increased prevalence of opioid dependence in pregnancy. Buprenorphine as maintenance treatment of opioid dependence during pregnancy has promise and may offer some benefits, but more research is needed, especially regarding induction of actively addicted women during pregnancy. For the present, methadone maintenance remains the standard of care for agonist treatment of opioid dependence in pregnancy against which other treatments must be compared.

REFERENCES

1. Substance Abuse and Mental Health Services Administration. Results from the 2010 National Survey on Drug Use and Health: summary of national findings [NSDUH Series H-41 HHS Publication No. (SMA) 11-46582011]. Rockville (MD): Substance Abuse and Mental Health Services Administration; 2011.
2. Brown HL, Britton KA, Mahaffey D, et al. Methadone maintenance in pregnancy: a reappraisal. Am J Obstet Gynecol 1998;179:459–63.
3. Substance Abuse and Mental Health Services Administration. Results from the 2009 National Survey on Drug Use and Health, vol. I. Summary of national findings (Office of Applied Studies, NSDUH Series H-38A, HHS Publication No. SMA 10-4586Findings). Rockville (MD): Substance Abuse and Mental Health Services; 2010.

4. CDC grand rounds: prescription drug overdoses—a U.S. Epidemic. MMWR Morb Mortal Wkly Rep 2012;61:10–3.

5. Centers for Disease Control and Prevention. Vital signs: overdoses of prescription opioid pain relievers–United States, 1999-2008. MMWR Morb Mortal Wkly Rep 2011;60:1487–92.

6. Finkelstein N, Kennedy C. Gender-specific substance abuse treatment. Rockville (MD): National Women's Resource Center for the Prevention and Treatment of Alcohol, Tobacco, and other Drug Abuse and Mental Illness and Substance Abuse and Health Services Administration and Health Resources and Services Administration; 1997.

7. National Pregnancy and Health Survey. Drug use among women delivering live births: 1992. Bethesda (MD): National Institute on Drug Abuse; 1997.

8. Rondinelli AJ, Ouellet LJ, Strathdee SA, et al. Young adult injection drug users in the United States continue to practice HIV risk behaviors. Drug Alcohol Depend 2009; 104(1–2):167–74.

9. Wu L-T, Ling W, Burchett B, et al. Gender and racial/ethnic differences in addiction severity, HIV risk, and quality of life among adults in opioid detoxification: results from the National Drug Abuse Treatment Clinical Trials Network. Subst Abuse Rehabil 2010;2010(1):13–22.

10. Kelly JJ, Davis PG, Henschke PN. The drug epidemic: effects on newborn infants and health resource consumption at a tertiary perinatal centre. J Paediatr Child Health 2000;36(3):262–4.

11. Soothill PW, Nicolaides KH, Campbell S. Prenatal asphyxia, hyperlacticaemia, hypoglycaemia, and erythroblastosis in growth retarded fetuses. Br Med J (Clin Res Ed) 1987;294:1051–3.

12. Bolnick JM, Rayburn WF. Substance use disorders in women: special considerations during pregnancy. Obstet Gynecol Clin North Am 2003;30(3):545–58, vii.

13. Jones HE, Heil SH, O'Grady KE, et al. Smoking in pregnant women screened for an opioid agonist medication study compared to related pregnant and non-pregnant patient samples. Am J Drug Alcohol Abuse 2009;35(5):375–80.

14. Green TC, Grimes Serrano JM, Licari A, et al. Women who abuse prescription opioids: findings from the Addiction Severity Index-Multimedia Version Connect prescription opioid database. Drug Alcohol Depend 2009;103:65–73.

15. Riley EP, Infante MA, Warren KR. Fetal alcohol spectrum disorders: an overview. Neuropsychol Rev 2011;21(2):73–80.

16. Sampson PD, Streissguth AP, Bookstein FL, et al. Incidence of fetal alcohol syndrome and prevalence of alcohol-related neurodevelopmental disorder. Teratology 1997; 56(5):317–26.

17. Larkby CA, Goldschmidt L, Hanusa BH, et al. Prenatal alcohol exposure is associated with conduct disorder in adolescence: findings from a birth cohort. J Am Acad Child Adolesc Psychiatry 2011;50(3):262–71.

18. Kahlert C, Rudin C, Kind C. Sudden infant death syndrome in infants born to HIV-infected and opiate-using mothers. Arch Dis Child 2007;92(11):1005–8.

19. Hayford S, Epps R, Dahl-Regis M. Behavior and development patterns in children born to heroin-addicted and methadone-addicted mothers. J Natl Med Assoc 1988; 80(11):1197–200.

20. Rutherford HJ, Williams SK, Moy Sheryl, et al. Disruption of maternal parenting circuitry by addictive process: rewiring reward and stress systems. Front Psychiatry 2011;2:37.

21. Broussard CS, Rasmussen SA, Reefhuis J, et al. Maternal treatment with opioid analgesics and risk for birth defects. Am J Obstet Gynecol 2011;204(4):314.

22. Jones HE, Jannson LM, O'Grady KE. Maternal treatment with opioid analgesics and risk for birth defects: additional considerations. Am J Obstet Gynecol 2011;205(3): e12.

23. Epstein RA, Ray WA, Bobo WV, et al. Increasing first trimester use of opioid analgesics. Journal of Women's Health 2011;(20)10:1403–4.

24. Alto WA, O'Connor AB. Management of women treated with buprenorphine during pregnancy. Am J Obstet Gynecol 2011;205:302–8.

25. Morse B, Genshan S, Hutchins E. Screening for substance abuse during pregnancy: improving care, improving health. Arlington (VA): National Center for Education in Maternal and Child Health; 1997.

26. Burns E, Gray R, Smith LA, Brief screening questionnaires to identify problem drinking during pregnancy: a systematic review. Addiction 2010;105(4):601–14.

27. Yonkers KA, Gotman N, Kershaw T, et al. Screening for prenatal substance use: development of the substance use risk profile-pregnancy scale. Obstet Gynecol 2010;116(4):827–33.

28. Sokol R, Martier S, Ager J. The T-ACE questions: Practical prenatal detection of risk drinking. Am J Obstet Gynecol 1989;160(4):863–8.

29. Russell M. New assessment tools for risk drinking during pregnancy. Alcohol Health and Research World 1994;18(1):55–61.

30. Saunders JB, Aasland OG, Babor TF, et al. Development of the Alcohol Use Disorders Identification Test (AUDIT): WHO collaborative project on early detection of persons with harmful alcohol consumption—II. Addiction 1993;88(6):791–804.

31. Ewing HM. Born Free project. Martinez (CA): Contra Costa County.

32. Weiner L, Rosetti H, Edelin K. Behavioral evaluation of fetal alcohol education for physicians. Alcohol Clin Exp Res 1982;6(2):230–3.

33. Roberts SC, Nuru-Jeter A. Women's perspectives on screening for alcohol and drug use in prenatal care. Womens Health Issues 2010;20(3):193–200.

34. Zahradnik A, Otto C, Crackau B, et al. Randomized controlled trial of a brief intervention for problematic prescription drug use in non-treatment-seeking patients. Addiction 2009;104(1):109–17.

35. Chaudhury R, Jones HE, Wechsberg W, et al. Addiction Severity Index composite scores as predictors for sexual-risk behaviors and drug-use behaviors in drug-using pregnant patients. Am J Drug Alcohol Abuse 2010;36(1):25–30.

36. Stine S, Heil SH, Kaltenbach K, et al. Characteristics of opioid-using pregnant women who accept or refuse participation in a clinical trial: screening results from the MOTHER study. Am J Drug Alcohol Abuse 2009;35:429–33.

37. Winklbaur B, Kopf N, Ebner N, et al. Treating pregnant women dependent on opioids is not the same as treating pregnancy and opioid dependence: a knowledge synthesis for better treatment for women and neonates. Addiction 2008;103:1429–40.

38. Benningfield M, Arria AM, Kaltenbach K, et al. Co-occurring psychiatric symptoms are associated with increased psychological, social, and medical impairment in opioid dependent pregnant women. Am J Addict 2010;19:416–21.

39. Chen C, Lin H. Prenatal care and adverse pregnancy outcomes among women with depression: a nationwide population-based study. Can J Psychiatry 2011; 56(5):273–80.

40. Fitzsimmons H, Tuten M, Vaidya V. Mood disorders affect drug treatment success of drug-dependent pregnant women. J Subst Abuse Treat 2007;32:19–25.

41. Klinger G, Merlob P. Selective serotonin reuptake inhibitor induced neonatal abstinence syndrome. Isr J Psychiatry Relat Sci 2008;45(2):107–13.

42. Sulkowski MS, Mast EE, Seeff LB, et al. Hepatitis C virus infection as an opportunistic disease in persons infected with human immunodeficiency virus. Clin Infect Dis 2000;30(Suppl 1):77–84.

43. McCance-Katz EF. Treatment of opioid dependence and coinfection with HIV and hepatitis C virus in opioid-dependent patients: the importance of drug interactions between opioids and antiretroviral agents. Clin Infect Dis 2005;41(Suppl 1):S89–95.

44. Batkis MF, Treisman GJ, Angelino AF. Integrated opioid use disorder and HIV treatment: rationale, clinical guidelines for addiction treatment, and review of interactions of antiretroviral agents and opioid agonist therapies. AIDS Patient Care STDs 2010;24(1):15–22.

45. Goler N, Armstrong MA, Taillac CJ, et al. Substance abuse treatment linked with prenatal visits improves perinatal outcomes: a new standard. J Perinatol 2008;28(9): 597–603.

46. Terplan M, Lui S. Psychosocial interventions for pregnant women in outpatient illicit drug treatment programs compared to other interventions. Cochrane Database Syst Rev 2007;4:CD006037.

47. Peirce J, Petry NM, Stitzer ML, et al. Effects of lower-cost incentives on stimulant abstinence in methadone maintenance treatment: a National Drug Abuse Treatment Clinical Trials Network study. Arch Gen Psychiatry 2006;63(2):201–8.

48. Lott DC, Jencius S. Effectiveness of very low-cost contingency management in a community adolescent treatment program. Drug Alcohol Depend 2009;102(1–3): 162–5.

49. Gossop M, Stewart D, Marsden J. Attendance at Narcotics Anonymous and Alcoholics Anonymous meetings, frequency of attendance and substance use outcomes after residential treatment for drug dependence: a 5-year follow-up study. Addiction 2008;103(1):119–25.

50. Kaltenbach K, Berghella V, Finnegan L. Opioid dependence during pregnancy. Effects and management. Obset Gynecol Clin North Am, 1998;25(1):139–51.

51. Kaltenbach K, Silverman N, Wapner R. Methadone maintenance during pregnancy. In: State methadone treatment guidelines, Center for Substance Abuse Treatment 1992. Rockville (MD): US Department of Health and Human Services; 1992. p. 85–93.

52. Jones HE, Kaltenbach K, Heil SH, et al. Neonatal abstinence syndrome after methadone or buprenorphine exposure. New Engl J Med 2010;363(24):2320–31.

53. Finnegan L, Wapner R. Narcotic addiction in pregnancy. In: Neibyl J, editor. Drug use in pregnancy. Philadelphia: Lea and Febiger; 1987. p. 203–22.

54. Rayburn WF, Bogenschutz M. Pharmacotherapy for pregnant women with addiction. Am J Obstet Gynecol 2004;191:1885–97.

55. Nanovskaya T, Deshmukh S, Brooks M, et al. Transplacental transfer and metabolism of buprenorphine. J Pharmacol Exp Ther 2002;300(1):26–33.

56. Johnson RE, Chutuape MA, Strain EC, et al. Comparison of levomethadyl acetate, buprenorphine, and methadone for opioid dependence. N Eng J Med 2000;343: 1290–7.

57. Center for Substance Abuse Treatment. Clinical guidelines for the use of buprenorphine in the treatment of opioid addiction. In: Treatment improvement protocol (TIP) series 402004. Rockville (MD): Department of Health and Human Services; 2004.

58. Jones HE, Martin PR, Heil SH, et al. Treatment of opioid-dependent pregnant women: clinical and research issues. J Subst Abuse Treat 2008;35(3):245–59.

59. Lintzeris N, Nielsen S. Benzodiazepines, methadone and buprenorphine: interactions and clinical management. Am J Addict 2010;19(1):59–72.

60. Amato L, Minozzi S, Vecchi S, et al. Benzodiazepines for alcohol withdrawal. Cochrane Database Syst Rev 2010;3:CD005063.

61. White JM. Pleasure into pain: the consequences of long-term opioid use. Addict Behav 2004;29(7):1311–24.

62. Alford DP, Compton P, Samet JH. Acute pain management for patients receiving maintenance methadone or buprenorphine therapy. Ann Intern Med 2006;144(2): 127–34.

63. Gevirtz C, Frost EA, Bryson EO. Perioperative implications of buprenorphine maintenance treatment for opioid addiction. Int Anesthesiol Clin 2011;49(1):147–55.

64. Bryson EO, Lipson S, Gevirtz C. Anesthesia for patients on buprenorphine. Anesthesiol Clin 2010;2010(28):611–7.

65. Heil SH, Jones HE, Arria A, et al. Unintended pregnancy in opioid-abusing women. J Subst Abuse Treat 2011;40(2):199–202.

66. Lindemalm S, Nydert P, Svensson JO, et al. Transfer of buprenorphine into breast milk and calculation of infant drug dose. J Hum Lact 2009;25:199–205.

67. American Academy of Pediatrics. Committee on Drugs. The transfer of drugs and other chemicals into human milk. Pediatrics 2001;108:776–89.

68. Backes CH, Backes CR, Gardner D, et al. Neonatal abstinence syndrome: transitioning methadone-treated infants from an inpatient to an outpatient setting. J Perinatol 2011. [Epub ahead of print].

69. Abdel-Latif ME, Pinner J, Clews S, et al. Effects of breast milk on the severity and outcome of neonatal abstinence syndrome among infants of drug-dependent mothers. Pediatrics 2006;117(6):e1163–9.

70. Zelson C, Rubio E, Wasserman E. Neonatal narcotic addiction: 10 year observation. Pediatrics 1971;48(2):178–89.

71. Jansson L, Velez M, Harrow C. The opioid-exposed newborn: assessment and pharmacologic management. J Opioid Manag 2009;5(1):47–55.

72. The American Academy of Pediatrics, Committee on Drugs. Neonatal drug withdrawal. Pediatrics 1998;101:1079–88.

73. Kraft WK, Dysart K, Greenspan JS, et al. Revised dose schema of sublingual buprenorphine in the treatment of the neonatal opioid abstinence syndrome. Addiction 2011;106(3):574–80.

74. Poon CY. Update on the pharmacologic management of neonatal abstinence syndrome. J Perinatol 2011;31(11):692–701.

75. Coyle M, Ferguson A, Lagasse L, et al. Diluted tincture of opium (DTO) and phenobarbital versus DTO alone for neonatal opiate withdrawal in term infants. J Pediatr 2002;140(5):561–4.

76. Agathe A, Kim GR, Mathias KB, et al. Clonidine as an adjunct therapy to opioids for neonatal abstinence syndrome: a randomized, controlled trial. Pediatrics 2009; 123(5):849–56.

77. O'Grady MJ, Hopewell J, White MJ. Management of neonatal abstinence syndrome: a national survey and review of practice. Arch Dis Child Fetal Neonatal Ed 2009;94(4): F249–52.

Training the Next Generation of Providers in Addiction Medicine

Ernest Rasyidi, MD[a],*, Jeffery N. Wilkins, MD[b], Itai Danovitch, MD[b]

KEYWORDS

- Addiction • Psychiatry • Physician training • Primary care • Addiction medicine
- Addiction psychiatry • Patient-centered medical home

KEY POINTS

- Most medical students and residents will receive inadequate addiction medicine training.
- Formal addiction medicine training within the medical field has been most closely tied to psychiatry.
- At the medical school level, formal addiction education typically occurs in the context of psychiatric didactics and clerkships.
- Attempts at improvement need to revolve around integration of addiction medicine education into nonpsychiatric specialties.
- Case-based learning has emerged as an effective medium for imparting a rich array of medical knowledge during the didactic years.
- There is a need to bolster addiction medicine training for primary care residencies with explicit recommended requirements as well as suggestions on how to develop primary care residencies that could meet these requirements.
- Within the United States there exists a profound discrepancy between the significant public health problem of substance abuse and access to treatment for addicted individuals.

THE CHALLENGE IN ADDICTION MEDICINE TRAINING

Despite decades of evidence demonstrating the need for improved training of physician trainees, most medical students and residents will receive inadequate addiction medicine training and will, therefore, lack core clinical competencies required for working with patients addicted to alcohol, drugs of abuse, prescription drugs, and tobacco.

Studies have demonstrated the annual cost of alcohol abuse at $191.6 billion, drug abuse at $151.4 billion, and tobacco use at $167.8 billion for a total annual cost of $510.8 billion.[1] Focusing on alcohol use, the 2010 National Survey on Drug Use and

The authors have nothing to disclose.
[a] Department of Psychiatry and Behavioral Neurosciences, Cedars-Sinai Medical Center, 6214 Drexel Avenue, Los Angeles, CA 90048, USA; [b] Department of Psychiatry and Behavioral Neurosciences, Cedars-Sinai Medical Center, 8700 Beverly Boulevard, Los Angeles, CA 90048, USA
* Corresponding author.
E-mail address: Ernest.Rasyidi@cshs.org

Psychiatr Clin N Am 35 (2012) 461–480
http://dx.doi.org/10.1016/j.psc.2012.04.001
0193-953X/12/$ – see front matter Published by Elsevier Inc.

Health demonstrates that 51.8% of US individuals aged 12 years and older, or 131.3 million people, identify themselves as current drinkers, with nearly one fourth (23.1%) aged 12 or older reporting binge drinking at least once in the past 30 days. Thus, 58.6 million people report binge drinking while another 6.7%, or 16.9 million individuals report heavy drinking (of note, only approximately 10% of the heavy drinkers receive treatment).[2] Of course, these costs do not define or estimate the personal and family tragedies that are a part of the addiction process. Primary care physicians are well positioned to join others in mitigating the addiction process in their patients, particularly in performing the Screening, Brief Intervention and Referral for Treatment (SBIRT) model discussed here.

THE CURRENT STATE OF ADDICTION MEDICINE TRAINING

Formal addiction training within the medical field has been most closely tied to psychiatry, dating back to the National Institute on Drug Abuse (NIDA) Career Teacher program initiation in the 1970s. Psychiatry has set forth some of the clearest training guidelines and training evaluation standards throughout the subsequent four decades. Psychiatry has also maintained a streamlined path toward board certification by the American Board of Psychiatry and Neurology as an addiction psychiatrist, having achieved American Board of Medical Specialties (ABMS) status as a subspecialty within psychiatry. Further, the training of addiction psychiatry fellows has been certified by the Accreditation Council for Graduate Medical Education (ACGME).

Addiction Problems are Outpacing Caregivers

Even with current training, the medical needs of persons with addiction problems in society far outpace the capacity for care by addiction psychiatrists, or psychiatrists specializing in addiction for that matter. In addition, medical care for addicted patients (eg, alcohol-induced liver, gastrointestinal, and neurologic disorders; addiction-related cardiovascular and infectious disorders; and lung and other diseases stemming from tobacco use) often requires interventions that better fit the medical training and experience of other medical specialties.

In 2008, the number of practicing physicians and surgeons was approximately 661,400, of whom 14,400 were physician specialists in addiction and, of these, approximately 6000, or fewer than 1% of all physicians, are addiction psychiatrists. Five percent of graduating medical student residency matches each year belongs to psychiatry, in contrast to more than one third of residency matches for fields defined as primary care (eg, family medicine, primary medicine, and pediatrics). Thus, as many experts have pointed out through the decades, there is a need for primary care physicians to have sufficient clinical competencies in addiction medicine. Yet, beginning with medical school education, there are no formal requirements for addiction medicine training. Rather, guidelines set general requirements that medical colleges can then apply to a broad array of diseases. The main accrediting body for medical schools in the United States is the American Association of Medical Colleges (AAMC), and medical school curricula are guided largely by the requirements and recommendations set forth by two branches of the AAMC, the Liaison Committee on Medical Education (LCME)[3] and Medical School Objectives Project (MSOP).[4] The LCME requires the curriculum to include "behavioral subjects," as well as education on "preventive, acute, chronic, continuing, [and] rehabilitative" care. These requirements are flexible, and although they could describe many of the areas addressed in treating alcohol misuse and smoking cessation, they could also apply to obesity and poorly managed diabetes. The MSOP cites the mental status exam as a required area of competency as well as an ability to formulate a treatment plan for common

Table 1	
Medical school addiction care training characteristics	
LCME	**MSOP**
153 schools	The ability to perform both a complete and an organ
75,000 students	system specific examination, including a mental
Behavioral subjects (Section ED-10)	status examination
Preventive, acute, chronic, continuing,	The ability to construct appropriate management
and rehabilitative care	strategies for patients with common conditions,
(Section ED-13)	both acute and chronic, including psychiatric
	conditions and those requiring short- and long-
	term rehabilitation

conditions, both medical and psychiatric. Though the MSOP criteria are slightly more concrete, there is still no explicit educational requirement for treating substance-related disorders (**Table 1**).

Residency Training in Addiction Medicine

Residency training provides little improvement over medical school with regard to training in addiction medicine. Whereas psychiatry residency has clear requirements for addiction medicine training, both in terms of duration and content, this is not the case across all other residency programs. Training programs are accredited by the ACGME, which puts forth the requirements for the various specialties. The other major regulatory body is the ABMS, which monitors and certifies "board certified" status in the colloquial sense. For psychiatric residency there is a minimum requirement of 1 month full-time equivalent with an experience focused on "detoxification, management of overdose, [and] maintenance pharmacotherapy" as well as behavioral interventions.[5] There is specific mention of the stages of change recovery model and self-help groups. This contrasts greatly with the core primary care specialties, which do not have explicit training requirements for addictions:

- For internal medicine, residents are required to have "opportunities for experience in psychiatry" among other specialties, but they are not mandated to have such rotations, especially for addictions.[6]
- In family medicine, residents must take "into account social, behavioral, economic, cultural, and biologic dimensions." Further, the ACGME requires that "behavioral counseling" be integrated into family medicine resident education,[7] though there is no stated requirement for exposure to addictions or substance use.
- In the pediatrics residency, the "comprehensive experience" is required to include "acute psychiatric, behavioral, and psychosocial problems" but with no specific mention of addiction[8] (**Table 2**).

Fellowships in Addiction Medicine

Up until now, only psychiatry has offered subspecialization fellowships in addiction medicine that have been recognized by the ACGME, and ABMS board certification in a psychiatric subspecialty in addiction medicine can be achieved by passing a post-training examination. Fellows may enroll after completion of any residency, though only those who have completed a psychiatric residency are eligible to sit for the American Board of Psychiatry and Neurology (ABPN) examination that is

Table 2 Residency addiction medicine training characteristics			
Psychiatry	**Internal Medicine**	**Family Medicine**	**Pediatrics**
182 programs	381 programs	452 programs	198 programs
5070 residents	23,268 residents	10,129 residents	8584 residents
1 month	No specific duration	No specific duration	No specific duration
Intoxication	Opportunities for experience in	Social and behavioral considerations	Psychiatric, behavioral, and psychosocial problems
Detoxification	psychiatry, but no requirement	Behavioral counseling	
Pharmacotherapy			
Behavioral therapy			

recognized by the ABMS.[9,10] Curriculum requirements include training on substance effects, management of intoxication and withdrawal, and pharmacologic and psychotherapeutic interventions. Core competency requirements set forth by the ABPN for addiction psychiatrists also include knowledge on evaluation and consultation for forensic populations, young adults, women, elderly, and medical professionals, among others.

American Board of Addiction Medicine

A new direction in the field of addiction medicine training was taken with the formation of the American Board of Addiction Medicine (ABAM) in 2007 (**Table 3**). The mission of ABAM to obtain ABMS certification of addiction medicine started with an earlier ASAM committee with that same charge. ABAM has now established ten new addiction medicine programs across the country, with many more under development. These programs are not currently ACMGE certified, though ABAM plans to initiate the application process for certification in 2013.[16] Physicians may apply only after completing an ACMGE accredited residency. Because of this requirement to have previously completed a residency, the ABAM programs are included in **Table 4**. The curriculum put forth by ABAM is comprehensive in scope, with explicit requirements for training in various levels of care; training in pharmacologic and behavioral interventions; and specific consideration for women, children, geriatric, and pain medicine populations. In addition, there is an emphasis on developing administrative and educational skills in the second year of training[17] (see **Table 4**). Currently, completion of an ABAM program could lead to ABAM certification but not to ABMS board certification. In addition, physicians from any ABMS recognized specialty are eligible for the ABAM exam if they have 1 year's full-time equivalent over the past 5 years in addiction-related work along with other continuing medical education (CME) and licensure criteria.[18]

CURRENT DEFICITS IN ADDICTION MEDICINE TRAINING

At the medical school level, formal addiction education typically occurs in the context of psychiatric didactics and clerkships. In curricula where this is the case, changes to psychiatric experiences, including shortening of the duration of required clerkships and a reliance on quantitative educational goals, leave many of the skills needed to treat addictions underpracticed, and, hence, underdeveloped.

Table 3
Select list of physician contributions to substance abuse treatment and physician training

1784; 1812	Benjamin Rush, MD 1784: Publishes pamphlet, "Inquiry into the Effects of Ardent Spirits on the Human Mind and Body." 1812: Published first textbook on "Medical Inquiries and Observations upon the Diseases of the Mind"; became known as the "Father of American Psychiatry."[11] Dr. Rush pioneered the therapeutic approach to addiction.[12,13] Before his work, drunkenness was viewed as a "choice" and, thus, a sin. Rush declared that it was the properties of alcohol, rather than the alcoholic's choice, that was the causal agent. He developed the conception of alcoholism as a form of medical disease and proposed that alcoholics should be weaned from their addiction via less potent substances.[14]
1849	Swedish physician Magnus Huss coins the term "alcoholismus chronicus" to describe chronic alcohol use disease. Historically, this is cited as the introduction of the term alcoholism.
1935	Alcoholics Anonymous (AA) founded by Dr. Bob H. Smith (surgeon) and Bill Wilson.
1935	State and US Public Health addiction treatment hospitals are established including at Lexington, KY and Fort Worth, TX. Birthplace of modern addiction clinical research where physicians Marie Nyswander, Jerome Jaffe, George E. Vaillant, and Patrick Hughes were all trained.
1949–1950	Minnesota Model of cooperation between 12-step–based treatment process and medical management emerges at Hazelden and its affiliation with Willmar State Hospital, coordinated by Nelson Bradley, MD.
1944–1967	American Medical Association and American Hospital Association pass resolutions that lead to hospital-based treatment of alcoholism.
1954	The New York City Medical Society on Alcoholism (NYCMSA) holds inaugural scientific meeting; in 1969, the society changes its name to American Medical Society on Alcoholism and in 1988 changes its name to the American Society of Addiction Medicine (ASAM).
1965	Vincent P. Dole, MD, a physician clinical research at the Rockefeller Institute, now Rockefeller University, and Marie Nyswander, MD, a psychiatrist and psychoanalyst, publish their landmark JAMA article introducing methadone treatment of opioid dependence.[15]
1971	National Institutes of Health (National Institute of Alcohol and Alcoholism [NIAAA] and National Institute on Drug Abuse [NIDA]) create the Career Teacher Program in the addictions including faculty development in 59 medical schools.
1972	California Society for the Treatment of Alcoholism and Other Drug Dependencies, later to become California Society of Addiction Medicine (CSAM), is founded; is supported by California Medical Association to educate and certify physicians in the addictions and launches certification program in 1982. In 1986, California Society's certification program is adopted by AMSA, later to become American Society of Addiction Medicine (ASAM); the California Society formally gives AMSA its certification examination.
1985	American Academy of Psychiatrists in Alcoholism and the Addictions is formed; later becomes the American Academy of Addiction Psychiatry (AAAP).
1991	American Board of Medical Specialties (ABMS) grants addiction psychiatry subspecialty status through the American Board of Psychiatry and Neurology; addiction psychiatry training programs are certified by Accreditation Council for Graduate Medical Education (ACGME).
2006	ASAM Board approves strategic plan to establish addiction medicine as an ABMS-recognized medical specialty; a medical specialty action group is formed to carry out this process.
2007	The American Board of Addiction Medicine (ABAM) is incorporated; its inaugural meeting occurs in April, 2008.
2011	Ten addiction medicine fellowship programs are certified by ABAM.

Table 4 Fellowship addiction medicine training characteristics	
ABPN	**ABAM[a]**
45 programs	10 programs
68 fellows	25 residents (estimated)
1–2 years	1–2 years
Inpatient, outpatient, medical, surgical, Intensive care unit, ED	Inpatient, outpatient, partial hospitalization program, intensive outpatient program, residential care
Genetic vulnerability	Prevention, screening
Pharmacotherapy	Pharmacotherapy
Psychotherapeutic modalities (cognitive–behavioral therapy, motivational enhancement therapy, group therapy)	Behavioral therapy
Special populations	Special populations
Continuity care	Medical comorbidities
	Psychiatric comorbidities
Teaching and supervision experiences	Administrative and educational training

[a] Not currently recognized by the American Board of Medical Specialties.

Clinical Skills

A study by Rosenthal and colleagues in 2005[19] sought to examine what might be the impact of trends toward shorter psychiatric clerkships on student evaluation methods. A clear relationship was shown between "shrinking" psychiatry clerkships and a heavier reliance on National Board of Medical Examiner (NBME) "shelf" examinations as a means of rotation evaluation. One finding that met statistical significance was the use of oral examination as part of the evaluation process. This occurred in only 4.5% of 4-week clerkships versus 42.9% in 8-week clerkships. The authors of the study express understandable concern that such a paradigm shift leads to overvaluing book learning and multiple-choice recognition at the expense of the clinical skills and professionalism assessed in oral examination.

When clerkships are shortened and shelf examinations are more prevalent, medical schools may attempt to ensure the quality of training by having explicit objective measures over the course of the rotation to make sure students are gaining adequate exposure to an appropriate variety of diagnoses and developing needed skills. However, a 2009 study by West and Nierenberg[20] found that even when medical students met required numbers of patient encounters during a psychiatric clerkship, nine of the ten learning targets for counseling skills were never met. Equally concerning, students reported that they "found a new source of information (eg, locating a Narcotics Anonymous list for a patient)" in fewer than 5% of patient encounters, "used cost conscious strategy" in 3.2% of patient encounters, and "utilized a critical pathway or national guideline (eg, researching evidence-based treatment for posttraumatic stress disorder [PTSD])" in only 1.6% of patient encounters. Though this study was geared at utilizing novel systems to evaluate the success and deficits of the clerkship as a whole, the implication it holds for addiction medicine training is concerning. Students were expected to see a minimum of two patients with a substance abuse diagnosis as part of the differential over the course of the clerkship. Even though this number was met, it appears that students were still lacking in the experiences and training crucial to the effective treatment of addictions, namely counseling, utilization of evidence-based treatments, and a thorough consideration of the financial costs of various treatments. This also shows that when addiction medicine training is linked to general psychiatric education in medical school, it will be subject to the same fluctuations in duration and quality that those experiences undergo.

Perceptions and Stigma of Addiction

In psychiatric residency, insufficient exposure to addiction populations, along with a lack of highly specialized faculty, leads to a discouraging training experience that allows stigma against addictions to continue. Renner and colleagues[21] showed in their 2009 study of 276 general psychiatry residents that trainees have generally poor perceptions of careers in addiction medicine. That study showed that this poor perception was due to cited concerns with the addiction medicine training experience, which included:

- "Not enough exposure to addiction patients"
- Working with "difficult" patients
- Lack of competent faculty
- Overemphasis on detoxification during training with a lack of exposure to long-term care.

Breaking down each of these major factors shows that even with the ACGME criteria for duration of addiction medicine training, residents still felt exposure to addiction patients was inadequate. It also shows that patients suffering from addiction continue to be viewed with stigma, being seen as entitled, manipulative, and demanding. This is significant when taken in the context that these views are often held by general psychiatry residents, who have decided to enter a profession treating historically stigmatized populations, those with mental illness. The concerns regarding lack of adequately trained faculty arise when training programs rely on general psychiatry faculty, with variable degrees of addiction medicine training and experience, to supervise and teach addiction rotations. In addition, the emphasis on acute detoxification over long-term care creates a skewed perception of addiction treatment. This may be a product of programs that lack a robust outpatient addiction treatment program. It may also be the result of a program that includes certain service needs such as a commitment to have residents help provide detoxification services to a busy medical center. Finally, this scenario may also be a product of a poor understanding of what good addiction medicine training can possibly achieve in terms of educational goals. Altogether, this lack of exposure to addiction populations in a sufficient range of settings and lack of highly trained faculty are the major deficits in psychiatric residency training.

Lack of Emphasis on Addiction Medicine Training in Nonpsychiatric Residencies

In nonpsychiatric residencies, examination of the ACGME requirements for core primary care specialties reveals a lack of emphasis on identifying and treating addictions, leaving large segments of the population potentially untreated. As discussed, there are no explicit requirements for addiction training in internal medicine, family medicine, or pediatric programs. Although the ACGME requirements for pediatrics specifically mentions several dozen conditions ranging from "sepsis . . . coma . . . status epilepticus . . . cystic fibrosis . . . and rheumatologic disorders," there is no mention of substance use, addiction, or even the words "alcohol" or "tobacco." Without making light of the seriousness of cystic fibrosis, this disease has an annual prevalence of about 1000 new cases each year, affecting a total of about 30,000 adults and children in the United States.[22] In comparison, data from the 2010 Monitoring the Future (MTF) study found that approximately 42% of young Americans have tried cigarettes by the 12th grade and 19% of 12th graders acknowledged being current smokers.[23] In addition, 71% of American youth admitted having consumed alcohol by 12th grade. Though the MTF study does not estimate the rates of substance use in terms of total numbers, the 2010 United States Census report listed more than 74 million people younger than age 18 years.[24] Thus, one could grossly extrapolate that roughly 31 million Americans have tried cigarettes and 52 million have tried alcohol by age 18. It is clear that merely relying on current training requirements would potentially leave the primary care physicians of tomorrow poorly equipped to treat large swaths of the population.

IMPROVING ADDICTION TRAINING MEDICINE IN MEDICAL SCHOOL

Recognizing the shortcomings of addiction medicine training in medical school, attempts at improvement need to revolve around integration of addiction education into nonpsychiatric specialties to ensure adequate exposure and an ability to approach addiction problems in a comprehensive fashion. Because addiction medicine training is often linked to psychiatry in medical school, some efforts have been made to bolster general psychiatry training to enhance education on addiction along with other psychiatric disorders. Another approach has been to remove addictions from the purely psychiatric domain and integrate it with other medical comorbidities via problem-based learning and revised curricula.

Mandatory Psychiatric Rotations

In terms of augmenting general psychiatric education, one study by Halperin documented improvement in addiction treatment skills with the addition of extra psychiatry clerkship time.[25] That study showed that implementation of a mandatory 2-week rotation during the fourth year of medical school, in addition to a required 4-week clerkship during the third year, could greatly improve the confidence of soon to graduate medical students in identifying and dealing with the types of psychiatric presentations encountered in outpatient settings. This 2-week rotation emphasized various general psychiatric goals, including the identification and treatment of substance abuse in medical settings, particularly when patients were not spontaneously identifying their substance use–related illness. This was accomplished through a focus on interview techniques to lower patients' defensiveness and avoidance of truth telling. The study showed that students were greatly encouraged by the rotation experience and that by placing the brief rotation in the fourth year, their practice habits would be changed by the rotation. This method may be successful in improving addiction medicine education, but it requires an increased allocation of curriculum time to general psychiatry, and in this particular study, occurred in a program that had already reduced its core clerkship to 4 weeks to allow more time for its pediatric clerkship.

Case-Based Learning

Given the competition between educational topics for space in the curriculum, case-based learning has emerged as an effective medium for imparting a rich array of medical knowledge during the didactic years. In one example, Paley and colleagues wrote in their 2009 report regarding the use of fetal alcohol spectrum disorders (FASDs) how carefully selected case reports can convey critical teaching points from a broad array of disciplines.[26] Student knowledge was effectively enhanced in areas from embryology and brain development, to core addiction medicine training topics including psychopharmacology, epidemiology, ethics, screening, and intervention. This technique can be especially useful as medical schools face the challenge of finding sufficient time in the curriculum for increasingly complex diseases.

Integration of Addiction Medicine Training

Another method to augment addiction medicine training beyond psychiatric education and disperse it across more of medical school training is the development of a curriculum seeking to integrate addictions into a broad array of medical specialties with clear educational goals appropriate for all future physicians, regardless of their subsequent specialization. In the 2010 article by Lande and colleagues[27] there is a clear description and summarization of Project MAINSTREAM, "a core addiction medicine curriculum designed to improve education of health professionals in substance abuse, for developing addiction medicine curricula and for gauging their professional growth."[(p127)] This initiative was developed in part by the Substance Abuse Mental Health Services Administration (SAMHSA) and aims to integrate certain core competencies into the first 2 years of medical education. The areas of competencies include screening, brief intervention, and referral to treatment (SBIRT, discussed more fully later in this article), as well as co-occurring disorders, legal and ethical issues, prescription drug abuse, and dealing with impaired health professionals. In addition, Project MAINSTREAM emphasizes integration of addiction medicine training into internal medicine, family medicine, and other primary care specialties. It encourages facilitation of this goal through recognition of addictions as of equal significance compared to other major medical illnesses, through development of faculty specifically trained in addiction medicine, and through the creation of appropriate organizational structures (eg, separate programs or divisions devoted to addictions) in academic training settings. This integrative approach facilitates addiction medicine training beyond the psychiatric clerkship and in concert with other major aspects of general medical education.

It is paramount that addiction becomes an important layer working with other specialties on a wide variety of cases. Given finite time in didactic years, it will be necessary for students to be able to learn from a multitude of specialties simultaneously. Also, if trends toward shrinking psychiatry clerkships continue, addictions will need to integrate into the curricula of internal medicine, family medicine, pediatrics, and emergency medicine, both as a reflection of the role addictions play in all these specialties as well as a means of ensuring adequate exposure in tomorrow's physicians.

IMPROVING ADDICTION MEDICINE TRAINING IN RESIDENCY

In residency the need to develop and satisfy objective measurable educational criteria must be balanced with the acquisition of subjective skills necessary to treat addictions effectively. Gaining comfort in working with addiction populations and a sense of mastery with treatment skills can occur only with consistent exposure. Enhancement of addiction medicine training in psychiatric residency has revolved around quantitative and qualitative efforts as well as structural changes to rotations.

Some initiatives reflect a need to develop objective measurements in conjunction with regulatory needs such as the ACGME requirements for "practice-based learning and improvement." Other efforts recognize the need to focus on the subjective aspects of addiction medicine training such as increasing empathy and addressing stigma. Finally, some programs have chosen to fundamentally redesign how addiction medicine training is administered and have aimed to integrate addiction training beyond a circumscribed rotation.

Addiction Medicine Training Scale

Sattar and colleagues wrote about the implementation of the Addiction Training Scale (ATS),[28] developed to help trainers identify deficits in residents' substance abuse training. This scale asks questions regarding competency in diagnosis, detoxification of all major substances, individual and group therapy, and 12-step and other treatment modalities. The authors found that the scale correlated with the confidence and preparedness that residents expressed in their ability to treat substance abuse populations. They then discussed how the next step would be to test whether this sense of confidence corresponded with actual performance capability. Despite this limitation, it is reasonable that a scale such as the ATS could help tailor training needs to individual residents by identifying areas of perceived weakness for additional focused training.

Reflection Techniques

An attempt to improve the subjective experience of resident training in addictions was studied by Ballon and Skinner.[29] In their 2008 report, they wrote about the implementation of reflection techniques in enhancing the quality of resident education during a 4-week rotation held during the post-graduate year 1. The major components of this technique included keeping a journal to reflect on their experiences during the addiction rotation (residents were informed that this journal was private and would not be reviewed by the coordinator); having weekly individual supervision sessions as well as group process meetings up to three times per month; protected time for journaling, reflection, and further reading; and finally a mandatory reflection paper due just before the end of the rotation. The authors concluded that this technique benefited resident education in multiple domains including breaking down negative attitudes, values, and beliefs regarding people suffering from addiction that the residents had held coming into the rotation; imparting the nature of addiction as a chronic illness; bolstering the residents' awareness of treatment modality options; and developing professional attitudes that enhance the care of addiction populations.

Integration of Addiction Medicine Training and Chief Residency

Another initiative to strengthen addiction medicine training during general psychiatry residency was studied by Iannucci and colleagues as the Massachusetts General Hospital/McLean program implemented structural changes to the curriculum over a 3-year course during the academic years beginning 2005 through 2007.[30] These changes included integrating addiction medicine training over all 4 years of residency by providing a wide array of training settings, from inpatient services to emergency room rotations and outpatient clinics. In addition, there was an intentional focus on both patients presenting with non-substance-abuse–related primary diagnoses subsequently found to have co-occurring disorders as well as specific substance abuse consultations. This curriculum culminated with two options during the fourth and final year of residency: a chief position specifically dedicated to addiction psychiatry, or further electives in addiction psychiatry. In both scenarios, supervision was specifically provided by the clinical director who was a board-certified addiction psychiatrist, or highly trained members of the addiction psychiatry staff. This deliberate effort is an understandable response to the recognition that appropriately trained faculty are key in providing an optimal training experience. The other major component of the chief resident experience was the implementation of opportunities to teach junior residents. This role is crucial in fostering a sense of efficacy and mastery in the addiction psychiatry chief resident, providing an opportunity of modeling to junior residents, and assisting in disseminating vital information and skills when specially trained faculty are in short supply.

Expanding the Scope of Addiction Medicine Training

Altogether, these moves reflect a need to bolster the ACGME criteria through concerted efforts to develop scales for monitoring education, to enhance subjective experiences, and to expand the training experience beyond the minimum criteria of a circumscribed rotation. Part of expanding the scope of addiction medicine training is the creation of teaching opportunities for senior residents to foster a sense of efficacy and confidence that is needed to cultivate further interest. Because unless residents have a better experience with addiction medicine training, they will be unlikely to pursue further exposure, and the major limiting factor of developing well trained faculty for future generations cannot be addressed.

Addiction Medicine Training in Primary Care Residencies

Outside of psychiatry, most of the published literature highlights the need to bolster addiction medicine training in primary care residencies with explicit recommended requirements as well as suggestions on how to develop primary care residencies that could meet these requirements. Additional literature documents some of the innovative programs that have been implemented to enrich addiction medicine training. One of the most articulate and comprehensive calls for integrating addiction medicine into primary care residency was written by O'Connor and colleagues in 2011.[31] In their article, the group identifies six core competencies that residents should be able to perform by the completion of primary care training, summarized in **Box 1**.

These recommendations go far beyond the previous standards of merely screening and referring, as they require a deeper understanding of the pathology at work as well as set standards for the initial stages of treatment. The group goes on to give

---

Box 1
Proposed primary care resident competencies

Describe the epidemiology and spectrum of addiction.

Screen and for and diagnose addiction.

Assess the medical, behavioral, and social consequences of addiction.

Use brief intervention and counseling approaches.

Use appropriate medications for addictions.

Refer patients to substance abuse treatment programs when indicated.

Data from O'Connor PG, Nyquist JG, McLellan AT. Integrating addiction medicine into graduate medical education in primary care: the time has come. Ann Intern Med 2011;154:56–9.

recommendations on how to successfully achieve these competencies, in part citing the Project Mainstream (www.projectmainstream.net) curriculum model previously mentioned. They also cite the need to treat addictions with the same importance as other common chronic conditions, such as cardiovascular disease, stating that effective teaching of the SBIRT model helps to fulfill ACGME competency requirements in domains such as patient care, systems-based practice, and practice-based learning and improvement. They reiterate previously discussed themes of enhancing faculty development if they are to serve as addiction medicine instructors as well as a need for effective administrative units (departments, divisions, and programs) in academic institutions. Finally, they touch on the need to address these competencies if the patient-centered "medical home" model, which relies on multidisciplinary teams of physicians, nurses, and others, is to ever be successful.

Chief Resident Immersion Training

One program that has resulted from the recognition that primary care providers will not only be on the front lines in the battle against addiction, but will also be needed to do much of the heavy lifting, is the Chief Resident Immersion Training (CRIT) program.[32,33] CRIT recognizes the relative dearth of resources in relation to need and focuses brief intensive training on chief residents from internal medicine, family medicine, and emergency medicine residencies. This 4-day course is held once a year and is limited to 22 attendees. The course includes didactic sessions, small group discussions, role play, journal clubs, and experiential learning via Alcoholics Anonymous (AA) meeting attendance and discussions with individuals in recovery. Chief residents who complete CRIT are expected to develop a substance use teaching project to implement on return to their home institution with guidance and support from CRIT faculty. The creation of a program that selects for chief residents is intentional. Chief residents play a key role in training future physicians and often move on to organizational leadership positions.[34] This program has been shown to be high yield, with data showing significant increase in knowledge; confidence; and preparedness to diagnose, manage, and teach. The value of training chief residents to maximize dissemination of information was also evident in the increase of substance use clinical and teaching practices in CRIT participants compared to control.

Thus, future initiatives at improving addiction medicine training in nonpsychiatric residencies will need to reflect an awareness of the need for explicit training objectives along with novel methods for disseminating this training. Psychiatry should play an important role in addiction training of other specialties promoting interdisciplinary exposure using trained addiction medicine educators (senior residents, fellows, and faculty) to collaborate with nonpsychiatrist physicians.

SCREENING, BRIEF INTERVENTION, AND REFERRAL MODEL FOR TRAINING OF RESIDENTS AND ESTABLISHED PRACTITIONERS

Screening, brief intervention, and referral for treatment (SBIRT) is a manual-based, just-in-time partial solution for providing physicians with a functional level of competence in their evaluation of alcohol and other substance abusing patients. SBIRT is a secondary and tertiary prevention protocol that can be performed by physicians in a few minutes; physicians use state-of-the-art clinical research screening tools that have been rigorously evaluated for their validity and reliability. The National Institute of Alcohol and Alcoholism (NIAAA) promotes SBIRT as its core activity in the NIAAA "Guide to Clinicians: Helping Patients Who Drink Too Much."[35] In the NIAAA guide, patients who are "at-risk" drinkers are identified first (secondary prevention), followed by identification of persons who meet criteria for an alcohol disorder (tertiary prevention). The screening tools employed in the NIAAA guide include the Alcohol Use Disorders Identification Test sponsored by the World Health Organization,[36] the Michigan Alcoholism Screening Test,[37] and the Drug Abuse Screening Test (DAST).[38] For an at-risk drinker, the physician begins by stating "You're drinking more than is medically safe. . .I strongly recommend that you cut down (or quit) and I am willing to help." For those meeting criteria for an alcohol disorder, the physician begins by stating "I believe that you have an alcohol use disorder. I strongly recommend that you quit drinking and I'm willing to help." The brief intervention component of SBIRT utilizes skillsets outlined in the evidence-based counseling methodology of motivational interviewing.[39] This methodology first clarifies patients' ambivalence toward their substance abuse through the patients' defining their own discrepancy between what it is they want to achieve if treatment is successful and how their substance abuse prevents or interferes with their desired achievement. Random assignment, controlled trials have demonstrated the efficacy of this approach.[40]

SAMHSA sponsors much of the health services research involving SBIRT, particularly in community settings.[41] Early applications of SBIRT included studies of trauma patients in emergency departments (EDs) and surgical trauma units. For example, trauma is directly associated to 40% of ED visits, half of which are further linked to alcohol use[42]; these numbers are even higher in Level I trauma centers.[43] In addition, SBIRT has been demonstrated at post-SBIRT follow-up to reduce alcohol consumption, decrease driving while intoxicated, and decrease hospitalizations due to repeat injury.[44] A major review of SBIRT evaluated SAMHSA-funded SBIRT screening programs across multiple sites through August 2007. Of the 459,599 patients who were screened, 23% were found to manifest a positive screen for active alcohol and other substance abuse. Sixteen percent received the SBIRT's brief intervention and 4% received a specialty referral. Outcome at 6 months demonstrated[45]:

- 39% decrease in alcohol use
- 68% decrease in illicit drug use
- Across-the-board improvements in general health, mental health, employment, housing, and criminal activity.

Whereas all physicians will benefit from SBIRT training, it is particularly suited for primary care physicians,[46] including family medicine physicians and pediatricians. Primary care physicians using SBIRT have the capacity to improve the treatment rate of individuals with an alcohol use disorder, currently only at about 10% of this population in the United States.[2] Successful identification of at-risk drinkers can reduce potential transitions to alcohol use disorders, while also potentially preventing subsequent alcohol-related automobile and other accidents/trauma. Recent studies have demonstrated that ED SBIRT-induced gains in reduced drinking and subsequent trauma significantly decay 3 months after the initial SBIRT session.[47,48] The association of this decay in SBIRT-induced behavioral change with significant attrition to follow-up strongly supports the prior recommendation by Bernstein and colleagues[49] that once patients have been identified in the ED it is important to transfer the ongoing treatment to an ongoing primary care process where follow-up is significantly enhanced and SBIRT-induced behavioral changes decay at a slower rate.[48]

FUTURE ROLES FOR PSYCHIATRISTS SPECIALIZING IN ADDICTION MEDICINE, INCLUDING ADDICTION PSYCHIATRISTS

Any discussion regarding the future direction of addiction medicine would be incomplete without considering the ramifications the patient-centered medical home (PCMH) model holds for all of medicine including specialties like addiction medicine.

Box 2
Principles of PCMH

A personal physician who provides first contact and continuity.

Physician-directed care, in which the personal physician takes responsibility for coordination of care among other members of the treatment team.

Whole-person orientation, taking into account acute and chronic conditions, preventive medicine, and end-of-life issues.

Personal physician–led coordination and/or integration of care across the spectrum. This can be achieved through utilization of specialists and subspecialists.

Improved access to care; this is typically achieved through restructuring of traditional appointment schedules to allow greater availability of same-day access while utilizing "new options for communication."

Adapted from American Academy of Pediatrics. The joint principles of the patient-centered medical home. Available at: http://practice.aap.org/public/pmo_document302_en.pdf. Accessed December 5, 2011.

The PCMH is one of the leading models being looked toward for future directions in the world of health care reform.[50,51] There are varying degrees of evidence that patients treated in this model have improved outcomes at lower costs to the health care system,[52–54] two core tenets essential to making universal health care in the United States a reality. Though this model dates back to the 1967 when it was developed by the pediatrics field as a means of creating a central archive for a child's medical record and subsequently expanding to a specific approach to providing health care,[55,56] it has gained momentum in recent years with the exponential increase in health care costs. The main defining elements of the PCMH model are summarized in the text that follows (**Box 2**).

A more thorough discussion of the PCMH model along with its merits and weaknesses is beyond the scope of this discussion, though the cited references serve as good starting points for those interested in further review. What is important to explore is how such a model would impact the role of psychiatrists specializing in addiction medicine and what sort of training would best equip them to work in such a model. Within this model there are two foreseeable roles for psychiatrists specializing in addiction:

1. Personal physician
2. Member of the treatment team coordinated by a personal physician.

A discussion of these two options will show that a role as a team member may be more feasible but will require particular strengths in administration and education.

THE PSYCHIATRIST SPECIALIZING IN ADDICTION MEDICINE AS PERSONAL PHYSICIAN

Many in clinical practice today would argue that psychiatrists specializing in addiction medicine and treating patients with alcohol dependence and major depression on a weekly basis are the de facto primary care physicians and that by referring to the internal medicine specialist once a month, they have the most frequent contact with the patient. Other subspecialties such as endocrinology have begun to explore the possibility of serving as the center of the PCMH model in lieu of a primary care physician. The argument is that some subspecialists see patients frequently over a long-term course as part of the management of certain chronic conditions (eg, diabetes, hepatitis, rheumatoid arthritis). The American College of Physicians has gone so far as to issue a statement recommending that subspecialist practices be recognized as medical homes as long as they are willing "to provide care consistent with the PCMH model."[57] However, the literature has shown some concerns associated with having a specialist serve as personal physician.[58] These include the ability of a specialist to provide the comprehensive care required of a personal physician in the PCMH model; the feasibility of restructuring a specialty practice to be consistent with the team approach; and ease of access needed, especially if the specialist serves as the personal physician for only some of the patients in the practice. In addition, given the deepening projected shortages of physicians, one would question the efficiency of allocating specialists in a primary care capacity.

THE PSYCHIATRIST SPECIALIZING IN ADDICTION MEDICINE AS PCMH TEAM MEMBER

The more likely role of tomorrow's psychiatrist specializing in addiction is an integral support member of the PCMH team under the coordination of a personal physician. Amiel and Pincus have written on how the general psychiatrist might be implemented in the PCMH model to satisfy the comprehensive care requirement.[59] In that article, the authors discuss the possibility of bringing psychiatry into a PCMH to serve those with relatively low-severity mental illness while brining general medicine into psychiatrically oriented patient homes for the more severely mentally ill. Beyond merely bringing the psychiatrist into the primary care clinic, the actual role and duties of the psychiatrist is likely to change drastically.

Similar to personal physicians assuming additional coordination and supervision duties at the expense of some direct patient contact, psychiatrists of the PCMH will need to be effective team leaders, educators, administrators, and liaisons.

- They will have less time in direct patient care and will instead be called upon to lead a team of nonphysician members in administering much of the direct patient care in relation to mental health services within the PCMH.
- They must be able to use their expert knowledge and training to continuously teach and supervise team members in diagnostic and therapeutic skills.
- They will also need to manage personnel, recognizing individual traits, tendencies, and deficits to ensure that patients are optimally matched with caregivers.
- Finally, they will serve as the bridge between the nonphysician behavioral health team members and the coordinating personal physician.

When one considers the vast numbers of underserved patients who potentially require treatment under some form of universal health coverage, along with the shortage of treatment providers, the health care system will have to improvise unconventional methods to meet that need. The most obvious way to achieve this will be by taking a physician who could hypothetically care for 100 patients directly and engaging him or her as a supervisor of five nonphysicians who could each treat 80 patients, allowing that one physician to treat 400 patients indirectly. Given the possibility of such a model becoming a prevalent one in the future, it will be imperative that the psychiatrist of tomorrow specializing in addiction medicine be trained not only in strong clinical skills, but also in effective leadership, education, managerial, and communication skills.

SUMMARY

Within the United States there exists a profound discrepancy between the significant public health problem of substance abuse and the access to treatment for addicted individuals. Part of the insufficient access to treatment is a function of relatively low levels or professional experts in addiction medicine. Part of the low levels of professional addiction experts is the result of inadequate addiction medicine training of medical students and residents. This article outlines deficits in addiction medicine training among medical students and residents, yet real change in the addiction medicine training process will always be subject to the complexity of producing alterations across multiple credentialing institutions as well as the keen competition between educators for "more time" for their particular subject. Other hurdles include the broad-based issue of stigma regarding alcoholism[60] and other substance abuse that likely impact all systems that regulate physician addiction medicine training. As noted in the discussion of psychiatry residency, even psychiatry residents manifest stigma regarding substance abusing patients.[21]

Five currently active processes may allow for fundamental change to the inertia in physician addiction medicine training while also potentially impacting stigma:

1. We appear to be at the beginning of the integration of addiction into traditional medicine through the formation of a legitimized addiction medicine subspecialty.
2. The training of primary care trainees and practitioners in the use of SBIRT is accelerating, thus creating another process of addiction integration into traditional medicine.
3. The PCMH is being established as a model for primary care
4. The Paul Wellstone and Pete Domenici Mental Health Parity and Addiction Equity Act of 2008 (MHPAEA) became effective for group health care plan years beginning on or after July 1, 2010; thereby, substance abuse benefits and cost are to be the same as general medical or surgical benefits.[61]
5. The equalizer is prescription drug abuse, which is increasing recognition of addiction among populations where it was previously ignored or denied.

The first three activities will create a medical office "experience" that is largely unknown but carries the power to change the perception of addiction: patients visiting their primary care physicians, who then screen them for addiction problems and give the same attention to treatment and prevention of addiction problems as they might give to treatment and prevention of cardiovascular disease and other medical issues.

The personal experience of the aforementioned medical scene by members of US society may also provide a very positive impact on psychiatrists, including those who specialize in addiction medicine. It is quite possible that the recognition of addiction medicine as a traditional medical subspecialty as well as the integration of addiction throughout medicine will precede any substantive change in the integration of mental health care with the rest of medicine. Yet, any integration of addiction within the entire field of medicine may open a path for mental health to follow. Psychiatrists, including those who are addiction experts, need to be a part of this new medical integration process. Being a part of new treatment models is why we proposed six future skillsets for psychiatrists who specialize in addiction (**Box 3**). The selection of these proposed skillsets anticipates an integrated health care team utilizing some form of a patient-centered approach—three are skillsets that are already required, while the last three address new skillsets that will be helpful in working with the integrative health care team model. Whatever form the future of addiction care takes, psychiatrists who specialize in addiction medicine can provide positive and core contributions as expert addiction and mental health consultants including:

1. How does one screen for major depression and/or an anxiety disorder and also determine a diagnosis?

Box 3
Skillset of tomorrow's addiction psychiatrist

1. Pharmacotherapy of addiction
2. Multiple psychotherapeutic modalities for addiction
3. High level of expertise in treating co-occurring disorders to treat patients refractory to general psychiatry and addiction medicine
4. Teaching ability to train and educate specialists and nonphysicians in SBIRT
5. Administrative ability to manage nonphysician PCMH members
6. Liaison skills to act as bridge between personal physicians and nonphysicians

---

2. In prescribing, what constitutes legitimate follow-up of patients on antidepressants and antianxiety agents, including how to avoid additional substance abuse problems when prescribing sedative-hypnotics?
3. When and how should patients be referred to a psychiatrist?

Finally, it is important to note that any of the potential changes described in this article need to influence only 10% of the approximately 17 million current heavy drinkers to seek treatment to equal the approximately 1.7 million heavy drinkers who are now in treatment, let alone any of the approximately 50 million current at-risk drinkers, virtually none of whom are in treatment. Among other social changes that will alter the future of addiction treatment, the integration of addiction into traditional medicine may go a long way in altering the current ratios of who seeks treatment and is willing to participate in treatment.

REFERENCES

1. Harwood H. U.S. Department of Health and Human Services. Updating estimates of the economic costs of alcohol abuse in the United States. Available at: http://pubs.niaaa.nih.gov/publications/economic-2000/alcoholcost.PDF. Accessed December 27, 2011.
2. Substance Abuse and Mental Health Services Administration. Results from the 2010 National Survey on Drug Use and Health: summary of national findings, NSDUH series H-41, HHS publication no. (SMA) 11-4658. Rockville (MD): Substance Abuse and Mental Health Services Administration; 2011.
3. Liaison Committee on Medical Education. Standards for accreditation of medical education programs leading to the M.D. degree. May 2011. Available at: http://www.lcme.org/functions.pdf. Accessed December 20, 2011.
4. American Association of Medical Colleges. Report I: learning objectives for medical student education, guidelines for medical schools. Medical School Objectives Project, January 1998. Available at: https://members.aamc.org/eweb/upload/Learning%20Objectives%20for%20Medical%20Student%20Educ%20Report%20I.pdf. Accessed December 20, 2011.
5. ACGME. Psychiatry residency requirements. Available at: http://www.acgme.org/acWebsite/downloads/RRC_progReq/400_psychiatry_07012007_u04122008.pdf. Accessed November 25, 2011.
6. ACGME. Internal medicine residency requirements. Available at: http://www.acgme.org/acWebsite/downloads/RRC_progReq/140_internal_medicine_07012009.pdf. Accessed November 25, 2011.

7. ACGME. Family medicine residency requirements. Available at: http://www.acgme. org/acWebsite/downloads/RRC_progReq/120pr07012007.pdf. Accessed November 25, 2011.

8. ACGME. Pediatric residency requirements. Available at: http://www.acgme.org/ acWebsite/downloads/RRC_progReq/320_pediatrics_07012007.pdf. Accessed November 25, 2011.

9. Polydorou S, Gunderson EW, Levin FR. Training physicians to treat substance use disorders. Curr Psychiatry Rep 2008;10(5):399–404.

10. Tontchev GV, Housel TR, Callahan JF, et al. Specialized training on addictions for physicians in the United States. Substance Abuse 2011;32:84–92.

11. Hellemans A, Bunch B. The timetables of science. New York: Simon & Schuster; 1988. p. 261.

12. Elster J. Strong feelings: emotion, addiction, and human behavior. Cambridge, MA: MIT Press; 1999. Available at: http://books.google.com/?id=63_19D3jPDgC&pg= PA131&lpg=PA131&dq=%22benjamin+rush%22+%22harry+levine%22. Accessed December 27, 2011.

13. Durrant R, Thakker J. Substance use & abuse: cultural and historical perspectives. Thousand Oaks, CA: SAGE Publications; 2003.

14. Rush B. Inquiry into the effects of ardent spirits upon the human body and mind. Philadelphia: Bartam; 1805.

15. Dole VP, Nyswander ME. A medical treatment for diacetylmorphine (heroin) addiction: a clinical trial with methadone hydrochloride. Jama 1965;193(8):646–50.

16. ABAM. "What's new." Available at: http://www.abam.net/whats-new/. Accessed November 25, 2011.

17. ABAM. Compendium of education objectives for addiction medicine residency training. Available at: http://www.abam.net/wp-content/uploads/2011/04/ABAM-Foundation-Compendium-of-Educational-Objectives-March-25-2011.pdf. Accessed November 25, 2011.

18. ABAM. Eligibility criteria booklet for 2012 exam. Available at: http://www.abam.net/ wp-content/uploads/2011/06/2012-Cert-App-Eligibility-Criteria-Final.pdf. Accessed November 25, 2011.

19. Rosenthal RH, Levine LE, Carlson DL, et al. The "shrinking" clerkship: characteristics and length of clerkship in psychiatry undergraduate education. Acad Psychiatry 2005;29:47–51.

20. West DA, Nierenberg DW. Student experiences with competency domains during a psychiatry clerkship. Acad Psychiatry 2009;33:204–11.

21. Renner JA, Karam-Hage M, Levinson M, et al. What do psychiatric residents think of addiction psychiatry as a career? Acad Psychiatry 2009;33:139–42.

22. Cystic Fibrosis Foundation. Available at: http://www.cff.org/AboutCF/. Accessed November 25, 2011.

23. Johnston LD, O'Malley PM, Bachman JG, et al. Monitoring the future national results on adolescent drug use: overview of key findings, 2010. Ann Arbor (MI): Institute for Social Research, The University of Michigan; 2011.

24. United States Census Bureau. Age and sex composition: 2010. 2010 Census Briefs. Suitland (MD): Bureau of the Census; 2011.

25. Halperin PJ. Psychiatry in medicine: five years of experience with an innovative required fourth-year medical school course. Acad Psychiatry 2006;30:120–5.

26. Paley B, O'Connor MJ, Baillie SJ, et al. Integrating case topics in medical school curriculum to enhance multiple skill learning: using fetal alcohol spectrum disorders as an exemplary case. Acad Psychiatry 2009;33:143–8.

27. Lande RG, Wyatt SA, Przekop PR. Addiction medicine: a model osteopathic medical school curriculum. J Am Osteopath Assoc 2010;110(3):127–32.
28. Sattar SP, Madison J, Markert RJ, et al. Addiction training scale: pilot study of a self-report evaluation tool for psychiatry residents. Acad Psychiatry 2004;28:204–8.
29. Ballon BC, Skinner W. "Attitude is a little thing that makes a big difference": reflection techniques for addiction psychiatry training. Acad Psychiatry 2008;32:218–24.
30. Iannucci R, Sanders K, Greenfield SF. A 4-year curriculum on substance use disorders for psychiatry residents. Acad Psychiatry 2009;33:60–6.
31. O'Connor PG, Nyquist JG, McLellan AT. Integrating addiction medicine into graduate medical education in primary care: the time has come. Ann Intern Med 2011; 154:56–9.
32. Alford DP, Bridden C, Jackson AH, et al. Promoting substance use education among generalist physicians: an evaluation of the Chief Resident Immersion Training (CRIT) program. J Gen Intern Med 2008;24(1):40–7.
33. CRIT. 2012 program brochure. Available at: http://www.bumc.bu.edu/care/files/2010/06/CRIT-Program-Brochure-2012.pdf. Accessed November 25, 2011.
34. Alpert JJ, Levenson SM, Osman CJ, et al. Does being a chief resident predict leadership in pediatric careers? Pediatrics 2000;105:984–8.
35. National Institute on Alcohol Abuse and Alcoholism. Clinician's guide. 2005 edition. Available at: http://pubs.niaaa.nih.gov/publications/Practitioner/CliniciansGuide2005/clinicians_guide.htm. Accessed December 27, 2011.
36. World Health Organization, Department of Mental Health and Substance Dependence. Alcohol use disorders identification test: guidelines for use in primary care. 2nd edition; 2001. Available at: http://whqlibdoc.who.int/hq/2001/who_msd_msb_01.6a.pdf. Accessed January 4, 2012.
37. Selzer ML. Michigan Alcohol Screening Test (MAST). Available at: http://www.ncadd-sfv.org/symptoms/mast_test.html. Accessed December 27, 2011.
38. Skinner HA. Drug Abuse Screening Test (DAST). Available at: http://www.drtepp.com/pdf/substance_abuse.pdf. Accessed January 4, 2012.
39. Miller WR, Rollnick S. Motivational interviewing: preparing people to change addictive behavior. New York: The Guildford Press, 1991.
40. Hettema J, Steele J, Miller WR. 2005. Motivational interviewing. Annu Rev Clin Psychol 2005;1:91–111.
41. Substance Abuse Mental Health Services Administration. Screening, brief intervention, and referral to treatment (SBIRT). Available at: http://www.samhsa.gov/prevention/sbirt/. Accessed November 25, 2011.
42. Nilsen P, Baird J, Mello MJ, et al. A systematic review of emergency care brief alcohol interventions for injury patients. J Subst Abuse Treat 2008;35:184–201.
43. Gentilello LM, Ebel BF, Wickizer TM, et al. Alcohol interventions for trauma patients treated in emergency departments and hospitals: a cost benefit analysis. Ann Surg 2005;241 (4):541–50.
44. Vaca FE, Winn D. The basics of alcohol screening, brief intervention and referral to treatment in the emergency department. West J Emerg Med 2007;8(3):88–92.
45. Madras BK, Compton WM, Avula D, et al. Screening, brief interventions, referral to treatment for illicit drug and alcohol use at multiple healthcare sites: comparison at intake and 6 months. Drug Alcohol Depend 2009;99(1–3):280–95.
46. Babor TF, Higgins-Biddle JF. Brief intervention for hazardous and harmful drinking: a manual for use in primary care. Geneva (Switzerland): World Health Organization. WHO/MSD/MSB/01.6b; 2001.
47. Kaner E, Beyer F, Dickinson H, et al. Effectiveness of brief alcohol interventions in primary care populations. Cochrane Database Syst Rev 2007;2:CD004148.

48. Aseltine RJ Jr, Academic ED SBIRT Research Collaborative. The impact of screening, brief intervention and referral for treatment in emergency department patients' alcohol use: a 3-, 6- and 12-month follow-up. Alcohol Alcohol 2010;45:514–9.
49. Bernstein E, Bernstein J, Levenson S. Project ASSERT: an ED-based intervention to increase access to primary care, preventive services, and the substance abuse treatment system. Ann Emerg Med 1997;30:182–9.
50. Larson EB, Reid R. The patient-centered medical home movement: why now? Jama 2010;303:1644–5.
51. Rittenhouse DR, Shortell SM. The patient-centered medical home: will it stand the test of health reform? Jama 2009;301:2038–40.
52. Saultz JW, Lochner J. Interpersonal continuity of care and care outcomes: a critical review. Ann Fam Med 2005;3:159–66.
53. Solberg LI, Asche SE, Fontaine P, et al. Trends in quality during medical home transformation. Ann Fam Med 2011; 9:515–21.
54. Bodenheimer T. Lessons from the trenches—a high-functioning primary care clinic. N Engl J Med 2011;365:5–8.
55. American Academy of Pediatrics. Preamble to patient-centered medical home joint principles. Available at: http://practice.aap.org/content.aspx?aid=2063. Accessed December 5, 2011.
56. American Academy of Family Physicians (AAFP), American Academy of Pediatrics (AAP), American College of Physicians (ACP), and American Osteopathic Association (AOA). Joint principles of the patient-centered medical home. Available at: http://practice.aap.org/public/pmo_document302_en.pdf. Accessed December 5, 2011.
57. American College of Physicians. Clarification document. Available at: http://www.acponline.org/advocacy/where_we_stand/medical_home/clarification.pdf. Accessed December 5, 2011.
58. Casalino LP, Rittenhouse DR, Gillies RR, et al. Specialist physician practices as patient-centered medical homes. N Engl J Med 2010;362:1555–8.
59. Amiel JM, Pincus HA. The medical home model: new opportunities for psychiatric services in the United States. Curr Opin Psychiatry 2011;24:562–8.
60. Pescosolido BA, Martin JK, Long JS, et al. A decade of change in public reactions to schizophrenia, depression, and alcohol dependence. Am J Psychiatry 2010;167:1321–30.
61. Obama administration issues rules requiring parity in treatment of mental, substance use disorders. US Department of Health and Human Services. News release, January 29, 2010. Available at: http://www.hhs.gov/news/press/2010pres/01/20100129a.html. Accessed December 27, 2011.

Advances in the Psychosocial Treatment of Addiction

The Role of Technology in the Delivery of Evidence-based Psychosocial Treatment

Lisa A. Marsch, PhD[a],*, Jesse Dallery, PhD[b]

KEYWORDS

- Addiction • Computer • Mobile • Psychosocial treatment • Technology

KEY POINTS

- Although there is strong empirical support for many psychosocial interventions targeting SUDs and related issues, they are rarely provided to those in need.
- Technology-based delivery platforms offer significant promise to increase the reach of evidence-based psychosocial interventions.
- There is a rapidly expanding research effort to translate evidence-based psychosocial interventions into technology-based platforms (eg, web, computer, mobile phone).
- Many technology-based delivery platforms can provide ubiquitous, on-demand access to therapeutic support, and delivery evidence-based treatments with high fidelity.
- Despite the promise of technology, more scientifically rigorous work is necessary to establish efficacy and effectiveness in diverse settings, tailor treatment based on the needs of the user, and isolate mechanisms of behavior change produced by technology-based interventions.

The substance abuse treatment field has made substantial gains in developing empirically supported psychosocial interventions for substance use disorders (SUDs) and co-occurring issues, such as psychiatric comorbidities and HIV risk behavior. Although medication is indicated to treat many SUDs (eg, opioid use disorders),

Disclosures: In addition to her academic affiliation, Dr Marsch is affiliated with HealthSim, LLC, the health-promotion software development organization that developed the web-based therapeutic education system referenced in this manuscript. Dr Marsch has worked extensively with her institutions to manage any potential conflict of interest.

[a] Center for Technology and Behavioral Health, Dartmouth Psychiatric Research Center, Department of Psychiatry, Dartmouth College, Rivermill Commercial Center, 85 Mechanic Street, Suite B4-1, Lebanon, NH 03766, USA; [b] Department of Psychology, University of Florida, PO Box 112250, Gainesville, FL 32611, USA
* Corresponding author.
E-mail address: Lisa.A.Marsch@Dartmouth.edu

Psychiatr Clin N Am 35 (2012) 481–493
doi:10.1016/j.psc.2012.03.009
0193-953X/12/$ – see front matter © 2012 Elsevier Inc. All rights reserved.

providing evidence-based psychosocial interventions (eg, prosocial life skills training, relapse prevention skills training, and HIV education) is often critical for medication treatment to be maximally effective. Furthermore, in many cases, psychosocial interventions are critical for generating important skills, attitudes, information, and motivation to promote a drug-free lifestyle. Providing evidence-based psychosocial interventions has been shown to meaningfully improve treatment outcomes, including drug abstinence, treatment retention, psychosocial functioning, and relapse prevention. A recent meta-analysis (n = 2340) demonstrated that nearly 2.5 times as many substance users who received evidence-based psychosocial treatment achieved posttreatment and/or clinically significant abstinence, compared with those who received non–evidence-based psychosocial treatment or no psychosocial treatment.[1]

We review the empirical support for an array of psychosocial treatment interventions targeting SUDs.[2-4] We discuss the barriers to widespread adoption of many evidence-based psychosocial treatments in current systems of care, and the promise of leveraging technology (eg, computers, web, mobile phones, emerging technologies) to enhance the reach of evidence-based treatments in a manner that provides "on-demand," ubiquitous access to therapeutic support in diverse settings. We conclude with a brief description of future directions for technology-based intervention research and dissemination.

EVIDENCE-BASED PSYCHOSOCIAL INTERVENTIONS: DEFINITION AND CHALLENGES ASSOCIATED WITH THEIR IMPLEMENTATION

For the purposes of this article, we restrict our definition of evidence-based therapies targeting SUDs to those supported by randomized, controlled studies, and that also have a technology-based counterpart. These interventions include the community reinforcement approach (CRA), cognitive–behavioral therapy (CBT) and skills training, motivational enhancement therapy (MET: and motivational interviewing [MI]), and contingency management (CM). We also discuss other psychosocial interventions for co-occurring issues (comorbidities), HIV reduction strategies for individuals with SUDs, as well as other, cutting-edge technology-based platforms that do not have a comparable, in-person counterpart (eg, neurocognitive remediation strategies). Although we discuss these interventions separately, they are generally compatible and often include overlapping active ingredients of behavior change.[5,6] Indeed, several psychosocial treatments have been shown to have additive effects when combined relative to when they are delivered alone.[7]

Although the evidence base for psychosocial interventions is strong, they are infrequently provided to individuals with SUDs, even in formal systems of care such as substance abuse treatment.[8,9] Cost is among the most significant barriers to providing evidence-based, behavior change interventions. These interventions are expensive to implement and require financial and staffing resources not available to the average community-based treatment program. They can also be complex and require considerable staff training to be properly applied. Even if evidence-based interventions are initiated by treatment programs, it may be difficult to ensure their fidelity. This may be because of the significant staff turnover in many programs and/or the high patient caseloads maintained by program counselors and their limited contact time with any 1 patient. In addition, travel to treatment programs may be a barrier to accessing evidence-based care for many patients, especially in rural areas. Thus, the limited compatibility of research-based interventions with treatment agency realities presents numerous operational barriers to the transfer of evidence-based practice into community-based settings.

Further, the majority (90%) of persons with SUDs are not in substance abuse treatment. Nearly 21 million Americans annually remain untreated for a SUD, suggesting that the current treatment system is inaccessible or unacceptable to most substance-abusing individuals.[10] Although evidence-based interventions targeting SUDs could be embedded within other systems of care, including an array of medical settings (eg, emergency rooms, primary care, health clinics) and/or criminal justice settings (eg, probation and parole, jails, prisons), they are infrequently provided in such settings. Challenges to delivering evidence-based care in these settings are similar to challenges to delivering these interventions in substance abuse treatment settings, and include limited training, time, and (sometimes) interest among providers to deliver such interventions. Because the availability of trained clinicians is limited and many individuals do not seek out traditionally delivered interventions, offering a "toolkit" of technology-based interventions as alternative or complementary therapeutic tools targeting SUDs and related issues holds promise to markedly impact these behavioral health issues.

HARNESSING TECHNOLOGY TO DELIVER EVIDENCE-BASED PSYCHOSOCIAL INTERVENTIONS

We briefly review the empirical support and conceptual underpinnings of psychosocial treatments and, for each intervention, we discuss how the intervention has been translated into a technology-based platform. Although a few technology-based programs reviewed have an accumulating body of empirical support from numerous randomized, controlled trials, some of these technology-based platforms are still in the development and early testing phases. Thus, the evidence base for these programs varies across programs and further work is still needed to test these interventions using scientifically rigorous research designs.[11]

The Community Reinforcement Approach

The CRA is grounded in research related to drug self-administration and a behavioral analysis of drug dependence. Drugs are viewed as competing successfully with more delayed prosocial reinforcers because of their more immediate reinforcing effects.[12,13] To address this, the skills training component of CRA teaches skills and encourages behaviors that increase nondrug sources of reinforcement (eg, prosocial activities) and shares many common elements with other evidence-based, CBT, and relapse prevention behavioral interventions for SUDs. CRA has been shown to be highly effective in the treatment of a variety of adult substance abusing populations.[14-16] CRA is also highly efficacious in adolescent populations.[17] Compared with a number of other behavioral therapy and family-based approaches, the adolescent CRA, which largely targets youth but also includes a parent component,[18] produced among the highest rates of abstinence (72% total days abstinent) and was demonstrated to be the most cost effective.[15]

Therapeutic Education System

The principles underlying CRA were translated into a technology-based intervention, the therapeutic education system, which is the first web-based psychosocial treatment program for individuals with SUDs evaluated in systematic scientific research. This interactive program is composed of 65 modules with an optional, computerized CM component (see below).[19] These modules include targeting cognitive behavioral skills (refusal skills, managing harmful thoughts, etc), improving psychosocial functioning (family/social relations, managing negative moods, etc), and reducing behavior that may place one at risk for HIV, hepatitis, or sexually transmitted infections. The therapeutic education system is self-directed, includes functionality to build individ-ualized treatment plans, assesses a patient's grasp of material, and adjusts the pace and level of repetition of material to promote skills mastery. It also includes interactive videos to help patients learn behaviors (eg, progressive muscle relaxation). Random-ized trials have found that the therapeutic education system[3,17,20]:

1. Produced outcomes superior to standard substance abuse treatment;
2. Improved objectively measured drug abstinence comparable with rates produced by highly trained clinicians delivering comparable therapy;
3. Improved HIV/prevention knowledge and intentions to reduce HIV risk behavior; and
4. Is highly acceptable to an array of SUD audiences.

Cognitive–Behavioral Therapy and Skills Training Therapies

Cognitive–behavioral approaches have been shown to be effective in a variety of drug-using populations, including cocaine[21] and alcohol users,[22] as well as in adolescents[23] and individuals with a variety of psychiatric disorders.[24] Broadly, these interventions seek to modify relations between environmental and cognitive anteced-ents of problem behavior ("risk factors") and problem behavior such as drug use. These interventions also focus on skills building, such as developing problem solving, coping, and refusal skills. The skills-building features of these interventions may be important in achieving abstinence from the target drug, as well as in addressing other co-occurring problems in patients' lives. Indeed, there is some evidence that effects of CBT and skills-building therapy are long lasting, and continued improvement is evident even 1 year posttreatment.[25,26]

A largely video-based, computer-delivered CBT intervention, the Computer-based Training in Cognitive Behavioral Therapy (or CBT4CBT) program, was developed by Carroll and colleagues.[27] This 6-session program employs key CBT content (e.g., understanding one's patterns of substance use; improving coping skills and decision-making skills). CBT4CBT was found to significantly enhance treatment outcomes when provided as an adjunct to traditional substance abuse treatment[25] and showed promise for cost effectiveness.[28] Participants also demonstrated significantly en-hanced coping skills from the CBT4CBT intervention.[29]

Motivational Interviewing and Motivational Enhancement Therapy

MI and MET are client-centered, semidirective methods designed to help individuals to explore and resolve ambivalence about change and reinforce behavior change.[30] MI is typically a brief intervention, usually 1 session in length, that may be provided as a stand-alone intervention or as part of the beginning of a treatment episode. MET uses MI principles, but is typically a slightly longer intervention (up to about 4 sessions).[6] A recent Cochrane review concluded that MI significantly impacts substance use compared with no treatment controls, but that effects decay over time.[31] Additional research has demonstrated that MI may be particularly effective in strengthening engagement in more intensive addiction treatment. Further, MET has been shown to generally be as effective as other common psychosocial treatments for SUDs.[32]

Several technology-delivered interventions have been developed to deliver MET and MI targeting SUDs. Ondersma and colleagues[33] developed the motivational enhancement system, initially designed to give feedback, assess readiness to change, explore the pros and cons of change, and encourage goal setting to postpartum women who reported substance use before pregnancy. This program has been shown to be highly acceptable and improve motivation to reduce substance use[33] as well as reduce actual substance use among postpartum women.[34] Ondersma and colleagues[35] demonstrated similar effects with a brief MET/MI intervention targeting smoking among pregnant women.

Another web-based MET/MI intervention has been shown to reduce drinking in several groups with problematic drinking, including heavy drinking college students and nondependent problem drinkers.[36–38] This program has also been recently modified for, and shown promise with, military populations.[39]

Contingency Management

Numerous studies over the past 25 years have established the broad applicability and versatility of CM procedures.[40–42] In this treatment, incentives are provided to individuals contingent on a target behavior (eg, biochemical confirmation of drug abstinence). These tangible incentives enable immediate, positive reinforcement (eg, recreational items, retail goods or services) for drug abstinence. Thus, the conceptual model underpinning this intervention is quite similar to CRA. CM interventions have been shown to promote abstinence from cocaine use,[43] cocaine use among methadone-maintained patients,[44] heroin use[45] and polydrug use.[46,47] CM has also been found to exert powerful and precise control of cigarette smoking in both adults and adolescents.[48,49] Further, CM has been provided along with CRA, and both components have been shown to independently contribute efficacy to the combined intervention.[7] Recently, CM has also been extended to promote medication adherence in a variety of populations, including promoting medication adherence among substance-abusing HIV patients.[50,51]

Internet-based contingency management interventions

Several researchers have leveraged technology for the delivery of evidence-based CM interventions targeting SUDs. Dallery and colleagues developed and evaluated an Internet-based CM intervention (Mōtiv8) targeting smoking cessation.[52,53] In this model, smokers use web-cameras to record themselves blowing into carbon monoxide (CO) detectors to provide objective evidence of smoking behavior or abstinence (by meeting targeted CO levels). Reinforcement (eg, incentives, money) was then delivered immediately to individuals who met targeted CO levels. Results have demonstrated that Internet-based CM can promote smoking cessation in heavy, rural, and adolescent smokers.[54] The Internet-based CM model has been extended to incorporate an up-front deposit by the participant.[55] The deposit can be earned back based on evidence of abstinence, and as such it may represent a feasible way to offset costs associated with CM interventions. The Internet-based CM model has also been extended to include group contingencies, where small groups of smokers work together to achieve cessation goals to receive incentives.[55] Participants provide encouragement, feedback, and so on via a discussion board integrated into the Mōtiv8 architecture. The group contingency model could aid in the sustainability of the intervention without an increase in costs.

Additionally, Silverman and colleagues[56,57] have applied a web-based CM intervention to provide incentives for drug abstinence and workplace performance among chronically unemployed individuals with SUDs in a therapeutic workplace. Briefly, to gain access to the workplace, each day patients were required to provide a urine specimen that tested negative for drugs (eg, cocaine, opiates, alcohol). If the specimen tested positive, they were not allowed to work that day. Those who gained entrance received basic skills education and job skills training, and at the end of the shift they received a voucher that could be exchanged for goods and services. This therapeutic workplace model[56,57] has strong empirical support and demonstrates how a technology-based system can produce long-lasting, sustainable effects.[58]

PSYCHOSOCIAL INTERVENTIONS FOR CO-OCCURRING ISSUES

Psychiatric comorbidity, including personality disorders, depression, anxiety, and family dysfunction, are prevalent among individuals with SUDs.[59] Providing employment, family counseling, psychiatric services, and patient education services (eg, prosocial life skills training) as part of treatment is often critical for treatment to be maximally effective. In 1 elegant and striking demonstration of the role of psychosocial interventions in methadone maintenance therapy,[60] patients were randomly assigned to receive:

1. Methadone only at doses of 60 mg or higher with no other services;
2. The same doses of methadone plus counseling; or
3. The same doses of methadone plus counseling and onsite medical/psychiatric, employment, and family therapy.

Results indicated that 69%, 41%, and 19% of patients in each of these three conditions had unremitting use of opiates or cocaine, respectively, demonstrating convincingly that the quantity and quality of psychotherapeutic interventions targeting co-occurring issues markedly impact patient outcomes.

Kay-Lambkin and colleagues[61] developed a computerized intervention targeting co-occurring depression and substance use (with a particular focus on alcohol and cannabis). This 9-session program highlights the relationship between these co-occurring issues and teaches CBT skills using an MI therapeutic style. This program has been shown to produce greater effects on depression and substance use relative to both a brief MI intervention and supportive counseling and to generally produce equivalent outcomes to comparable therapy delivered by clinicians.[61,62]

MOBILE PSYCHOSOCIAL INTERVENTIONS TARGETING SUDS

Although the development and scientific study of psychosocial treatment interventions targeting SUDs delivered on mobile phones is a less well developed area of research, early work in this field is promising. Marsch and colleagues[20] developed and evaluated a prototype of a mobile phone-based psychosocial support program for individuals in substance abuse treatment and showed that providing this mobile intervention, as a supplement to standard substance abuse treatment, markedly impacted treatment outcomes. In addition, Gustafson and colleagues[63] developed ACHESS, a mobile phone-based recovery support tool for individuals in recovery from SUDs. ACHESS provides tools for personalized monitoring and support to individuals in their recovery effort and may be a valuable relapse prevention aid.

HIV RISK REDUCTION

Substance abusing individuals engage in high-risk behaviors, such as sharing injection equipment and/or risky sexual behavior associated with drug use, including engaging in unprotected sex, sex with multiple partners, and sex work, that may place them at risk for infection with HIV and other infectious diseases.[64] Several studies have demonstrated that behavior therapies targeting substance use can reduce HIV risk behaviors.[65,66] A number of effective HIV prevention interventions for both adults and adolescents with SUDs exist, and typically target HIV-related sexual and drug-use behaviors.[67,68] Such programs are typically designed to increase accurate knowledge about HIV and teach skills that promote preventive actions that provide effective deterrents against infection, increase individuals' intentions to reduce risk behavior and communicate about condom use with partners, improve attitudes toward condom use and safer sex, increase individuals' self-efficacy/ability to effectively use condoms, and reduce their perceived invulnerability to HIV, because these variables are strongly predictive of progression to consistent condom use and safer sex.

Several technology-delivered HIV education and prevention programs have been developed for and evaluated with individuals with SUDs.[69] Several such programs have been shown to be highly acceptable and effective as part of substance abuse treatment in promoting high levels of HIV prevention knowledge and reductions in HIV risk behavior among injection drug users[70] as well as adolescents with SUDs.[71]

COMPUTERIZED NEUROCOGNITIVE REMEDIATION/EXECUTIVE FUNCTION THERAPY

The role of executive function and inhibitory cognitive control in the development and maintenance of addictive disorders has been increasingly well-established in addiction research. From this framework, addiction is viewed as an alteration of brain decision-making processes, where the impulsive choices and reduced cognitive control associated with drug use may be the result of the more impulsive brain system dominating the executive brain system (eg, planning, self-control).[8,72]

Neurocognitive remediation (sometimes called executive function therapy) is based on the assumption that, if cognitive functions associated with the executive system can be rehabilitated, self-control behavior may increase.[73] These interventions are delivered via computer and are designed to enhance cognitive skills through exercises that target problem-solving skills, attention, memory, and abstract reasoning. For example, in 1 study, cognitively impaired polysubstance abusers who received computerized cognitive rehabilitation showed improvements in cognitive performance tests and remained in treatment longer than those in a control condition.[74] In addition, interventions designed to enhance cognitive functioning among individuals with SUDs has been shown to enhance the efficiency of cognitive behavioral therapies (eg, relapse prevention).[75]

ADVANTAGES OF TECHNOLOGY TO DELIVER EVIDENCE-BASED INTERVENTIONS

Using technology (eg, computers, web, mobile devices) to deliver evidence-based interventions may enable widespread dissemination to an array of audiences in diverse settings. For example, web-based interventions can be offered in the home, community organizations, schools, emergency rooms, and health care providers' offices, as well as via mobile devices and online social networks. Technology has the potential to address the challenges associated with the delivery of science-based interventions, because it allows for complex interventions to be delivered at a low cost, without increasing demands on staff time or training needs. Technology-delivered interventions can also help ensure the fidelity of intervention delivery.

In addition, the temporal flexibility of technology-based interventions may allow for "on-demand," ubiquitous access to therapeutic support, thereby creating unprecedented models of intervention delivery and reducing barriers to accessing care. Further, the anonymity afforded by technology-based interventions may be appealing to individuals when addressing sensitive topics such as substance use and other risk behaviors.[76] Technology-based therapeutic tools may become increasingly important and clinically useful in light of the 2010 National Drug Control Strategy from the US Office of National Drug Control Policy, which places a strong emphasis of cost-effective care and on integrating treatment for SUDs into other areas of health care (outside formal treatment systems) where providers may have limited expertise in treating individuals with SUDs (mental health, infectious disease management, primary care).[77] Technology-based tools are well-positioned to meet this unmet need in this new model of care.

- Nearly 80% of Americans have Internet access.
- Eight-seven percent of Americans subscribe to mobile phone services.
- Over 46% Americans participate in online social networks.
- Worldwide, there are over 1.5 billion Internet users.
- The growth rate in worldwide users since 2000 has exceeded 340%.
- More than 92% of individuals worldwide subscribe to mobile phone services, with more than 4 billion mobile phone subscriptions worldwide, and an average growth rate of 24% per year.

Although youth remain the primary users of online social networks (e.g., 75% of persons aged 18–24 have an online social network site), adults are increasingly using online social networks. Indeed, the number of adults who have a social network site has quadrupled in the past 4 years, from 8% in 2005 to 46% in 2009.[78] Thus, the potential reach of innovative technological interventions offered on these platforms is enormous.

Additionally, although white Americans (80%) are more likely to use the Internet than African Americans (72%) or Hispanic Americans (61%), African Americans are the most active users of the mobile Internet (accessed via mobile devices). The rate of increase in the use of mobile devices to access the Internet among minority groups is twice the national average since 2007, for example, 141% increased use for African Americans versus the 73% average.[79] By offering interventions on a wide variety of platforms to optimally capitalize on the technology most frequently used by various target populations, technology-based interventions also offer great potential to eliminate the "digital divide" and address healthcare disparities that exist in many traditional models of care.[80]

EMERGING TECHNOLOGIES

Significant developments in technology continue to emerge and offer promise for integration into systems of health care.[81–83] Ubiquitous computing (ubicomp; also sometimes referred to as pervasive computing) and ambient intelligence are rapidly evolving fields in which human–computer interaction are embedded into everyday objects and activities.

Ubiquitous or pervasive computing typically refers to technologies that "weave themselves into the fabric of everyday life until they are indistinguishable from it,"[84] and generally involve miniaturized mobile or embedded information and communication technologies with some degree of "intelligence," network connectivity, and advanced user interfaces.[85] For example, ubiquitous computing technologies may allow for the unobtrusive and objective measurement of behavioral states and biological and environmental variables in real time (eg, via mobile computing devices and wearable sensors). Ubiquitous computing is thus composed of computational and wireless communication devices that are naturally integrated into human activity.

Ambient intelligence refers to a similar concept related to an intelligent environment or an intelligent service system surrounding individuals that anticipate, adapt to, and meet users' needs.[86]

Although these evolving technologies have only just started to be applied to the field of substance abuse and related disorders, they have significant potential for having a marked impact on the field. Indeed, as Boyer and associates[87] convincingly argue, these approaches could allow for real-time, unobtrusive psychophysiologic measurement, and on-demand, continuous access to tailored support, education, and interventions targeting substance abuse. For example, ubicomp tools may allow one to obtain real-time data of physiologic and environmental factors that precede and follow drug use (or abstinence) and provide in-the-moment interventions responsive to these factors.[85] Additionally, ambient intelligent environments, in which environments surrounding an individual could be used to reduce risk behavior, could be used as part of relapse prevention efforts.

SUMMARY

The clinical community has a growing array of psychosocial interventions with a strong evidence base available for the treatment of SUDs. Considerable opportunity exists for leveraging technology in the delivery of evidence-based interventions to promote widespread reach and impact of evidence-based care. Data from this line of research to date are promising, and underscore the potential public health impact of technology-based therapeutic tools.

To fully realize the potential of technology-delivered interventions, several areas of inquiry remain important. First, scientifically sound strategies should be explored to ensure technology-based interventions are optimally designed to produce maximal behavior change. Second, efficient and effective methods should be identified to integrate technology-based interventions into systems of care in a manner that is most responsive to the needs of individual users. Third, payment, privacy, and regulatory systems should be refined and extended to go beyond electronic medical records and telehealth/distance care models, and support the deployment of technology-based systems to enhance the quality, efficiency and cost-effectiveness of care. Fourth, the mechanisms underlying behavior change derived from technology-based treatments should be explicated, including new mechanisms that may be tapped via novel, technology-based tools.[5,6] Such work will be critical in isolating mechanisms that are useful in predicting treatment response, and in ensuring that key ingredients are present in technology-based interventions as they are made widely available.

REFERENCES

1. Dutra L, Stathopolou G, Basden S, et al. A meta-analytic review of psychosocial interventions for substance use disorders. Am J Psychiatry 2008;165:179–87.
2. Bickel WK, Christensen DR, Marsch LA. A review of computer-based interventions used in the assessment, treatment, and research of drug addiction. Subst Use Misuse 2011;46:4–9.
3. Marsch LA. The application of technology to the assessment, prevention and treatment of substance use disorders: an editorial. Substance Use Misuse 2011;46:1–3.
4. Moore BA, Fazzino T, Garnet B, et al. Computer-based interventions for drug use disorders: a systematic review. J Subst Abuse Treat 2011;40:215–23.
5. Moos RH. Theory-based processes that promote the remission of substance use disorders. Clin Psychol Rev 2007;27:537–51.
6. Moos, RH. Theory-based active ingredients of effective treatments for substance use disorders. Drug Alcohol Depend 2007;88:109–21.
7. Higgins ST, Sigmon SC, Wong CJ, et al. Community reinforcement therapy for cocaine-dependent outpatients. Arch Gen Psychiatry 2003;60:1043–52.
8. Bickel WK, Marsch LA. A future for the prevention and treatment of drug abuse: applications of computer-based interactive technology. In: Henningfield JE, Santora PB, Bickel WK, editors. Addiction treatment: science and policy for the twenty-first century. Baltimore: The John Hopkins University Press; 2007.

9. McLellan AT, Carise D, Kleber HD. Can the national addiction treatment infrastructure support the public's demand for quality care? J Subst Abuse Treat 2003;25:117–21.

10. Substance Use and Mental Health Services Administration (SAMHSA) Ooas. Results from the 2008 national survey on drug use and health: national findings (NSDUH Series H-34, DHHS Publication No. SMA 08-4343). Rockville (MD): Author; 2009.

11. Kiluk BD, Sugarman DE, Nich C, et al. A methodological analysis of randomized clinical trials of computer assisted therapies for psychiatric disorders: toward improved standards for an emerging field. Am J Psychiatry 2011;168:790–9.

12. Higgins ST, Budney AJ, Bickel WK, et al. Incentives improve outcome in outpatient behavioral treatment of cocaine dependence. Arch Gen Psychiatry 1994;51:568–76.

13. Hunt GM, Azrinm NH. A community-reinforcement approach to alcoholism. Behav Res Ther 1973;11:91–104.

14. Abbott PJ, Weller SB, Delaney HD, et al. Community reinforcement approach in the treatment of opiate addicts. Am J Drug Alcohol Abuse 1998;24:17–30.

15. Budney RK, Higgins S. A community reinforcement plus vouchers approach: treating cocaine addiction. Rockville (MD): NIDA; 1998.

16. Gross A, Marsch LA, Badger GJ, et al. A comparison between low magnitude voucher and buprenorphine medication contingencies in promoting abstinence from opioids and cocaine. Exp Clin Psychopharmacol 2006;14:148–56.

17. Dennis MD, Godley SH, Diamond G, et al. The cannabis youth treatment study: main findings from two randomized trials. J Subst Abuse Treat 2004;27:197–213.

18. Godley SH, Meyers RJ, Smith JE, et al. The adolescent community reinforcement approach (A-CRA). Cannabis Youth Treatment (CYT) Series. Volume 4. Rockville (MD): Center for Substance Abuse Treatment, Substance Abuse and Mental Health Services Administration; 2001.

19. Bickel WK, Marsch LA, Buchhalter AR, et al. Computerized behavior therapy for opioid-dependent outpatients: a randomized controlled trial. Exp Clin Psychopharmacol 2008;16:132–43.

20. Marsch LA. Computer-delivered psychosocial treatment for substance use disorders. Presentation in symposium on Neurobehavioral and Technological Mechanisms to Improve the Efficacy and Effectiveness of Substance Abuse Treatment (Aklin WM, Onken L, co-chairs). Washington, DC: American Psychological Association Annual Meeting; 2011.

21. Rohsenow DJ, Monti PM, Martin RA, et al. Brief coping skills treatment for cocaine abuse: 12 month substance abuse outcomes. J Consult Clin Psychol 2000;68:515–20.

22. Miller WR, Wilbourne PL. Mesa Grande: a methodological analysis of clinical trials of treatments for alcohol use disorders. Addiction 2002;97:265–77.

23. Kaminer Y, Slesnick N. Evidence-based cognitive-behavioral and family therapies for adolescent alcohol and other substance use disorders. In: Galanter M, editor. Recent developments in alcoholism, vol XVII: research on alcohol problems in adolescents and young adults. New York: Springer; 2005.

24. Barlow DH. Cognitive behavioral therapy for panic disorder: current status. J Clin Psychiatry 1997;58:32–6.

25. Carroll KM, Nich, C, Ball, SA, et al. One-year follow-up of disulfarim and psychotherapy for cocaine-alcohol users: sustained effects of treatment. Addiction 2000;95:1335–49.

26. Hall SM, Humfleet GL, Munoz RF, et al. Extended treatment of older cigarette smokers. Addiction 2009;104:1043–52.

27. Carroll KM, Ball SA, Martino S, et al. Computer-assisted delivery of cognitive-behavioral therapy for addiction: a randomized trial of CBT4CBT. Am J Psychiatry 2008;165:881–8.

28. Olmstead TA, Ostrow CD, Carroll KM. Cost-effectiveness of computer-assisted training in cognitive-behavioral therapy as an adjunct to standard care for addiction. Drug Alcohol Depend 2010;110:200–7.
29. Kiluk BD, Nich C, Babuscio T, et al. Quality versus quantity: acquisition of coping skills following computerized cognitive-behavioral therapy for substance use disorders. Addiction 2010;105:2120–7.
30. Miller WR, Rollnick S. Motivational interviewing: preparing people for change. New York: Guilford Press; 2002.
31. Smedslund G, Berg RC, Hammerstrøm KT, et al. Motivational interviewing for substance abuse. Cochrane Database Syst Rev 2011;5:CD008063.
32. Stephens RS, Roffman RA, Curtin L. Comparison of extended versus brief treatments for marijuana use. J Consult Clin Psychol 2000;68:898–908.
33. Ondersma SJ, Chase SK, Svikis DS, et al. Computer-based brief motivational intervention for perinatal drug use. J Subst Abuse Treat 2005;28:305–12.
34. Ondersma SJ, Svikis DS, Schuster CR. Computer-based brief intervention: a randomized trial with postpartum women. Am J Prev Med 2007;32:231–8.
35. Ondersma SJ, Svikis DS, Lam PK, et al. A randomized trial of computer-delivered brief intervention and low-intensity contingency management for smoking during pregnancy. Nicotine Tob Res 2012;14:351–60.
36. Hester RK, Delaney HD, Campbell W. The college drinker's check-up: outcomes of two randomized clinical trials of a computer-delivered intervention. Psychol Addict Behav 2012;26:1–12.
37. Hester RK, Delaney HD. Behavioral Self-Control Program for Windows: results of a controlled clinical trial. J Consult Clin Psychol 1997;65:686–93.
38. Hester RK, Squires DD, Delaney HD. The Drinker's Check-up: 12-month outcomes of a controlled clinical trial of a stand-alone software program for problem drinkers. J Subst Abuse Treat 2005;28:159–69.
39. Pemberton MR, Williams J, Herman-Stahl M, et al. Evaluation of two web-based alcohol interventions in the U.S. military. J Stud Alcohol Drugs 2011;72:480–9.
40. Kidorf M, Stitzer ML. Contingent access to clinic privileges reduces drug abuse in methadone maintenance patients. In: Higgins ST, Silverman K, editors. Motivating behavior change among illicit-drug abusers: contemporary research on contingency management interventions. Washington, DC: American Psychological Association Books; 1999. p. 221–41.
41. Stitzer ML, Bigelow GE. Contingent reinforcement for reduced carbon monoxide levels in cigarette smokers. Addict Behav 1982;7:403–12.
42. Robles E, Silverman K, Stitzer ML. Contingency management therapies. In: Strain EC, Stitzer ML, editor. Methadone treatment for opioid dependence. Baltimore: The Johns Hopkins University Press; 1999. p. 196–222.
43. Higgins ST, Budney AJ, Bickel WK, et al. Incentives improve outcome in outpatient behavioral treatment of cocaine dependence. Arch Gen Psychiatry 1994;51:568–76.
44. Silverman K, Higgins ST, Brooner RK, et al. Sustained cocaine abstinence in methadone maintenance patients through voucher-based reinforcement therapy. Arch Gen Psychiatry 1996;53:409–15.
45. Silverman K, Wong CJ, Higgins ST, et al. Increasing opiate abstinence through voucher-based reinforcement therapy. Drug Alcohol Depend 1996;41:157–65.
46. Downey KK, Helmus TC, Schuster CR. Treatment of heroin-dependent poly-drug abusers with contingency management and buprenorphine maintenance. Exp Clin Psychopharmacol 2000;8:176–84.

47. Piotrowski NA, Tusel DJ, Sees KL, et al. Contingency contracting with monetary reinforcers for abstinence from multiple drugs in a methadone program. Exp Clin Psychopharmacol 1999;7:399–411.

48. Dallery J, Glenn IM, Raiff BR. An Internet-based abstinence reinforcement treatment for cigarette smoking. Drug Alcohol Depend 2007;86:230–8.

49. Reynolds B, Dallery J, Shroff P, et al. A web-based contingency management program with adolescent smokers. J Appl Behav Anal 2008;41:597–601.

50. Rosen MI, Dieckhaus K, McMahon TJ, et al. Improved adherence with contingency management. AIDS Patient Care STDs 2007;21:30–40.

51. Sorenson JL, Haug NA, Delucchi KL, et al. Voucher reinforcement improves medication adherence in HIV-positive methadone patients: a randomized trial. Drug Alcohol Depend 2007;88:54–63.

52. Dallery J, Glenn IM. Effects of an Internet-based voucher reinforcement program for smoking abstinence: a feasibility study. J Appl Behav Anal 2005;38:349–57.

53. Dallery J, Glenn IM, Raiff BR. An Internet-based abstinence reinforcement treatment for cigarette smoking. Drug Alcohol Depend. 2007;86:230–8.

54. Dallery J, Raiff BR. Contingency management in the 21st century: technological innovations to promote smoking cessation. Substance Use Misuse 2011;46:10–22.

55. Dallery J, Meredith S, Glenn I. A deposit contract method to deliver abstinence reinforcement for cigarette smoking. J Appl Behav Anal 2008;41:609–15.

56. Silverman K, Wong CJ, Grabinski MJ, et al. A web-based therapeutic workplace for the treatment of drug addiction and chronic unemployment. Behav Modif 2005;29: 417–63.

57. Silverman K, Wong CJ, Needham M, et al. A randomized trial of employment-based reinforcement of cocaine abstinence in injection drug users. J Appl Behav Anal 2007;40:387–410.

58. DeFulio A, Donlin WD, Wong CJ, et al. Employment-based abstinence reinforcement as a maintenance intervention for the treatment of cocaine dependence: a randomized controlled trial. Addiction 2009;104:1530–8.

59. Brooner RK, King VL, Kidorf M, et al. Psychiatric and substance use comorbidity among treatment-seeking opioid abusers. Arch Gen Psychiatry 1997;54:71–80.

60. McLellan AT, Arndt IO, Metzger DS, et al. The effects of psychosocial services in substance abuse treatment. JAMA 1993;269:1953–9.

61. Kay-Lambkin FJ, Baker AL, Lewin TJ, et al. Computer-based psychological treatment for comorbid depression and problematic alcohol and/or cannabis use: a randomized controlled trial of clinical efficacy. Addiction 2009;104:378–88.

62. Kay-Lambkin FJ, Baker AL, Kelly B, et al. Clinician-assisted computerised versus therapist-delivered treatment for depressive and addictive disorders: a randomised controlled trial. Med J Aust 2011;195:S44–50.

63. Gustafson DH, Shaw BR, Isham A, et al. Explicating an evidence-based, theoretically informed, mobile technology-based system to improve outcomes for people in recovery for alcohol dependence. Subst Use Misuse 2011;46:96–111.

64. Bogart LM, Kral AH, Scott A, et al. Sexual risk among injection drug users recruited from syringe exchange programs in California. Sex Transm Dis 2005;32:27–34.

65. Avants SK, Margolin A, Usubiaga MH, et al. Targeting HIV-related outcomes with intravenous drug users maintained on methadone: a randomized clinical trial of harm reduction group therapy. J Subst Abuse Treat 2004;26:67–78.

66. Margolin A, Avants SK, Warburton LA, et al. A randomized clinical trial of a manual-guided risk reduction intervention for HIV-positive injection drug users. Health Psychol 2003;22:223–8.

67. Auerbach JD, Kandathil SM. Overview of effective and promising interventions to prevent HIV infection. World Health Organization Technical Report Series 2006;938:43–78.
68. Holtgrave DR. Strategies for preventing HIV transmission. JAMA 2009;302:1530–1.
69. Noar SM. Computer technology-based interventions in HIV prevention: state of the evidence and future directions for research. AIDS Care 2011;23:525–33.
70. Marsch LA, Bickel WK. The efficacy of computer-based HIV/AIDS education for injection drug users. Am J Health Behav 2004;28:316–27.
71. Marsch LA, Grabinski MJ, Bickel WK, et al. Computer-assisted HIV prevention for youth with substance use disorders. Substance Use Misuse 2011;46:46–56.
72. Bechara A. Decision making, impulse control, and loss of willpower to resist drugs: a neurocognitive perspective. Nat Neurosci 2005;8:1458–63.
73. Bickel WK, Christensen DR, Marsch LA. A review of computer-based interventions used in the assessment, treatment, and research of drug addiction. Subst Use Misuse 2011;46:4–9.
74. Grohman K, Fals-Stewart W, Donnelly K. Improving treatment response of cognitively impaired veterans with neuropsychological rehabilitation. Brain Cogn 2006;60:203–4.
75. Pedrero-Perez EJ, Rojo-Mota G, Ruiz-Sanchez de Leon JM, et al. Cognitive remediation in addictions treatment. Rev Neurol 2011;52:163–72.
76. Des Jarlais DC, Paone D, Miliken J, et al. Audio-computer interviewing to measure HIV risk behaviour among injecting drug users: a quasi-randomised trial. Lancet 1999;353:1657–61.
77. NDCP. 2010 national drug control strategy. Available at: http://www.whitehousedrugpolicy.gov/. Accessed 2010.
78. Lenhart A. The democratization of online social networks. Available at: http://pewinternet.org/Presentations/2009/41-The-Democratization-of-Online-Social-Networks.aspx. Accessed November 10, 2009.
79. Horrigan J. Wireless internet use. Pew Internet & American Life Project, 2009. Available at: http://pewinternet.org/Reports/2009/12-Wireless-Internet-Use.aspx. Accessed November 10, 2009.
80. Gibbons MC. eHealth solutions for healthcare disparities. New York: Springer Science + Business Media, LLC; 2007.
81. Boyer EW, Smelson D, Fletcher R, et al. Wireless technologies, ubiquitous computing and mobile health: application to drug abuse treatment and compliance with HIV therapies. J Med Toxicol 2010;6:212–6.
82. Favela J, Tenton M, Gonzalez VM. Ecological validity and pervasiveness in the evaluation of ubiquitous computing technologies for health care. International Journal of Human-Computer Interaction 2010;26:414–44.
83. Orwat C, Graefe A, Faulwasser T. Towards pervasive computing in health care: a literature review. BMC Med Inform Decis Mak 2008;8:1–18.
84. Weiser M. The computer for the 21st century. Scientific American 1991;September:94–104.
85. Johnson K, Isham A, Shah DV, et al. Potential roles for new communication technologies in treatment of addiction. Curr Psychiatry Rep 2011;13:390–7.
86. Rodriguez MD, Favela J, Preciado A, et al. Agent-based ambient intelligence for healthcare. AI Communications 2005;18:201–16.
87. Boyer EW, Smelson D, Fletcher R, et al. Wireless technologies, ubiquitous computing and mobile health: application to drug abuse treatment and compliance with HIV therapies. J Med Toxicol 2010;6:212–6.

The Genetic Basis of Addictive Disorders

Francesca Ducci, MD, PhD[a], David Goldman, MD[b],*

KEYWORDS

• Substance use disorder • Heritability • *MAOA* • *COMT* • *HTR2B*

KEY POINTS

• Addictive disorders are etiologically complex conditions that result from multiple genetic and environmental risk factors. Heritability estimates for addictions range between 0.4 (hallucinogens) to 0.7 (cocaine).

• Genetic and environmental influences modulating risk of substance use disorders change developmentally and across the lifespan.

• Genes involved in vulnerability to addictions include both substance-specific genes and genes that act on common pathways involved in addiction to different agents and propensity to other psychiatric disorders. Substance-specific genes include genes for metabolic enzymes involved in the metabolism of the substance (eg, *ALDH2, ADH1B for alcohol*) as well as genes encoding gatekeeper molecules such as drug receptors (eg, nicotinic receptors, *OPRM1*).

• Genes influencing diverse aspects of addiction neurobiology including anxiety, impulsivity, and reward, including genes such as monoamine oxidase A (*MAOA*), the serotonin transporter (*SLC6A4*) and catechol-Omethyl transferase (*COMT*), have been implicated in the shared genetic liability between addictions and other psychiatric diseases.

• At this early stage at which genome-wide association studies have primarily been applied to relatively small addiction samples, more than 95% of the genetic variance remains unaccounted for, indicating that most of the genetic risk factors for addiction have not been discovered yet.

• The identification of the genetic determinants of addiction is important to improve our ability to predict risk, predict treatment response, develop new treatments, and understand better the effects of the environment. This potential is already exemplified by the use of an *OPRM1* variant to predict treatment response to naltrexone in alcoholism.

Addictions, including substance use disorders (SUDs), are multistep conditions that, by definition, require exposure to an addictive agent. The wide variety of

The authors have nothing to disclose.
[a] Institute of Psychiatry, Psychological Medicine, Kings College, Box P063, De Crespigny Park, London SE5 8AF, UK;   [b] Laboratory of Neurogenetics, National Institute on Alcohol Abuse and Alcoholism, National Institutes of Health, 5625 Fishers Lane, Rockville, MD 20852, USA
* Corresponding author.
E-mail address: david.goldman@mail.nih.gov

addictive agents encompasses drugs, foods, sex, video-gaming, and gambling. Any of these agents may lead to an "addicted state" through neurobiologic pathways partially overlapping with those involved in addiction to psychoactive substances.[1] Millions of people are exposed to addictive agents each year, for instance, in the course of medical care for treatment of pain. The vast majority do not become addicted, even if temporary tolerance and dependence are elicited. The probability of initial use and the probability of progression toward a pathologic pattern of use are influenced by intrinsic factors (eg, genotype, sex, age, age at first use, preexisting addictive disorder, or other mental illness), extrinsic factors (eg, drug availability, peer influences social support, childhood adversity, parenting style, socioeconomic status), and the nature of the addictive agent (eg, psychoactive properties, pharmacokinetics, mode of use or administration). The relative importance of these factors varies across the lifespan and at different stages of addiction. For example, peer influences and family environment are most important for exposure and initial pattern of use, whereas genetic factors and psychopathology play a more salient role in the transition to problematic use.[2]

In individuals who are vulnerable to addiction, repetitive exposure to the agent induces long-lasting neuroadaptive changes that further promote drug-seeking behaviors and ultimately lead to persistent and uncontrolled patterns of use that constitute addiction. These neuroadaptive changes are the bases for tolerance, craving, and withdrawal and lead to a motivational shift.[3] Motivation to drug-seeking behavior is initially driven by impulsivity and positive reward. In contrast, compulsivity and negative affect dominate the terminal stages of the pathology. Addictions are in a sense "end-stage" diagnoses because at the time diagnosis is made potentially irreversible neuroadaptive change have occurred—changes that were preventable at an early point of the trajectory of the illness.

The use and abuse of legal and illegal psychoactive substances is a worldwide public health priority with repercussions on the individuals, their families, and society. According to the World Health Organization (WHO), alcohol subtracts 69.4 million of disability-adjusted life years (DALYs)[4]; tobacco, 59.1 million; and illicit drugs, 12.2 million.[5] From an economic perspective, the cost of substance use and SUDs in the United States is approximately $484 billion/year, which is comparable to the cost of diabetes ($131.7 billion/year) and cancer ($171.6 billion/year).[6]

HERITABILITY OF ADDICTIONS

Evidence from family, adoption, and twin studies converges on the relevance of genetic factors in the development of addictions including SUDs and gambling.[7–13] Weighted mean heritabilities for addictions computed from several studies of large cohorts of twins are shown in **Fig. 1**.[14] Heritability is lowest for hallucinogens (0.39) and highest for cocaine (0.72).

Heritability estimates are usually higher for addiction than for substance use; however, "no pathologic drug use" and "initiation of use" are also heritable, indicating that genetic influences play a role also in initiation.[10,12,15]

Mode of Inheritance

The identification of specific genes and functional loci moderating vulnerability has been challenging because of the genetic complexity of addictive disorders. This complexity derives from multiple sources including incomplete penetrance, phenocopies, variable expressivity, gene–environment interactions, genetic heterogeneity, polygenicity, and epistasis.

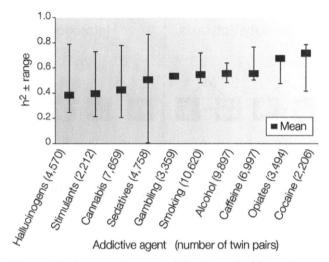

Fig. 1. Heritability (weighted means and ranges) of 10 addictive disorders: hallucinogens, cannabis, stimulants, sedatives, opiates, and cocaine dependence or abuse; alcohol dependence; smoking; caffeine consumption or heavy use; pathologic gambling. Weighted heritability (h^2) means were computed using data from large surveys of adult twins. (*Adapted from* Goldman D, Oroszi G, Ducci F. The genetics of addictions: uncovering the genes. Nat Rev Genet 2005;6(7):521–32.)

Twin studies can to some extent disentangle the roles of genetic heterogeneity and polygenicity–epistasis. As shown in **Fig. 2**,[14] under the epistatic model, combinations of genetic variants, each represented as a puzzle piece, determine phenotypes.

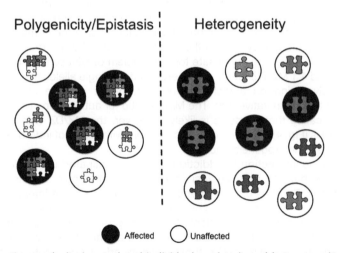

Fig. 2. Genetic complexity in unrelated individuals: epistasis and heterogeneity. Each risk allele is represented as a puzzle piece of different color or shape. Black circles indicate affected individuals and empty circles denote unaffected individuals. (*Adapted from* Goldman D, Oroszi G, Ducci F. The genetics of addictions: uncovering the genes. Nat Rev Genet 2005;6(7):521–32.)

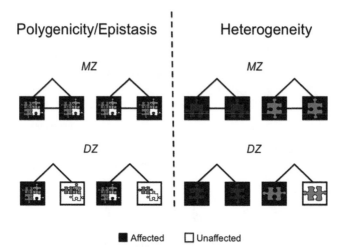

Fig. 3. Genetic complexity and twin concordance: epistasis and heterogeneity. Each risk allele is represented as a puzzle piece of different color or shape. Members of twin pairs are represented by squares. Black squares indicate affected individuals and empty squares denote unaffected individuals. (*Adapted from* Goldman D, Oroszi G, Ducci F. The genetics of addictions: uncovering the genes. Nat Rev Genet 2005;6(7):521–32.)

In contrast, under the genetic heterogeneity model, different genetic variants lead to the same phenotype in different individuals, but a single genetic variant can suffice. In twin studies epistasis leads to high monozygotic/dizygotic (MZ/DZ) concordance ratios, as shown in **Fig. 3**.

Because MZ twins share all alleles and DZ twins only on average half, epistatic models predict higher MZ/DZ concordance ratios. If a multigene combination is required, the MZ/DZ ratio is higher, and it is very high if a multilocus epistatic combination is required. The odds that DZ twins will inherit a combination of alleles is 0.5 raised to the power of the number of alleles involved in the combination, $(0.5)^n$. Multiple combinations may lead to the same phenotype, but for multilocus interactions this is less likely to compensate for the problem of joint probability to produce exactly 2:1 and 4:1 MZ/DZ ratios, as are expected for single alleles acting dominantly or recessively acting on a dichotomous trait, or for multiple alleles additively contributing to a quantitative trait. The MZ/DZ ratio for autism appears to be as high as 50:1, indicating that epistasis is likely. However, the MZ/DZ twin concordance ratios for SUDs (**Fig. 4**) converge on 2:1, consistent with alleles of individual effect and with the genetic heterogeneity model.

Gene × gene interaction in addiction has been evaluated using identified loci. However, the paucity of such loci identified so far would be insufficient for generalizations. Perhaps only by chance, the few gene × gene interaction studies performed so far in addiction are consistent with the genetic heterogeneity model and gene–gene additivity. In alcoholism, the protective effects of missense variants in *ADH1B* (*Arg48*) and *ALDH2* (*Lys487*) are additive,[16] which is perhaps not the expected result because these variants affect consecutive steps in the alcohol metabolic pathway and mediate propensity to alcohol-induced flushing. An additive effect on risk for alcoholism comorbid with other SUDs has been reported for functional loci mapping within the serotonin 3B receptor (*HTR3B*) and serotonin transporter (*SLC6A4*) genes.[17,18] In nicotine addiction, two variants associated

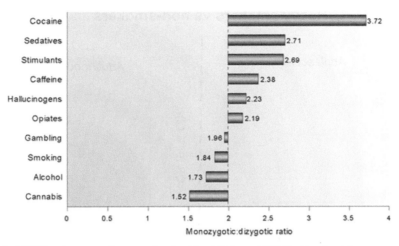

Fig. 4. MZ/DZ twin concordance ratios for 10 addictions. MZ/DZ ratios tend to converge on two, inconsistent with the epistatic model (see text). (*Adapted from* Goldman D, Oroszi G, Ducci F. The genetics of addictions: uncovering the genes. Nat Rev Genet 2005;6(7):521–32.)

with smoking appear to act additively.[19] These nicotine addiction risk variants map in the *CHRNA5–CHRNA3–CHRNB4* nicotinic acetylcholine receptor subunit cluster and in the *TTC12–ANKK1–DRD2* cluster, which includes *DRD2*, a dopamine receptor important in nicotine reward. In a community sample of 5000 Finns, the alleles most significantly associated with smoking were *CHRNA5 Asp398Asn* and an intronic variation within *TTC12* (rs10502172). Adolescent carriers of three to four risk alleles at these two loci (20% of the population) had a threefold increase in odds of smoking regularly and 2.5-fold increased odds of occasionally smoking as compared to noncarriers, who constitute 9% of the population. Carriers of one or two risk alleles were at intermediate risk. A similar stepwise increase in risk with allele dosage was observed in adulthood, and again consistent with additivity (**Fig. 5**).

The polygenic nature of addiction has implications for the manner in which genetic predictors may eventually be used in treatment and genetic counseling. The loci detected so far, including *CHRNA5 Asp398Asn*, which has a verified role in smoking, have little predictive value. However, as more genetic risk variants for addiction are discovered and personalized genotyping and sequencing become widespread, there will be increased efforts to use multilocus genetic risk scores to predict vulnerability.[20]

Changes in Gene Effects Across the Lifespan

Genetic and environmental influences modulating risk of SUDs change developmentally and across the lifespan. In a longitudinal twin study, Kendler and colleagues[21] found that gene effects in alcohol, cannabis, and nicotine addictions were low in early adolescence but their relative importance gradually grew in adulthood. In contrast, the effect of family environment declined from childhood to adulthood. A possible explanation is that as they mature, people have increasing latitude to shape their choices and social environments, thus increasing the relative importance of genotype.[22] Another explanation is that some genetic factors are important only after repetitive exposure to addictive agents. Also, some alleles may only alter responses of the adult brain. Genetic variation within

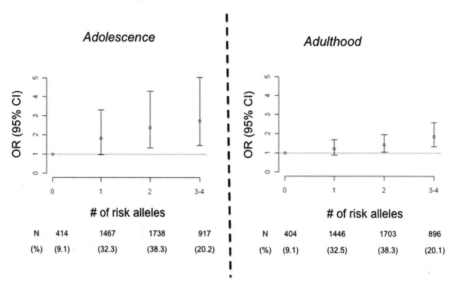

Fig. 5. Additive effects of the *TTC12–ANKK1–DRD2* and *CHRNA5–CHRNA3–CHRNB4* gene clusters on smoking behavior in adolescence and adulthood. Risk of heavy smoking increases linearly with the number of risk alleles at the two loci. Odds ratios (OR) and 95% confidence intervals (CI). (*Adapted from* Ducci F, Kaakinen M, Pouta A, et al. TTC12–ANKK1–DRD2 and CHRNA5–CHRNA3–CHRNB4 influence different pathways leading to smoking behavior from adolescence to mid-adulthood. Biol Psychiatry 2011;69(7):650–60.)

the *CHRNA5–CHRNA3–CHRNB4* gene cluster appears to have a stronger effect on smoking behavior in adulthood than in adolescence and moderated the risk of developing a severe pattern of smoking in subjects who had already initiated nicotine use.[19] In contrast, the *TTC12–ANKK1–DRD2* and *MAOA* appears to influence personality characteristics such as novelty seeking and impulsivity that promote substance initiation.[19]

Shared and Unshared Inheritance

Several addictive disorders tend to co-occur in the same individual.[23–25] Studies on genetically informative samples (eg, adoptive or twin studies) can measure the relative contribution of genes and environment to this comorbidity by evaluating the frequency of cross-transmission.[26] Twin studies reveal an overlap between genetic influences for alcoholism and illicit drug use disorders [27,28] and between alcoholism and smoking.[29] Kendler and colleagues[30] explored the effect of shared genetic influences on addiction to alcohol, caffeine, nicotine, cannabis, and cocaine in a portion of the Virginia twin sample including 5000 participants. In this study genetic risk could not be explained by one factor acting across all substances. Rather, two shared factors were found: an illicit agent factor mainly explaining vulnerability to cannabis and cocaine dependence and a licit agent factor mainly explaining vulnerability to alcohol, caffeine, and nicotine.

SUDs are frequently comorbid with other mental illnesses including internalizing disorders, such as depression and anxiety, and externalizing disorders, such as conduct disorder (CD), antisocial personality disorder, borderline personality disorder, and attention-deficit/hyperactivity disorder (ADHD).[24,25,31] Twin studies indicate shared genetic influences between SUDs and externalizing disorders.[27,28,32] Longitudinal studies have shown that CD and ADHD are important risk factors for addiction.[33] In contrast, twin studies have failed to reveal a shared genetic vulnerability between addiction and internalizing disorder, and it has been suggested that anxiety and depression are more commonly a consequence rather than a risk factor for addiction, being related to neuroadaptation and withdrawal.[34,35] However, longitudinal studies have shown that some anxiety disorders and anxiety-related personality traits such as panic disorder, social phobia, and increased harm avoidance predict subsequent alcohol problems in adolescents and young adults.[36]

Overall, twin studies predict that genes involved in vulnerability to SUDs include both substance-specific genes and genes that act on common pathways involved in addiction to different agents and propensity to other psychiatric disorders. Substance-specific genes include genes for metabolic enzymes (*ALDH2*, *ADH1B*) as well as genes encoding gatekeeper molecules such as drug receptors (eg, nicotinic receptors, *OPRM1*). On the other hand, genes influencing diverse aspects of addiction neurobiology including anxiety, impulsivity, and reward, including genes such as monoamine oxidase A (*MAOA*), the serotonin transporter (*SLC6A4*), and catechol-*O*-methyl transferase (*COMT*), have been implicated in the shared genetic liability between addictions and other psychiatric diseases.

INTERPLAY BETWEEN GENETIC AND ENVIROMENTAL FACTORS

The gene (**nature**) versus environment (**nurture**) debate represented a misguided and polarizing, dichotomy. Genetic and environmental factors interact in complex ways[37] but there are two main types of violations of gene–environment independence: gene × environment interaction and gene × environment correlation.

Gene × environment correlation (rGE) occurs when genotype correlates (r) with probability of exposure to an environmental factor. Twin studies can address the existence of rGE by measuring the "genetics of the environment." A gene-based example of rGE is the effect of *CHRNA5 Asn398* to increase risk of lung cancer.[38] This functional allele is associated with heavy smoking, thereby leading to increased exposure to carcinogens.

Gene × environment interaction (G × E) occurs when the effect of the environmental exposure on an outcome is modified by genotype (for review see Ref.[39]). Stressors occurring early in life, such as childhood adversity, are well known risk factors for addiction and comorbid conditions, including antisocial personality disorder (ASPD), CD, borderline personality disorder, and anxiety disorders. However, not all people exposed to early trauma develop psychopathology, indicating differences in resiliency. Functional loci that contribute to interindividual differences in stress resiliency include monoamine oxidase A (*MAOA*),[40] the serotonin transporter (*SLC6A4*),[41] *COMT*,[42] the corticotrophin-releasing hormone receptor 1 gene, neuropeptide Y,[43] *FKBP5*,[44] the glucocorticoid receptor (GR) gene (*NR3C1*),[45] and the adenylate cyclase activating polypeptide 1 (pituitary) receptor type gene (*ADCYAP1R1*).[46]

Intermediate Phenotypes

One strategy to discover gene effects in etiologically complex diseases such as addiction is the deconstruction of phenotypes into elements that are etiologically less complex. Intermediate phenotypes access mediating mechanisms of genetic and environmental influences. Heritable intermediate phenotypes that are disease associated are termed **endophenotypes.**[47]

Alcohol-induced flushing is a protective alcohol-related endophenotype influenced by alleles mediating variation in alcohol metabolism. Low response to alcohol is an endophenotype predictive of alcoholism risk.[48–50] In humans, level of response is due mainly to pharmacodynamic variation in response[51] rather than variation in metabolism. Low response to alcohol has been associated with genetic variation in the serotonin transporter gene (*SLC6A4*) and in the gene encoding the subunit a6 of the γ-aminobutyric acid receptor A (*GABRA6*).[52] Other addiction-relevant intermediate phenotypes include electrophysiologic, neuropsychological, neuroendocrinologic, and, more recently, neuroimaging measures. Neuroimaging accesses neuronal mechanisms underlying emotion, reward, and craving and has thereby enabled linkage of genes to neuronal networks relevant in addiction (for review see Ref.[53]). For example, amygdala activation after exposure to emotional imagery and stressful stimuli captures interindividual differences in emotional response.[54] As discussed in the text that follows, amygdala activation is influenced by *SLC6A4* and *MAOA*. On the other hand, task-elicited activation of the prefrontal cortex accesses prefrontal cognitive function that is impaired in several psychiatric diseases including addictions and has been linked to genetic variation within *COMT* and *MAOA*. Activation of the ventral striatum and other brain areas during positive reward allows exploration of reward circuits[55] enabling the observation that the *OPRM1 Asn398Asp* variant associated with altered naltrexone treatment response also modulates reward processes in the ventral striatum.[56] Effect sizes of genetic variants on intermediate phenotypes appear to be larger than effects on complex disease phenotypes, potentially reflecting proximity to gene action, measurement properties, and specificity.[43,57]

Gene Identification

Candidate gene and genome-wide analyses are increasingly integrated to identify genetic variations influencing addiction. In the former, genes known to influence the pathogenesis or treatment of addictions are selected, for example, based on discoveries in animal pharmacobehavioral and genetic studies or based on what is known about the pharmacokinetics and pharmacodynamics of the drug. In genome-wide studies, the genome is interrogated in a hypothesis-free way.

Candidate Genes

Alcohol-metabolizing genes: ADH1B and ALDH2

Polymorphisms in the genes encoding for the alcohol-metabolizing enzymes such as the alcohol dehydrogenase IB (ADH1B) and aldehyde dehydrogenase 2 (ALDH2) influence alcohol consumption and risk of alcohol use disorders. ADH1B and ALDH2 catalyze consecutive steps in alcohol metabolism. In adults, these enzymes play an important role although several other enzymes also catalyze these metabolic steps, including catalase, cytochrome P450, and other enzymes in the ADH and ALDH gene families. ADH oxidizes ethanol to acetaldehyde, which is then converted to acetate by ALDH. Acetaldehyde is toxic and adducts with both proteins and DNA. Both acetaldehyde and alcohol are recognized as mutagens. Acetaldehyde is a potent releaser of histamine, and thereby triggers flushing, an aversive reaction characterized by headache, nausea, palpitations, and flushing of the skin. Ordinarily, acetaldehyde is rapidly converted to acetate, and levels of acetaldehyde are very low even after alcohol ingestion. However, if aldehyde dehydrogenase is blocked by disulfiram (a medication used to help alcoholics maintain abstinence) then flushing is observed after ingestion of small quantities of alcohol. The acetaldehyde accumulation can lead

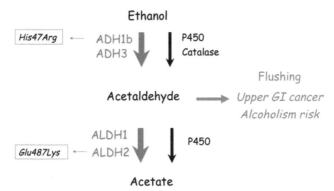

Fig. 6. Functional polymorphisms in ethanol metabolism: *ADH1B His48Arg* and *ALDH2 Glu487Lys*. Higher activity of *ADH1B*, conferred by *Arg48*, or lower activity of *ALDH2*, conferred by *Lys487*, leads to accumulation of acetaldehyde after alcohol consumption and the flushing reaction.

to increased risk of upper gastrointestinal (GI) cancer, and cancer risk is greatly augmented by pharmacologic blockade of aldehyde dehydrogenase or natural genetic variation.[58] As shown in **Fig. 6**, there are two common enzyme variants of ADH1B and ALDH2 that lead to alcohol-induced flushing, that are protective against alcoholism, and that play a role in the risk of upper GI cancer associated with alcohol consumption (**Fig. 7**).

At the *ADH1B His48Arg* locus (rs1229984), the *His48* allele directly leads to increased catalytic efficiency of *ADH1B*. Indeed, the rate of oxidation of ethanol to acetaldehyde is increased 100-fold in *His48/His48* homozygotes compared to *Arg48/Arg48* homozygotes. At the *ALDH2 Glu487Lys* locus (rs671), the *Lys487* allele dominantly inactivates ALDH2. Higher ADH1B activity or lower ALDH2 activity lead to accumulation of acetaldehyde and flushing following consumption of small quantities of alcohol. In East Asian populations in which both *His48* and *Lys487* are highly abundant, and in Jewish populations in which *His48* is abundant, many individuals carry genotypes protective against alcoholism. Recently, the protective effect of the *His48 ADH1B* variant on alcohol dependence was also demonstrated in European and African populations.[59] Following up the connection of acetaldehyde to mutation, both the *ADH1B* and *ALDH2* flushing alleles have been associated with enhanced risk of cancers of the oropharynx and esophagus.[58] As seen in **Fig. 7**, rates of upper GI cancer are higher in parts of the world where the *ALDH2 Lys487* allele is abundant.

The *ADH1B* and *ALDH2* polymorphisms are ancient, occurring on characteristic and highly diverged haplotypes. It is unlikely that either generic variant was selected to high frequency to reduce the likelihood of alcoholism after the introduction of alcohol into these populations, which probably occurred well after the spread of the polymorphisms. It has been hypothesized that *Arg48* and/or *Lys487* were selected to high frequencies in East Asian populations because they alter susceptibility to protozoal infections of the gut, including amebiasis.[60] These infections are sometimes treated with metronidazole, which potently inhibits aldehyde dehydrogenase.[60]

Genes-Moderating Monoamines

Monoamines including serotonin (5-hydroxytryptamine, 5-HT), norepinephrine (NE), and dopamine (DA) are modulators of emotionality, cognition, and reward. Therefore,

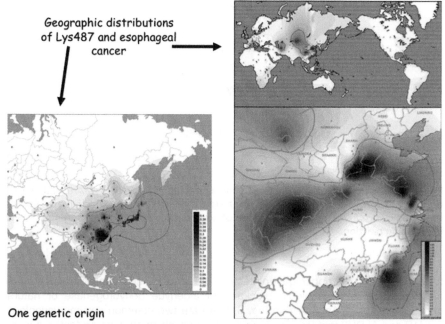

Geographic distributions of Lys487 and esophageal cancer

One genetic origin

Fig. 7. Geographic distributions of *ALDH2 Lys487* and esophageal cancer. The *Lys487* allele is highly abundant in Southeast Asia but virtually absent in Europeans, Africans, and Amerindians. Southeast Asia is also an epidemiologic hotspot for esophageal cancer, consistent with genetic epidemiologic studies that have connected risk of esophageal cancer to moderate consumption of alcohol in carriers of the *Lys487* allele. Acetaldehyde is a carcinogen.[58] (*Adapted from* Li H, Borinskaya S, Yoshimura K, et al. Refined geographic distribution of the oriental ALDH2*504Lys (nee 487Lys) variant. Ann Hum Genet 2009;73(Pt 3):335–45; with permission.)

it is unsurprising that genes regulating monoamines such as catechol-*O*-methyltransferase (*COMT*) and the serotonin transporter (*SLC6A4*) have been implicated in vulnerability to several psychiatric diseases, including addictions.

COMT metabolizes dopamine and norepinephrine and others catechols. COMT plays an important role in the regulation of dopamine in the prefrontal cortex, where the dopamine transporter is less expressed.[61,62] *COMT* knockout mice have increased levels of dopamine in this brain region.[63,64] The *COMT* gene has two promoters that control the transcription of two different mRNAs and encode a soluble, cytoplasmic protein (S-COMT) and a membrane-bound form (MB-COMT) which—in humans—has 50 additional amino acid residues at the N-terminus. S-COMT predominates in most tissues, accounting for 95% of total COMT activity.[65] In brain, where MB-COMT activity is much higher,[66] this enzyme is located in the cell body, axons, and dendrites of cortical neurons.[67] *Val158Met* is a common functional single nucleotide substitution of COMT,[68] replacing methionine for valine at codon 158 of MB-COMT and at codon 108 of S-COMT. Via its effect on enzyme stability[69,70] the *Met158* allele is three- to fourfold less active.[71] Because of its higher activity, the *Val158* allele was predicted to lower dopamine level in the frontal cortex. Congruent with this hypothesis, the *Val158* allele has been associated with inefficient frontal lobe function evaluated with different psychological and neuroimaging methodologies.[72–74] Also, in

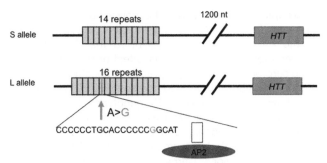

Fig. 8. The serotonin-transporter–linked polymorphic region. The human serotonin transporter promoter has a common VNTR termed *HTTLPR*. The major alleles within this VNTR, namely *L* (long) and *S* (short), differ in number of copies of a 20-bp to 23-bp imperfect repeat. The *L* allele, which leads to increased transcription efficiency, has 16 copies of the repeat and the *S* allele has 14 copies. Further, a relatively common, functional A > G SNP within the *L* allele leads to an *LG* allele functionally equivalent to the *S* allele. (*Data from* Lesch KP, Bengel D, Heils A, et al. Association of anxiety-related traits with a polymorphism in the serotonin transporter gene regulatory region. Science 1996;274(5292):1527–31; and Hu XZ, Lipsky RH, Zhu G, et al. Serotonin transporter promoter gain-of-function genotypes are linked to obsessive compulsive disorder. Am J Hum Genet 2006;78(5):815–26.)

a pharmacogenetic study, the COMT inhibitor tolcapone improved executive function in *val/val* homozygotes, but not in individuals homozygous for the *met* allele, indicating that this drug might correct the higher COMT activity, and consequent lower dopamine level, of *Val* carriers.[75] On the other hand, *Met158*, although associated with better cognitive performance, is associated with decreased stress resilience and increased anxiety. This allele has been associated with increased anxiety in women,[76] which might be explained because *COMT* promoters are down-regulated by estrogens.[77] The *Met* allele has also been associated with increased pain–stress response and a lower pain threshold,[42,78] and with increased amygdala reactivity to unpleasant stimuli.[79] Results from studies exploring the association between *COMT* and addiction are mixed. Some studies failed to find evidence for an associations[80]; some indicate *Val158* as the risk alleles and others indicate the *Met158* alleles as the risk allele. The *Val158* allele was found to be in excess among methamphetamine, nicotine, and polysubstance addicts.[80–82] On the other hand, in addicted populations with high frequencies of internalizing disorders, such as late-onset alcoholics in Finland[83] and Finnish social drinkers,[84] increased risk appeared to be conferred by the *Met158* allele.

SLC6A4

The serotonin transporter (SLC6A4) regulates synaptic levels of serotonin, a neurotransmitter involved in the regulation of mood, appetite, and impulse control. Reflecting these diverse actions, serotonin-specific reuptake inhibitors are the most commonly prescribed category of medications for mental illness. The serotonin transporter gene *SLC6A4* has a common variable number tandem repeat (VNTR) in its promoter region (*HTTLPR*) (**Fig. 8**) that is the most frequently studied locus in psychiatric genetics.

The major alleles within this VNTR differ in the number of copies of a 20- to 23-bp imperfect repeated sequence. The *L* allele, which leads to increased transcriptional efficiency, has 16 copies of the repeat and the S allele has 14 copies.[85] Further, there is a relatively common, functional A > G single-nucleotide polymorphism (SNP) within the L allele,[86] the L_G allele being equivalent to the S allele in transcriptional efficiency.[86] Further supporting the functional effect of HTTLPR, this locus has been shown to regulate serotonin transporter expression in postmortem brain[87] and in vivo using single-photon emission computed tomography (SPECT) imaging[88] although not in all studies.[89] Low-transcribing HTTLPR genotypes have been inconsistently associated with anxiety, depression, and alcoholism. However, the effects of this locus on complex behavior appear stronger if environmental exposure is also considered. HTTLPR moderated the impact of stressful life events on risk of depression and suicidal behavior.[90] Carriers of the low-transcribing S allele exhibited more depression and suicidality after stressful life events than L individuals with two copies of the allele.[90] Although a meta-analysis failed to support this G × E interaction,[91] other metanalyses have, and multiple lines of evidence support a role for HTTLPR regulation of emotion and response to stress. In particular, HTTLPR has been shown to influence the activity of the amygdala, a brain region that regulates emotional response to environmental changes and that is involved in the pathogenesis of depression and anxiety. Both adults[41] and children[92] carrying the low-activity s allele displayed increased amygdala reactivity to fearful stimuli, reduced amygdala volume,[93] and enhanced functional coupling between the amygdala and the ventromedial prefrontal cortex,[94] a brain region that ordinarily represses amygdala activation. In addition, HTTLPR appears to predict stress-induced cortisol release.[95] HTT gene × environment interactions have also been observed in animal models. The rhesus macaque has an orthologous polymorphism (rh-5HTTLPR) in the promoter region of serotonin transporter gene. In these animals, early life stress exposure led to dyscontrolled behavior and enhanced stress response later in life (for review see Ref.[96]). Consistent with findings in humans, rh-5HTTLPR influenced alcohol consumption and stress response, depending on rearing conditions. Carriers of the low-expression serotonin transporter genotype that were separated from their mothers at an early age displayed higher stress reactivity and ethanol preference.[97] Similarly to humans,[95] the combined effect of rh-HTTLPR and environment on stress reactivity appeared to be mediated by the hypothalamic–pituitary–adrenal (HPA) axis.

GENOME-WIDE ASSOCIATION STUDIES

As compared to candidate gene studies, genome-wide association studies (GWAS) have the advantage of covering the entire genome in an hypothesis-free way, and the methodology is powerful for detecting relatively common alleles (minor allele frequency [MAF] >5%) of moderate effect. As discussed later, the impact of less common variants cannot be studied by using the current GWAS arrays and requires sequencing strategies. Another advantage of GWAS is that the same genotyping arrays are obtained in different samples facilitating the combination of results from different studies in meta-analyses. This is a crucial aspect because extremely large study samples are necessary to be able to detect the small effects of many common variant on complex diseases. Of note in GWAS, up to 5 million SNPs can be simultaneously tested raising the issue of false positives due to multiple testing. To achieve an effective P value of .05, the genome-wide significance threshold is usually set at approximately 10^{-8}.

GWAS for addictions is at a relatively early stage. Several addictions have yet to be evaluated by GWAS and the samples that have been studied thus far have either not been very large (<10,000), or have been flawed by cross-site or cross-country heterogeneity, less than optimal phenotyping, and an insufficient number of subjects

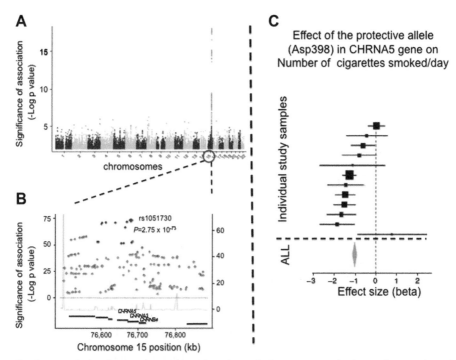

Fig. 9. Association between smoking (number of cigarettes smoked per day, CPD) and genetic variation within the *CHRNA5–CHRNA3–CHRNB4* gene-cluster on c15q25. (*A*) In the Manhattan plot, level of significance (–Log *P* value) of association to SNPs covering 22 autosomes is shown. SNPs reaching genome-wide significance ($P<10^{-8}$) are in green. (*B*) The chromosome 15 region contains the *CHRNA5–CHRNA3–CHRNB4* gene cluster. (*C*) The most significant SNP within this region is rs1051730, which correlates highly with *Asp398Asn*. (*Data from* Liu JZ, Tozzi F, Waterworth DM, et al. Meta-analysis and imputation refines the association of 15q25 with smoking quantity. Nat Genet 2010;42(5):436–40; Hong LE, Gu H, Yang Y, et al. Association of nicotine addiction and nicotine's actions with separate cingulate cortex functional circuits. Arch Gen Psychiatry 2009;66(4):431–41.)

with extreme phenotypes. So far, the strongest, and confirmed, locus detected by GWAS is for the *CHRNA5–CHRNA3–CHRNB4* gene cluster on chromosome 15q25.[38,98–102] This region harbors a locus-altering propensity to nicotine addiction. Nicotinic acetylcholine receptors (nAChRs) are pentameric cholinergic receptors that form ligand-gated ion channels. They are key mediators of the effect of nicotine on the central nervous system. Neuronal subtypes of nAChRs include various homomeric or heteromeric combinations of 12 different nicotinic subunits: $\alpha2$ through $\alpha10$ and $\beta2$ through $\beta4$. The *CHRNA5–CHRNA3–CHRNB4* gene cluster encodes for the $\alpha5$, $\alpha3$, and $\beta4$ subunits. Association of genetic variation within this region to smoking behavior was initially discovered using a candidate gene approach[99,100] but was subsequently replicated by GWAS. GWAS detect a highly significant peak on chromosome 15q25 corresponding to the region where these three genes are located (**Fig. 9**).

In this region, at least one functional locus responsible for the statistical signal is a nonsynonymous (aspartic acid, Asp [D] to asparagine, Asn [N]; rs16969968) SNP at codon 398 of *CHRNA5*. The *Asn398* allele has been associated with nicotine

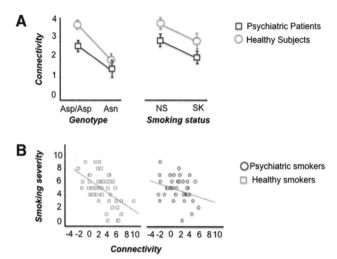

Fig. 10. Impact of psychiatric disease status, smoking behavior, and *Asp398Asn* influence on dorsal anterior cingulate–right ventral striatum functional connectivity. (*A*) *Asn398* carriers as compared to *Asp398/Asp398* homozygotes displayed reduced connectivity. Independently from genotype effect, reduced connectivity was also found in smokers (SK) vs nonsmokers (NS) and in psychiatric patients as compared to healthy participants. (*B*) Nicotine craving was negatively correlated with functional connectivity of dorsal anterior cingulate–ventral striatum in both smokers with and without psychiatric illnesses. (*Adapted from* Hong LE, Hodgkinson CA, Yang Y, et al. A genetically modulated, intrinsic cingulate circuit supports human nicotine addiction. Proc Natl Acad Sci U S A 2010;107(30):13509–14.)

dependence/heavy smoking,[99,100] pleasurable response to smoking,[101] smoking quantity,[38] smoking persistence, increased susceptibility to develop lung cancer and vascular disease among smokers,[38,103,104] serum cotinine levels among current smokers,[105] and smoking cessation.[106] According to a recent meta-analysis, each copy of the risk allele accounts only for approximately 0.5% of the variance in number of cigarettes smoked/day, reflecting the crude nature of the phenotype being studied[107] (see **Fig. 9**C). Potentially explaining the neural pathways by which the *Asp398Asn* locus alters propensity to nicotine addiction, the *Asn398* allele was found to predict the strength of a brain circuit connecting the anterior cingulate to the ventral striatum[107] (**Fig. 10**A). The anterior cingulate is a component of the limbic system involved in emotional modulation, and the ventral striatum is a principle reward region of the brain. Strength of this circuit itself was associated with smoking status and severity of smoking (see **Fig. 10**B), and this genotype predicted the circuit strength in both smokers and nonsmokers.[108]

In vitro studies have shown that $(\alpha 4\beta 2)_2\alpha 5$ receptors that differed only by the asparagine 398 amino acid displayed altered response to nicotine agonist compared with receptors containing aspartic acid.[109] Further studies showed that *Asn398* lowers Ca permeability and increases short-term desensitization in $(\alpha 4\beta 2)_2\alpha 5$, but does not alter the receptor sensitivity to activation.[110]

Other genetic loci implicated by GWAS in smoking behavior include the cytochrome P450, family 2, subfamily A, polypeptide 6 (*CYP2A6*). The CYP2A6 enzyme converts nicotine to cotinine and accounts for 70% of initial nicotine metabolism. Functional polymorphisms within *CYP2A6* have been associated with number of cigarette smoked per day. Variation within the dopamine β-hydroxylase (*DBH*) gene has been associated with smoking cessation.[111]

For alcoholism, GWAS has been even less successful than for smoking. No alcohol dependence GWAS has yielded a finding of genome-wide significance.[112–115] A large meta-analysis of GWAS on alcohol consumption was recently conducted in 12 population-based samples of European ancestry, totaling 26,316 individuals. The most significant associated marker, namely rs6943555, mapped to the autism susceptibility candidate 2 gene (*AUTS2*). Rs6943555 was found to moderate *AUTS2* expression in human postmortem brain from the prefrontal cortex. Differences in expression of *AUTS2* were found in whole-brain extracts of mice selected for differences in voluntary alcohol consumption.[116] Recently, multiple genome-wide significant loci for resting electroencephalogram (EEG) were identified by GWAS,[117] illustrating the potential power of combining GWAS with the endophenotype strategy. GWAS of neuroimaging responses relevant to addiction such as those exploring impulsivity and reward are under way.

RARE AND COMMON VARIANTS

The focus of genetic studies of addiction, as well as other common disorders, has been common genetic variants with MAF greater than 1%, and usually greater than 5%. The idea behind these studies is the common disease/common variant (CD/CV) hypothesis according to which common alleles of ancient origin and with small to moderate effect lead to susceptibility to common disorders. However, recent evidence suggests that rare variants of stronger effect might substantially contribute to the genetic vulnerability to common diseases (for review see Ref.[118]). For schizophrenia and autism, multiple risk rare variants with moderate to large effect sizes have been already reported.[119,120] Some of these variants appear to be associated with severe forms of disease and are thought to be of recent origin or de novo in sporadic cases. The contribution of rare variants in addictions is largely unknown. However, recent advances in sequencing technologies have opened the way for extensive searches for rare variants. The ability to detect and connect rare variants to behavior can be maximized by the study of genetically related individuals in families and founder populations that offers the advantage of reduced genetic and environmental heterogeneity as compared to mixed outbred populations and by sequencing individuals who are phenotypically extreme.

Rare genetic variants relevant to addiction have been found within the serotonin receptor 2B gene (*HTR2B*) and *MAOA*, and several of the functional *CYP26* alleles are also rare or uncommon. Both *HTR2B* and *MAOA* influence impulsivity and behavioral control and findings for these genes in humans remarkably parallel animal models.

MAOA is an X-linked gene encoding monoamine oxidase A, a mitochondrial enzyme that metabolizes monoamine neurotransmitters including norepinephrine, dopamine, and serotonin. *MAOA* knockout mice have higher levels of serotonin, norepinephrine, and to lesser extent dopamine, and manifest increased aggressive/impulsive behaviour and stress reactivity.[121] In 1993, Brunner and colleagues[122] reported a Dutch pedigree with eight males affected by borderline mental retardation and impulsive behaviors such as aggression, arson, attempted rape, fighting, and exhibitionism (**Fig. 11**A). Affected individuals were hemizygous for a stop-codon in the eighth exon of *MAOA* leading to a complete and selective deficiency of MAOA activity. Consistently with an X-linked recessive pattern of transmission, heterozygous women were unaffected. This stop codon variant has not been found in other populations. More recently, a common *MAOA* polymorphism influencing *MAOA* transcription was discovered.[123] This locus, termed the *MAOA*-linked polymorphic

A: Rare allele: Brunner syndrome

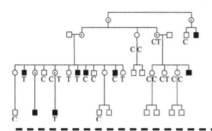

• MAOA C936T STOP codon found in one pedigree

• No MAOA activity

• Abnormal monoamine metabolites level

• Mental retardation

• Impulsive aggressive behavior

B: Common allele (*MAOA-LPR*)

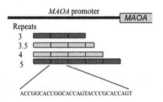

•Reduced MAOA expression with the 3-repeat allele that has a frequency of 30%

•Abnormal monoamine metabolites level

•Reduced stress resiliency

•Antisocial behaviors and addiction in subject exposed to childhood trauma

Fig. 11. Rare and common *MAOA* variants. (*A*) Dutch pedigree with eight males affected by Brunner syndrome, X-linked behavioral dyscontrol caused by an *MAOA* stop codon (C936T). (*B*) The *MAOA*-linked polymorphic region (*MAOA–LPR*) is a common 30-bp VNTR located approximately 1.2 kb upstream from the *MAOA* start codon and within the transcriptional control region. The three-repeat allele is transcribed less efficiently, leading to lower *MAOA* enzyme activity and behavioral consequences. ([*A*] *Adapted from* Brunner HG, Nelen M, Breakefield XO, et al. Abnormal behavior associated with a point mutation in the structural gene for monoamine oxidase A. Science 1993;262(5133):578–80.)

region (*MAOA–LPR*), is a VNTR located approximately 1.2 kb upstream from the *MAOA* start codon and within the gene's transcriptional control region[123] (see **Fig. 11**B). Alleles at this VNTR have a different number of tandem copies of a 30-bp sequence, with the three- and four-repeat alleles being by far the most common. Alleles with four repeats are transcribed more efficiently than alleles with three copies, leading to higher *MAOA* enzyme activity.[123]

Supporting the in vivo functional impact of this locus. *MAOA–LPR* was found to predict serotonin 1A receptor availability.[124] In a longitudinally studied cohort of boys, Caspi and colleagues[125] found an interactive effect between *MAOA–LPR* and childhood adversity on vulnerability to develop conduct disorder, an important risk factor for addiction. In this study, maltreated boys carrying the *MAOA* low-activity genotype were more likely to develop antisocial problems than boys with the high-activity genotype. This result has been confirmed by a meta-analysis of eight independent studies.[126] Results testing for *MAOA* × childhood adversity interaction in women are mixed. A recent study conducted in a sample of Native American women with extremely high rates of antisocial personality disorder and exposure to childhood adversity has reported results that parallel those observed in men. In this study, the effect of childhood sexual abuse on risk of developing alcoholism and antisocial personality disorder was influenced by *MAOA–LPR* genotype.[40] Sexually abused women homozygous for the low-activity *MAOA–LPR* allele had high rates of both disorders, and heterozygous women displayed an intermediate risk pattern.

However, in the absence of childhood sexual abuse, there was no relationship between *MAOA* genotype and these disorders.

Remarkably, and as was also the case with the serotonin transporter, an ortholo-gous *MAOA* VNTR is found in the rhesus macaque. As in humans, the lower activity allele predicts aggressive behavior in these animals, and the association is dependent on maternal separation.[127]

Interaction between *MAOA* on risk for antisocial behavior and impulsivity has also been reported for testosterone[128] and alcohol consumption.[129,130]

HTR2B

An *HTR2B* stop codon was linked to severe impulsive aggression, ASPD, and alcoholism, with an effect that appeared to be modulated by stress, alcohol consumption, and hormones. Unlike the *MAOA* stop codon, the *HTR2B* stop codon is recurrent, being found in at least 100,000 individuals, but population-restricted.

The *HTR2B* gene, located on chromosome 2 (2q36.3–q37.1), encodes the sero-tonin 2B receptor, a G protein–coupled receptor. Serotonin 2B receptors are widely expressed in the human brain. A rare *HTR2B* variant, namely Q20*, is associated with severe impulsivity and criminal violence in the Finnish population.[131] The stop codon has an allele frequency of 1.2% among Finns, but is specific to this founder. The variant was discovered by sequencing individuals displaying extremely severe impulsive and aggressive behavior. The sequencing sample consisted of population-matched controls and violent offenders who underwent psychiatric evaluation for the extreme nature of their crimes (homicides, assaults, arsons). The variant was enriched in individuals with a history of impulsive, nonpremeditated, violence. Carriers of the stop codon who had committed violent crimes did so while inebriated with alcohol, indicating that impulsive aggression could be the result of a *HTR2B* stop codon by alcohol interaction. Carriers of the stop codon were cognitively within the normal range, except for a potential difference in working memory, which is known to reflect frontal lobe function. In line with studies on humans, mice with the *htr2b* gene knocked out were more novelty seeking and impulsive. For example, in a delay discounting task, $htr2b^{-/-}$ mice were less able to tolerate delay in order to receive a larger reward.[131]

CLASSIFICATION AND TREATMENT OF ADDICTIONS

Current nosology of addictions limits both clinicians and researchers. The diagnoses are syndromic (based on clusters of symptoms and clinical course rather than etiologically based).[132] In addition, diagnoses are categorical, assuming a cutoff between normal and abnormal, although many of the problems associated with addiction are found in people who fall below the disease-associated threshold.[133] As discussed, twin studies have detected evidence of etiologic factors shared with other psychiatric diseases[28] and linking normal (personality) and abnormal variations (psychopathology).[19,32] The identification of specific genes and environmental factors altering vulnerability and ability to recover would seem to represent a first step to develop an etiologically based nosology and to individualize treatment. In this reconceptualization of addiction, neuroimaging and neuropsychological measures would be combined with genotype to help define new diagnostic categories encom-passing both premorbid vulnerability and addiction-induced neurobiologic change. Such a sea change in addiction diagnosis and management would require the collection of behavioral and genetic measures and their use against a research foundation that is today largely nonexistent. However, one of the first examples of pharmacogenetic prediction of treatment response in the addictions is a common functional missense variant of the μ-opioid receptor (*OPRM1 Asn40Asp*). As mentioned, this variant also appears to be associated with altered reward function.[56] In several studies, naltrexone, a μ-opioid receptor antagonist, was observed to augment abstinence and good therapeutic outcome in recovering alcoholics. Carriers of the *Asp40* allele were highly likely to show clinical improvement when treated with this drug.[134,135] Similarly, *CHRNA5 Asn398Asp*[106] and DBH have been reported to influence smoking cessation treatment, and would seem to indicate the existence of subgroups of addicted patients identifiable via genetic testing.

SUMMARY

Addictions are common, chronic, and relapsing diseases that develop through a multistep process. The impact of addictions on morbidity and mortality is high worldwide. Twin studies have shown that the heritability of addictions ranges from 0.39 (hallucinogens) to 0.72 (cocaine). Twin studies indicate that genes influence each stage from initiation to addiction, although the genetic determinants may differ. Addictions are by definition the result of gene × environment interaction. These disorders, which are in part volitional, in part inborn, and in part determined by environmental experience, pose the full range of medical, genetic, policy, and moral challenges. Gene discovery is being facilitated by a variety of powerful approaches, but is in its infancy. It is not surprising that the genes discovered so far act in a variety of ways: via altered metabolism of drug (the alcohol and nicotine metabolic gene variants), via altered function of a drug receptor (the nicotinic receptor, which may alter affinity for nicotine but as discussed may also alter circuitry of reward), and via general mechanisms of addiction (genes such as monoamine oxidase A and the serotonin transporter that modulate stress response, emotion, and behavioral control). Addiction medicine today benefits from genetic studies that buttress the case for a neurobiologic origin of addictive behavior, and some general information on familially transmitted propensity that can be used to guide prevention. A few well-validated, specific predictors such as *OPRM1*, *ADH1B*, *ALDH2*, *CHRNA5*, and *CYP26* have been identified and can provide some specific guidance, for example, to understand alcohol-related flushing and upper GI cancer risk (*ADH1B* and *AKLDH2*), variation in nicotine metabolism (*CYP26*), and, potentially, naltrexone treatment response (*OPRM1*). However, the genetic predictors available are few in number and account for only a small portion of the genetic variance in liability, and have not been integrated into clinical nosology or care.

REFERENCES

1. Reuter J, Raedler T, Rose M, et al. Pathological gambling is linked to reduced activation of the mesolimbic reward system. Nat Neurosci 2005;8(2):147–8.
2. Merikangas KR, Avenevoli S. Implications of genetic epidemiology for the prevention of substance use disorders. Addict Behav 2000;25(6):807–20.
3. Roberts AJ, Koob GF. The neurobiology of addiction: an overview. Alcohol Health Res World 1997;21(2):101–6.
4. World Health Organization (WHO). Management of substance abuse. Available at: http://www.who.int/substance_abuse/facts/alcohol/en/index.html. Accessed March 7, 2012.
5. World Health Organization (WHO). Management of substance abuse: the global burden. Available at: http://www.who.int/substance_abuse/facts/global_burden/en/. Accessed March 7, 2012.

6. Office of National Drug Control Policy (ONDCP). The economic costs of drug abuse in the United States 1992–1998. NCJ-190636, 2001. Available at: www.drugabuse.gov/about/welcome/aboutdrugabuse/magnitude. Accessed March 7, 2012.
7. Bierut LJ, Dinwiddie SH, Begleiter H, et al. Familial transmission of substance dependence: alcohol, marijuana, cocaine, and habitual smoking: a report from the Collaborative Study on the Genetics of Alcoholism. Arch Gen Psychiatry 1998;55(11):982–8.
8. Heath AC, Bucholz KK, Madden PA, et al. Genetic and environmental contributions to alcohol dependence risk in a national twin sample: consistency of findings in women and men. Psychol Med 1997;27(6):1381–96.
9. Kendler KS, Karkowski L, Prescott CA. Hallucinogen, opiate, sedative and stimulant use and abuse in a population-based sample of female twins. Acta Psychiatr Scand 1999;99(5):368–76.
10. Kendler KS, Karkowski LM, Neale MC, et al. Illicit psychoactive substance use, heavy use, abuse, and dependence in a US population-based sample of male twins. Arch Gen Psychiatry 2000;57(3):261–9.
11. Kendler KS, Prescott CA. Caffeine intake, tolerance, and withdrawal in women: a population-based twin study. Am J Psychiatry 1999;156(2):223–8.
12. Li MD, Cheng R, Ma JZ, et al. A meta-analysis of estimated genetic and environmental effects on smoking behavior in male and female adult twins. Addiction 2003;98(1):23–31.
13. Tsuang MT, Lyons MJ, Eisen SA, et al. Genetic influences on DSM-III-R drug abuse and dependence: a study of 3,372 twin pairs. Am J Med Genet 1996;67(5):473–7.
14. Goldman D, Oroszi G, Ducci F. The genetics of addictions: uncovering the genes. Nat Rev Genet 2005;6(7):521–32.
15. Kendler KS, Karkowski LM, Corey LA, et al. Genetic and environmental risk factors in the aetiology of illicit drug initiation and subsequent misuse in women. Br J Psychiatry 1999;175:351–6.
16. Thomasson HR, Edenberg HJ, Crabb DW, et al. Alcohol and aldehyde dehydrogenase genotypes and alcoholism in Chinese men. Am J Hum Genet 1991;48(4):677–81.
17. Enoch MA, Gorodetsky E, Hodgkinson C, et al. Functional genetic variants that increase synaptic serotonin and 5-HT3 receptor sensitivity additively predict alcohol and drug dependence. Biol Psychiatry 2010;67(9):91s.
18. Ducci F, Enoch MA, Yuan Q, et al. HTR3B is associated with alcoholism with antisocial behavior and alpha EEG power—an intermediate phenotype for alcoholism and co-morbid behaviors. Alcohol 2009;43(1):73–84.
19. Ducci F, Kaakinen M, Pouta A, et al. TTC12–ANKK1–DRD2 and CHRNA5–CHRNA3–CHRNB4 influence different pathways leading to smoking behavior from adolescence to mid-adulthood. Biol Psychiatry 2011;69(7):650–60.
20. Ripatti S, Tikkanen E, Orho-Melander M, et al. A multilocus genetic risk score for coronary heart disease: case-control and prospective cohort analyses. Lancet 2010;376(9750):1393–400.
21. Kendler KS, Schmitt E, Aggen SH, et al. Genetic and environmental influences on alcohol, caffeine, cannabis, and nicotine use from early adolescence to middle adulthood. Arch Gen Psychiatry 2008;65(6):674–82.
22. Kendler KS, Jacobson KC, Gardner CO, et al. Creating a social world: a developmental twin study of peer-group deviance. Arch Gen Psychiatry 2007;64(8):958–65.
23. Grant BF, Stinson FS, Dawson DA, et al. Co-occurrence of 12-month alcohol and drug use disorders and personality disorders in the United States: results from the National Epidemiologic Survey on Alcohol and Related Conditions. Arch Gen Psychiatry 2004;61(4):361–8.

24. Grant BF, Stinson FS, Dawson DA, et al. Prevalence and co-occurrence of substance use disorders and independent mood and anxiety disorders: results from the National Epidemiologic Survey on Alcohol and Related Conditions. Arch Gen Psychiatry 2004;61(8):807–16.

25. Kessler RC, Crum RM, Warner LA, et al. Lifetime co-occurrence of DSM-III-R alcohol abuse and dependence with other psychiatric disorders in the National Comorbidity Survey. Arch Gen Psychiatry 1997;54(4):313–21.

26. Goldman D, Bergen A. General and specific inheritance of substance abuse and alcoholism. Arch Gen Psychiatry 1998;55(11):964–5.

27. Hicks BM, Krueger RF, Iacono WG, et al. Family transmission and heritability of externalizing disorders: a twin-family study. Arch Gen Psychiatry 2004;61(9):922–8.

28. Kendler KS, Prescott CA, Myers J, et al. The structure of genetic and environmental risk factors for common psychiatric and substance use disorders in men and women. Arch Gen Psychiatry 2003;60(9):929–37.

29. Han C, McGue MK, Iacono WG. Lifetime tobacco, alcohol and other substance use in adolescent Minnesota twins: univariate and multivariate behavioral genetic analyses. Addiction 1999;94(7):981–93.

30. Kendler KS, Myers J, Prescott CA. Specificity of genetic and environmental risk factors for symptoms of cannabis, cocaine, alcohol, caffeine, and nicotine dependence. Arch Gen Psychiatry 2007;64(11):1313–20.

31. Ducci F, Enoch MA, Funt S, et al. Increased anxiety and other similarities in temperament of alcoholics with and without antisocial personality disorder across three diverse populations. Alcohol 2007;41(1):3–12.

32. Krueger RF, Hicks BM, Patrick CJ, et al. Etiologic connections among substance dependence, antisocial behavior, and personality: modeling the externalizing spectrum. J Abnorm Psychol 2002;111(3):411–24.

33. Sher KJ, Bartholow BD, Wood MD. Personality and substance use disorders: a prospective study. J Consult Clin Psychol 2000;68(5):818–29.

34. Kendler KS, Heath AC, Neale MC, et al. Alcoholism and major depression in women. A twin study of the causes of comorbidity. Arch Gen Psychiatry 1993;50(9):690–8.

35. Prescott CA, Aggen SH, Kendler KS. Sex-specific genetic influences on the comorbidity of alcoholism and major depression in a population-based sample of US twins. Arch Gen Psychiatry 2000;57(8):803–11.

36. Zimmermann P, Wittchen HU, Hofler M, et al. Primary anxiety disorders and the development of subsequent alcohol use disorders: a 4-year community study of adolescents and young adults. Psychol Med 2003;33(7):1211–22.

37. Ducci F, Roy A, Shen PH, et al. Association of substance use disorders with childhood trauma but not African genetic heritage in an African American cohort. Am J Psychiatry 2009;166(9):1031–40.

38. Thorgeirsson TE, Geller F, Sulem P, et al. A variant associated with nicotine dependence, lung cancer and peripheral arterial disease. Nature 2008;452(7187): 638–42.

39. Caspi A, Moffitt TE. Gene-environment interactions in psychiatry: joining forces with neuroscience. Nat Rev Neurosci 2006;7(7):583–90.

40. Ducci F, Enoch MA, Hodgkinson C, et al. Interaction between a functional MAOA locus and childhood sexual abuse predicts alcoholism and antisocial personality disorder in adult women. Mol Psychiatry 2008;13(3):334–47.

41. Hariri AR, Mattay VS, Tessitore A, et al. Serotonin transporter genetic variation and the response of the human amygdala. Science 2002;297(5580):400–3.

42. Zubieta JK, Heitzeg MM, Smith YR, et al. COMT val158met genotype affects mu-opioid neurotransmitter responses to a pain stressor. Science 2003;299(5610): 1240–3.

43. Zhou Z, Zhu G, Hariri AR, et al. Genetic variation in human NPY expression affects stress response and emotion. Nature 2008;452(7190):997–1001.

44. Binder EB, Bradley RG, Liu W, et al. Association of FKBP5 polymorphisms and childhood abuse with risk of posttraumatic stress disorder symptoms in adults. JAMA 2008;299(11):1291–305.

45. Desrivieres S, Lourdusamy A, Muller C, et al. Glucocorticoid receptor (NR3C1) gene polymorphisms and onset of alcohol abuse in adolescents. Addict Biol 16(3):510–3.

46. Ressler KJ, Mercer KB, Bradley B, et al. Post-traumatic stress disorder is associated with PACAP and the PAC1 receptor. Nature 2011;470(7335):492–7.

47. Goldman D, Ducci F. Deconstruction of vulnerability to complex diseases: enhanced effect sizes and power of intermediate phenotypes. Scientific World Journal. Review 2007;2(7):124–30.

48. Heath AC, Madden PA, Bucholz KK, et al. Genetic differences in alcohol sensitivity and the inheritance of alcoholism risk. Psychol Med 1999;29(5):1069–81.

49. Rodriguez LA, Wilson JR, Nagoshi CT. Does psychomotor sensitivity to alcohol predict subsequent alcohol use? Alcohol Clin Exp Res 1993;17(1):155–61.

50. Schuckit MA, Smith TL, Kalmijn J, et al. Response to alcohol in daughters of alcoholics: a pilot study and a comparison with sons of alcoholics. Alcohol Alcohol 2000;35(3):242–8.

51. Schuckit MA. Biological, psychological and environmental predictors of the alcoholism risk: a longitudinal study. J Stud Alcohol 1998;59(5):485–94.

52. Hu X, Oroszi G, Chun J, et al. An expanded evaluation of the relationship of four alleles to the level of response to alcohol and the alcoholism risk. Alcohol Clin Exp Res 2005;29(1):8–16.

53. Meyer-Lindenberg A, Weinberger DR. Intermediate phenotypes and genetic mechanisms of psychiatric disorders. Nat Rev Neurosci 2006;7(10):818–27.

54. Hariri AR, Drabant EM, Munoz KE, et al. A susceptibility gene for affective disorders and the response of the human amygdala. Arch Gen Psychiatry 2005;62(2):146–52.

55. Peters J, Bromberg U, Schneider S, et al. Lower ventral striatal activation during reward anticipation in adolescent smokers. Am J Psychiatry 2011;168(5):540–9.

56. Ramchandani VA, Umhau J, Pavon FJ, et al. A genetic determinant of the striatal dopamine response to alcohol in men. Mol Psychiatry 2011;16(8):809–17.

57. Ducci F, Goldman D. Genetic approaches to addiction: genes and alcohol. Addiction 2008;103(9):1414–28.

58. Brooks PJ, Goldman D, Li TK. Alleles of alcohol and acetaldehyde metabolism genes modulate susceptibility to oesophageal cancer from alcohol consumption. Hum Genomics 2009;3(2):103–5.

59. Bierut LJ, Goate AM, Breslau N, et al. ADH1B is associated with alcohol dependence and alcohol consumption in populations of European and African ancestry. Mol Psychiatry 2012;17(4):445–50.

60. Goldman D, Enoch MA. Genetic epidemiology of ethanol metabolic enzymes: a role for selection. World Rev Nutr Diet 1990;63:143–60.

61. Lewis DA, Melchitzky DS, Sesack SR, et al. Dopamine transporter immunoreactivity in monkey cerebral cortex: regional, laminar, and ultrastructural localization. J Comp Neurol 2001;432(1):119–36.

62. Mazei MS, Pluto CP, Kirkbride B, et al. Effects of catecholamine uptake blockers in the caudate-putamen and subregions of the medial prefrontal cortex of the rat. Brain Res 2002;936(1–2):58–67.

63. Giakoumaki SG, Roussos P, Bitsios P. Improvement of prepulse inhibition and executive function by the COMT inhibitor tolcapone depends on COMT Val158Met polymorphism. Neuropsychopharmacology 2008;33(13):3058–68.

64. Yavich L, Forsberg MM, Karayiorgou M, et al. Site-specific role of catechol-O-methyltransferase in dopamine overflow within prefrontal cortex and dorsal striatum. J Neurosci 2007;27(38):10196–209.

65. Jeffery DR, Roth JA. Characterization of membrane-bound and soluble catechol-O-methyltransferase from human frontal cortex. J Neurochem 1984;42(3):826–32.

66. Rivett AJ, Francis A, Roth JA. Distinct cellular localization of membrane-bound and soluble forms of catechol-O-methyltransferase in brain. J Neurochem 1983;40(1): 215–9.

67. Chen J, Song J, Yuan P, et al. Orientation and cellular distribution of membrane-bound catechol-O-methyltransferase in cortical neurons: implications for drug development. J Biol Chem 2011;286(40):34752–60.

68. Lachman HM, Papolos DF, Saito T, et al. Human catechol-O-methyltransferase pharmacogenetics: description of a functional polymorphism and its potential application to neuropsychiatric disorders. Pharmacogenetics 1996;6(3):243–50.

69. Scanlon PD, Raymond FA, Weinshilboum RM. Catechol-O-methyltransferase: thermolabile enzyme in erythrocytes of subjects homozygous for allele for low activity. Science 1979;203(4375):63–5.

70. Weinshilboum R, Dunnette J. Thermal stability and the biochemical genetics of erythrocyte catechol-O-methyl-transferase and plasma dopamine-beta-hydroxylase. Clin Genet 1981;19(5):426–37.

71. Chen J, Lipska BK, Halim N, et al. Functional analysis of genetic variation in catechol-O-methyltransferase (COMT): effects on mRNA, protein, and enzyme activity in postmortem human brain. Am J Hum Genet 2004;75(5):807–21.

72. Egan MF, Goldberg TE, Kolachana BS, et al. Effect of COMT Val108/158 Met genotype on frontal lobe function and risk for schizophrenia. Proc Natl Acad Sci U S A 2001;98(12):6917–22.

73. Goldberg TE, Egan MF, Gscheidle T, et al. Executive subprocesses in working memory: relationship to catechol-O-methyltransferase Val158Met genotype and schizophrenia. Arch Gen Psychiatry 2003;60(9):889–96.

74. Malhotra AK, Kestler LJ, Mazzanti C, et al. A functional polymorphism in the COMT gene and performance on a test of prefrontal cognition. Am J Psychiatry 2002; 159(4):652–4.

75. Gogos JA, Morgan M, Luine V, et al. Catechol-O-methyltransferase-deficient mice exhibit sexually dimorphic changes in catecholamine levels and behavior. Proc Natl Acad Sci U S A 1998;95(17):9991–6.

76. Enoch MA, Xu K, Ferro E, et al. Genetic origins of anxiety in women: a role for a functional catechol-O-methyltransferase polymorphism. Psychiatr Genet 2003; 13(1):33–41.

77. Jiang H, Xie T, Ramsden DB, et al. Human catechol-O-methyltransferase down-regulation by estradiol. Neuropharmacology 2003;45(7):1011–8.

78. Diatchenko L, Slade GD, Nackley AG, et al. Genetic basis for individual variations in pain perception and the development of a chronic pain condition. Hum Mol Genet 2005;14(1):135–43.

79. Smolka MN, Schumann G, Wrase J, et al. Catechol-O-methyltransferase val158met genotype affects processing of emotional stimuli in the amygdala and prefrontal cortex. J Neurosci 2005;25(4):836–42.

80. Tammimaki AE, Mannisto PT. Are genetic variants of COMT associated with addiction? Pharmacogenet Genomics 2010;20(12):717–41.

81. Vandenbergh DJ, Rodriguez LA, Miller IT, et al. High-activity catechol-O-methyl-transferase allele is more prevalent in polysubstance abusers. Am J Med Genet 1997;74(4):439–42.
82. Jugurnauth SK, Chen CK, Barnes MR, et al. A COMT gene haplotype associated with methamphetamine abuse. Pharmacogenet Genomics 2011;21(11):731–40.
83. Tiihonen J, Hallikainen T, Lachman H, et al. Association between the functional variant of the catechol-O-methyltransferase (COMT) gene and type 1 alcoholism. Mol Psychiatry 1999;4(3):286–9.
84. Kauhanen J, Hallikainen T, Tuomainen TP, et al. Association between the functional polymorphism of catechol-O-methyltransferase gene and alcohol consumption among social drinkers. Alcohol Clin Exp Res 2000;24(2):135–9.
85. Lesch KP, Bengel D, Heils A, et al. Association of anxiety-related traits with a polymorphism in the serotonin transporter gene regulatory region. Science 1996; 274(5292):1527–31.
86. Hu XZ, Lipsky RH, Zhu G, et al. Serotonin transporter promoter gain-of-function genotypes are linked to obsessive-compulsive disorder. Am J Hum Genet 2006; 78(5):815–26.
87. Little KY, McLauglin DP, Ranc J, et al. Serotonin transporter binding sites and mRNA levels in depressed persons committing suicide. Biol Psychiatry 1997; 41(12):1156–64.
88. Heinz A, Jones DW, Mazzanti C, et al. A relationship between serotonin transporter genotype and in vivo protein expression and alcohol neurotoxicity. Biol Psychiatry 2000;47(7):643–9.
89. Shioe K, Ichimiya T, Suhara T, et al. No association between genotype of the promoter region of serotonin transporter gene and serotonin transporter binding in human brain measured by PET. Synapse 2003;48(4):184–8.
90. Caspi A, Sugden K, Moffitt TE, et al. Influence of life stress on depression: moderation by a polymorphism in the 5-HTT gene. Science 2003;301(5631):386–9.
91. Risch N, Herrell R, Lehner T, et al. Interaction between the serotonin transporter gene (5-HTTLPR), stressful life events, and risk of depression: a meta-analysis. JAMA 2009;301(23):2462–71.
92. Szekely E, Herba CM, Arp PP, et al. Recognition of scared faces and the serotonin transporter gene in young children: the Generation R Study. J Child Psychol Psychiatry 2011;52(12):1279–86.
93. Pezawas L, Meyer-Lindenberg A, Drabant EM, et al. 5-HTTLPR polymorphism impacts human cingulate-amygdala interactions: a genetic susceptibility mechanism for depression. Nat Neurosci 2005;8(6):828–34.
94. Heinz A, Braus DF, Smolka MN, et al. Amygdala-prefrontal coupling depends on a genetic variation of the serotonin transporter. Nat Neurosci 2005;8(1):20–1.
95. Mueller A, Armbruster D, Moser DA, et al. Interaction of serotonin transporter gene-linked polymorphic region and stressful life events predicts cortisol stress response. Neuropsychopharmacology 2011;36(7):1332–9.
96. Barr CS, Newman TK, Becker ML, et al. The utility of the non-human primate: model for studying gene by environment interactions in behavioral research. Genes Brain Behav 2003;2(6):336–40.
97. Barr CS, Newman TK, Lindell S, et al. Interaction between serotonin transporter gene variation and rearing condition in alcohol preference and consumption in female primates. Arch Gen Psychiatry 2004;61(11):1146–52.
98. Berrettini W, Yuan X, Tozzi F, et al. Alpha-5/alpha-3 nicotinic receptor subunit alleles increase risk for heavy smoking. Mol Psychiatry 2008;13(4):368–73.

99. Bierut LJ, Madden PA, Breslau N, et al. Novel genes identified in a high-density genome wide association study for nicotine dependence. Hum Mol Genet 2007; 16(1):24–35.

100. Saccone SF, Hinrichs AL, Saccone NL, et al. Cholinergic nicotinic receptor genes implicated in a nicotine dependence association study targeting 348 candidate genes with 3713 SNPs. Hum Mol Genet 2007;16(1):36–49.

101. Sherva R, Wilhelmsen K, Pomerleau CS, et al. Association of a single nucleotide polymorphism in neuronal acetylcholine receptor subunit alpha 5 (CHRNA5) with smoking status and with 'pleasurable buzz' during early experimentation with smoking. Addiction 2008;103(9):1544–52.

102. Stevens VL, Bierut LJ, Talbot JT, et al. Nicotinic receptor gene variants influence susceptibility to heavy smoking. Cancer Epidemiol Biomarkers Prev 2008;17(12):3517–25.

103. Amos CI, Wu X, Broderick P, et al. Genome-wide association scan of tag SNPs identifies a susceptibility locus for lung cancer at 15q25.1. Nat Genet 2008;40(5):616–22.

104. Hung RJ, McKay JD, Gaborieau V, et al. A susceptibility locus for lung cancer maps to nicotinic acetylcholine receptor subunit genes on 15q25. Nature 2008;452(7187): 633–7.

105. Timofeeva MN, McKay JD, Smith GD, et al. Genetic polymorphisms in 15q25 and 19q13 loci, cotinine levels, and risk of lung cancer in EPIC. Cancer Epidemiol Biomarkers Prev 2011;20(10):2250–61.

106. Munafo MR, Johnstone EC, Walther D, et al. CHRNA3 rs1051730 genotype and short-term smoking cessation. Nicotine Tob Res 2011;13(10):982–8.

107. Neiswanger K, Hill SY, Kaplan BB. Association and linkage studies of the TAQI A1 allele at the dopamine D2 receptor gene in samples of female and male alcoholics. Am J Med Genet 1995;60(4):267–71.

108. Hong LE, Hodgkinson CA, Yang Y, et al. A genetically modulated, intrinsic cingulate circuit supports human nicotine addiction. Proc Natl Acad Sci U S A 2010;107(30): 13509–14.

109. Bierut LJ, Stitzel JA, Wang JC, et al. Variants in nicotinic receptors and risk for nicotine dependence. Am J Psychiatry 2008;165(9):1163–71.

110. Kuryatov A, Berrettini W, Lindstrom J. Acetylcholine receptor (AChR) alpha5 subunit variant associated with risk for nicotine dependence and lung cancer reduces (alpha4beta2)alpha5 AChR function. Mol Pharmacol 2011;79(1):119–25.

111. Thorgeirsson TE, Gudbjartsson DF, Surakka I, et al. Sequence variants at CHRNB3–CHRNA6 and CYP2A6 affect smoking behavior. Nat Genet 2010;42(5):448–53.

112. Treutlein J, Cichon S, Ridinger M, et al. Genome-wide association study of alcohol dependence. Arch Gen Psychiatry 2009;66(7):773–84.

113. Lind PA, Macgregor S, Vink JM, et al. A genomewide association study of nicotine and alcohol dependence in Australian and Dutch populations. Twin Res Hum Genet 2010;13(1):10–29.

114. Bierut LJ, Agrawal A, Bucholz KK, et al. A genome-wide association study of alcohol dependence. Proc Natl Acad Sci U S A 2010;107(11):5082–7.

115. Edenberg HJ, Koller DL, Xuei X, et al. Genome-wide association study of alcohol dependence implicates a region on chromosome 11. Alcohol Clin Exp Res 2010; 34(5):840–52.

116. Schumann G, Coin LJ, Lourdusamy A, et al. Genome-wide association and genetic functional studies identify autism susceptibility candidate 2 gene (AUTS2) in the regulation of alcohol consumption. Proc Natl Acad Sci U S A 2011;108(17):7119–24.

117. Hodgkinson CA, Enoch MA, Srivastava V, et al. Genome-wide association identifies candidate genes that influence the human electroencephalogram. Proc Natl Acad Sci U S A 2010;107(19):8695–700.
118. Uher R. The role of genetic variation in the causation of mental illness: an evolution-informed framework. Mol Psychiatry 2009;14(12):1072–82.
119. Sebat J, Lakshmi B, Malhotra D, et al. Strong association of de novo copy number mutations with autism. Science 2007;316(5823):445–9.
120. Stefansson H, Rujescu D, Cichon S, et al. Large recurrent microdeletions associated with schizophrenia. Nature 2008;455(7210):232–6.
121. Cases O, Seif I, Grimsby J, et al. Aggressive behavior and altered amounts of brain serotonin and norepinephrine in mice lacking MAOA. Science 1995;268(5218):1763–6.
122. Brunner HG, Nelen M, Breakefield XO, et al. Abnormal behavior associated with a point mutation in the structural gene for monoamine oxidase A. Science 1993;262(5133):578–80.
123. Sabol SZ, Hu S, Hamer D. A functional polymorphism in the monoamine oxidase A gene promoter. Hum Genet 1998;103(3):273–9.
124. Mickey BJ, Ducci F, Hodgkinson CA, et al. Monoamine oxidase A genotype predicts human serotonin 1A receptor availability in vivo. J Neurosci 2008;28(44):11354–9.
125. Caspi A, McClay J, Moffitt TE, et al. Role of genotype in the cycle of violence in maltreated children. Science 2002;297(5582):851–4.
126. Taylor A, Kim-Cohen J. Meta-analysis of gene-environment interactions in developmental psychopathology. Dev Psychopathol 2007;19(4):1029–37.
127. Newman TK, Syagailo YV, Barr CS, et al. Monoamine oxidase A gene promoter variation and rearing experience influences aggressive behavior in rhesus monkeys. Biol Psychiatry 2005;57(2):167–72.
128. Sjoberg RL, Ducci F, Barr CS, et al. A non-additive interaction of a functional MAO-A VNTR and testosterone predicts antisocial behavior. Neuropsychopharmacology 2008;33(2):425–30.
129. Tikkanen R, Sjoberg RL, Ducci F, et al. Effects of MAOA-genotype, alcohol consumption, and aging on violent behavior. Alcohol Clin Exp Res 2009;33(3):428–34.
130. Tikkanen R, Ducci F, Goldman D, et al. MAOA alters the effects of heavy drinking and childhood physical abuse on risk for severe impulsive acts of violence among alcoholic violent offenders. Alcohol Clin Exp Res 2010;34(5):853–60.
131. Bevilacqua L, Doly S, Kaprio J, et al. A population-specific HTR2B stop codon predisposes to severe impulsivity. Nature 2010;468(7327):1061–6.
132. Kupfer DJ, First MB, Regier DA, editors. A research agenda for DSM-V. Washington, DC: American Psychiatric Association; 2002.
133. Caetano R, Cunradi C. Alcohol dependence: a public health perspective. Addiction 2002;97(6):633–45.
134. Anton RF, Oroszi G, O'Malley S, et al. An evaluation of mu-opioid receptor (OPRM1) as a predictor of naltrexone response in the treatment of alcohol dependence: results from the Combined Pharmacotherapies and Behavioral Interventions for Alcohol Dependence (COMBINE) study. Arch Gen Psychiatry 2008;65(2):135–44.
135. Oslin DW, Berrettini W, Kranzler HR, et al. A functional polymorphism of the mu-opioid receptor gene is associated with naltrexone response in alcohol-dependent patients. Neuropsychopharmacology 2003;28(8):1546–52.

Neurobiology of Addiction
Insight from Neurochemical Imaging

Nina B.L. Urban, MD, MSc[a,b,*], Diana Martinez, MD[a,b]

KEYWORDS

- PET • SPECT • Dopamine • Reward system • Psychostimulants
- Neuroimaging

KEY POINTS

- Factors that determine who becomes addicted include genetic, developmental, and environmental risk factors.
- PET and SPECT imaging use radioligands that are specific for a given brain receptor, and labeled with a traceable radionuclide, allowing quantification of these receptors in humans in vivo.
- The mesolimbic and mesocortical dopamine pathways are crucial in drug reward and addiction. Imaging studies investigate vulnerability to addiction through dopamine-receptor and -transporter binding, as well as exploring dopamine transmission via pharmacologic challenge and depletion studies.
- Both dopamine receptors and dopamine release in areas of the striatum are reduced in cocaine, methamphetamine, heroin, and alcohol dependence, possibly related to treatment refractoriness.
- With the development of new radioligands, neuroimaging exploration of other neurotransmitter systems and their role in addiction has begun as well.

Drug addiction is a chronically relapsing disorder characterized by:[1]

1. Compulsion to seek and take the drug
2. Loss of control in limiting intake
3. Appearance of negative emotional symptoms as well as physical withdrawal symptoms when the drug cannot be accessed.

The authors have nothing to disclose.
[a] Department of Psychiatry, Division of Substance Abuse, Columbia University, New York, NY 10032, USA; [b] Department of Psychiatry, New York State Psychiatric Institute, 1051 Riverside Drive, Unit 31, New York, NY 10032, USA
* Corresponding author. Department of Psychiatry, New York State Psychiatric Institute, 1051 Riverside Drive, Unit 31, New York, NY 10032.
E-mail address: nu2118@columbia.edu

Psychiatr Clin N Am 35 (2012) 521–541
http://dx.doi.org/10.1016/j.psc.2012.03.011
0193-953X/12/$ – see front matter © 2012 Elsevier Inc. All rights reserved.

Much of the current neurobiological drug abuse research is focused on understanding the molecular mechanisms mediating the transition to the loss of behavioral control over drug-seeking and drug-taking, and the neuroadaptive changes that occur in the brain. The aim of this article is to summarize the contributions of neurochemical imaging studies to a better understanding of the neurobiology of addiction.

THE NEUROCIRCUITRY OF REWARD IN ADDICTION

Drugs of abuse mimic or enhance the actions of neurotransmitters, the endogenous chemical messengers in the nervous system, at receptors for these neurotransmitters. Opioids are presumed to be habit-forming because of actions at opiate receptors, and nicotine because of action at nicotinic acetylcholine receptors. Phencyclidine acts at N-methyl-D-aspartate (NMDA) and sigma receptors, and also blocks dopamine reuptake.[2] Δ^9-Tetrahydrocannabinol (THC) binds to endocannabinoid receptors.[3,4] Although amphetamine and cocaine do not act directly at dopamine receptors, they are reinforcing because they increase the concentration of dopamine at the dopamine receptors of the nucleus accumbens and frontal cortex.[5]

It has become clear that the acute administration of most drugs of abuse increases dopamine transmission in the basal ganglia,[5] and that dopamine transmission in this brain region plays a crucial role in mediating the reinforcing effects of these drugs.[6-8] The mesolimbic dopamine pathway is made up of dopaminergic cells in the ventral tegmental area (VTA) projecting into the nucleus accumbens (NAc), located in the ventral striatum, and is considered crucial for drug reward.[9] The mesostriatal (dopamine cells of the substantia nigra projecting to the dorsal striatum) and mesocortical (dopamine cells of the VTA projecting to the frontal cortex) pathways are also recognized in contributing to predicting drug reward (anticipation) and addiction.[10] The time course of dopamine signaling is also a key factor, where the fastest time course predominantly has a role in reward and attributing value to predicted outcomes of behavior, while steady activation of dopamine release plays a role in providing an enabling effect on specific behavior-related systems.[11] The mode of dopamine cell firing (phasic vs tonic) also differently modulates the rewarding, conditioning effects, or drugs (predominantly phasic) versus the changes in executive function that occur in addiction (predominantly tonic).[12]

IMAGING BRAIN RECEPTORS

The studies discussed in this article use positron emission tomography (PET) or single-photon emission computed tomography (SPECT) to image specific receptors and changes in neurotransmitters that occur in addiction. PET and SPECT use agonists and antagonists that are specific for a given brain receptor, and are labeled with a radionuclide (usually carbon-11 [^{11}C] or fluorine-18 [^{18}F] for PET and iodine-123 [^{123}I] for SPECT), which allow quantification of these receptors in human brain imaging studies (for an in-depth review of these imaging techniques, please see Refs.[13,14]). Briefly stated, PET and SPECT use radiotracers such that the radionuclide is incorporated into the receptor-specific molecule, which allows detection of the radiotracer with specialized scanners by virtue of its radioactive signal, as it binds to the receptors in the brain. The main outcome measure used in these imaging studies is the "binding potential" (BP), which depends on both the density of the receptor and its affinity for the radiotracer. BP is generally measured as either BP_{ND} (BP relative to the free fraction of radiotracer in the nondisplaceable, ie, not receptor specific, brain tissue) or BP_P (BP relative to the free fraction of radiotracer in the arterial plasma).[15]

In addition to imaging brain receptors, some radiotracers can be used to image the change in the levels of neurotransmitters within the brain.

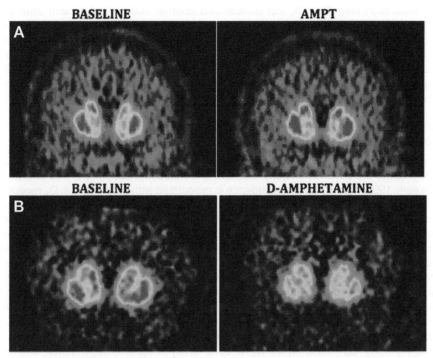

Fig. 1. Coronal slices of PET scans with [^{11}C]raclopride at the level of the striatum. (*A*) D_2 binding potential in the striatum before (baseline) and after AMPT. After depletion of endogenous dopamine, more D_2 receptors are available for the radioligand to bind to, resulting in a stronger signal. (*B*) Striatal D_2 binding at baseline and after *d*-amphetamine (0.3 mg/kg IV), leading to greater release of endogenous dopamine, resulting in displacement of [^{11}C]raclopride and a weaker signal.

Pharmacologic Challenges to Measure Dopamine Release

In addiction, the radiotracers most frequently used to image changes in dopamine transmission are [^{11}C]raclopride for PET and [^{123}I]iodobenzamide (IBZM) for SPECT, which bind to the D_2 family of receptors (referred to as D_2 for simplicity). These radiotracers bind to the D_2 receptors, but they are also sensitive to changes in level of endogenous dopamine in the brain.[16–21] For example, the administration of α-methyl paratyrosine (AMPT), which inhibits tyrosine hydroxylase and reduces endogenous levels of dopamine in the brain, results in a greater percentage of D_2 receptors being available to bind to the radiotracer because fewer are presumably occupied by dopamine.[22–26] Thus, by scanning subjects before and after the administration of AMPT, the percent of D_2 receptors that are occupied by dopamine at baseline can be measured. Alternatively, the administration of a drug (often stimulants such as methylphenidate or amphetamine) that significantly increases extracellular dopamine also reduces the percentage of D_2 receptors available to bind to the radiotracer, as it competes with endogenous dopamine.[16,21,27] The comparison of BP before and after stimulant administration (ΔBP), in the same individual, provides an indirect measure of presynaptic dopamine release, although the exact mechanism is still a matter of investigation.[28] These phenomena are depicted in **Fig. 1**, which shows an individual subject's [^{11}C]raclopride scan at baseline and after AMPT administration (see **Fig. 1**A, top panels) and another subject before and after the administration of a psychostimulant (d-amphetamine, 0.3 mg/kg) (see **Fig. 1**B, bottom panels). The administration of AMPT results in an increase in D_2 receptor BP (due to a decrease in endogenous dopamine), whereas the administration of a stimulant reduces [^{11}C]raclopride BP (due to an increase in endogenous dopamine, see **Fig. 1**B). Using these methods, imaging studies have been able to investigate changes in dopamine in addition to the changes in brain receptors that occur in addiction.

STIMULANT ABUSE AND DOPAMINE RECEPTORS
Cocaine

The drugs of abuse that have been studied most frequently with PET or SPECT imaging are the psychostimulants cocaine and methamphetamine. It was shown in the early 1990s that cocaine dependence is associated with a decrease in D_2 receptor binding when compared to matched control subjects.[29] Subsequent studies have consistently shown decreases in D_2 receptor BP of 11% to 15% in cocaine-dependent individuals compared to control subjects.[30–32] Two PET imaging studies scanned cocaine-dependent subjects after 3 months of abstinence, and both showed persistently lower D_2 receptor BP with [^{11}C]raclopride.[30,33] These findings suggest that the decrease in D_2 receptor BP is either long lasting or not reversible. Importantly, an imaging study in rhesus monkeys exposed to cocaine showed that D_2 receptor availability is decreased by 15% to 20% already after 1 week of cocaine self-administration, and that this decrease can persist even up to 1 year of abstinence, suggesting that the decrease in D_2 receptors is long lasting but reversible.[34] Only one imaging study has measured the D_1 receptor family in cocaine dependence, and this study showed no difference compared to control subjects.[35] Thus, the change in dopamine receptor availability associated with cocaine dependence appears to affect primarily the D_2 receptor family.

Methamphetamine

Imaging studies of the D_2-receptor in methamphetamine dependence have shown similar results. Three studies found a decrease in striatal D_2 receptor BP of about 10% to 15% in methamphetamine-dependent subjects compared to controls.[36–38] These studies also investigated the behavioral correlates of the decrease in BP. Lee and colleagues[37] showed an inverse relationship between BP and impulsiveness, in which lower BP was associated with greater impulsivity, which is consistent with an imaging study in rodents.[39] The study of Volkow and colleagues[36] found that D_2 receptor BP correlates with metabolic rate in the orbitofrontal cortex, which could reflect alterations in the dopamine-mediated striatal regulation of orbitofrontal activity via the striato–thalamo–cortical pathways.

Dopamine Receptors in Other Addictions

The decrease in striatal D_2-receptors was first described in cocaine abusers, and initially it was thought to result from chronic cocaine exposure. However, imaging studies have now demonstrated that decreased striatal D_2 receptor binding occurs in a number of addictions, such as heroin,[40] alcohol dependence,[41–44] tobacco,[45] and even obesity.[46,47] Thus, it is now thought that low D_2 receptor binding serves as a biomarker for addictive behavior, and may reflect a propensity to depend on pharmacologic stimulation to experience reward.[48,49] Depending on the addictive potential of each abused substance, only a relatively small percentage of individuals exposed to drugs will become addicted (eg, 15% over 10 years of cocaine use; 10%

lifetime risk for alcohol dependence[50]). Factors that determine who becomes addicted include genetic (50% of risk), developmental (the risk is higher in adolescence), and environmental (eg, drug access, stress) risk factors.[51]

Low Dopamine Receptor Binding May Predispose to Addiction

Imaging studies have also been used to investigate the vulnerability to addiction. In nonhuman primates, social status has been shown to affect dopamine D_2 receptor BP in the brain.[52] Low status was associated with decreased D_2 receptor BP compared to high social status monkeys, and was also associated with an increased propensity to self-administer cocaine.[52] Also in humans, one imaging study showed that volunteers with lower social status had lower values for [^{11}C]raclopride BP compared to subjects of high social status and support.[53] Imaging studies have also investigated the effect of a family history of addiction and D_2 receptors. Two studies have shown that volunteers with a family history of addiction (cocaine and alcohol), who are not addicted themselves, have higher D_2 receptor binding compared to subjects with no family history.[54] Because subjects with a strong family history of addiction would be expected to have a higher risk for dependence, these findings suggest that increased D_2 receptor BP may be protective.[54] Lastly, Volkow and colleagues have shown that high striatal D_2 binding in healthy controls is predictive of an unpleasant reaction to the administration of intravenous methylphenidate, and that low D_2 binding was associated with a pleasurable experience.[55,56] Thus, taken together these studies indicate that low D_2 receptor binding is associated with increased social stress, increased impulsivity, and an increased positive response to drugs of abuse, factors that have been shown to be risk factors for addiction.

STIMULANT ABUSE AND STRIATAL DOPAMINE TRANSMISSION

As described, PET or SPECT imaging with a D_2 antagonist radiotracer and a pharmacologic challenge that releases presynaptic dopamine (ΔBP) can be used to image changes in the level of endogenous dopamine in the striatum. Brain imaging studies in humans have shown that drug-induced increases in dopamine in the striatum are associated with the subjective experience of reward, that is, the experience of euphoria or feeling "high."[57] In addition, these studies have not been limited to the stimulant drugs. In humans, stimulants,[58,59] nicotine,[60] alcohol,[61,62] and marijuana[63] increase dopamine in dorsal and ventral striatum, which is consistent with animal studies showing that most drugs of abuse increase dopamine release from the presynaptic neurons in the striatum, regardless of their primary mechanism of action.[64] In addition, some of these studies have reported that participants who display the greatest dopamine increases with the drug also report the most intense "high" or "euphoria."[57,59]

These studies were performed in nonaddicted human volunteers, and support the hypothesis that increased striatal dopamine release is generally associated with the positive and reinforcing effects of drug of abuse. However, imaging studies in chronic drug users show that striatal dopamine release is altered in addiction. Volkow and colleagues,[31] using [^{11}C]raclopride displacement to measure dopamine release, previously found that cocaine dependence is associated with blunted dopamine release in response to a stimulant challenge (intravenous methylphenidate) compared to matched controls. In addition, the cocaine-dependent subjects also reported a decrease in the positive effects of the stimulant compared to the control subjects. Using SPECT and an amphetamine challenge (0.3 mg/kg IV), Malison and colleagues[65] performed a similar study in cocaine abusers and controls and reported only a 1% change in radiotracer binding in the cocaine abusers compared to a 10%

decrease in the control subjects. Lastly, Wu and colleagues[66] used the levodopa analogue 6-[^{18}F]-fluoro-L-3,4-dihydroxyphenylalanine (FDOPA), which provides a measure of presynaptic dopamine activity (ie, dopamine synthesis), to show that cocaine-dependent subjects who had been abstinent 11 to 30 days had lower uptake compared to controls. These findings taken together strongly support the hypothesis that cocaine dependence is associated with a decrease in presynaptic dopamine release, measured as presynaptic dopamine release and presynaptic stores of dopamine in the striatum.

Cocaine Self-Administration

Our group previously performed a similar study using PET to image dopamine release in cocaine abusers. In this study, non-treatment–seeking cocaine-dependent subjects were scanned with [^{11}C]raclopride and an amphetamine challenge to measure presynaptic dopamine release.[67] After the PET scans, the cocaine-dependent subjects performed cocaine self-administration sessions to investigate the relationship between dopamine release and a laboratory model of cocaine-seeking behavior. Participants were given five choices between low-dose smoked cocaine and an alternative positive reinforcer (money), and the choices were weighted toward the money. As in previous studies, the cocaine abusers had blunted dopamine release compared to the controls subjects. However, this study also showed that, within the cocaine-abusing subjects, low stimulant-induced dopamine release in the ventral striatum was associated with more choices for cocaine over money, and suggest that low dopamine release is associated with compulsive cocaine use.[67]

STIMULANT ABUSE, DOPAMINE TRANSMISSION, AND RESPONSE TO TREATMENT
Cocaine

More recently, our group investigated this finding in the clinical setting.[33] The goal of this study was to investigate whether blunted striatal dopamine transmission predicted response to treatment that uses positive reinforcement to reduce cocaine use. Treatment-seeking cocaine-dependent subjects underwent PET scans using [^{11}C]raclopride to image baseline dopamine D_2 receptor binding and stimulant-induced presynaptic dopamine release. After the scans, the subjects were enrolled in 24 weeks of treatment using contingency management combined with community reinforcement, which is a behavioral treatment that uses monetary vouchers to induce abstinence from cocaine,[68,69] and that is similar to the choice presented in the laboratory in our previous study.[67] The results of this study showed that both baseline D_2 receptor BP and presynaptic dopamine release (ΔBP) were lower in the subjects who relapsed compared to those who were able to respond to treatment (this finding is illustrated in **Fig. 2**). Importantly, the treatment responders did not differ from the control comparison group in either outcome measure (D_2 receptor BP or stimulant-induced ΔBP), suggesting that this group had intact striatal dopamine transmission.

Methamphetamine

A recent study by Wang and colleagues[38] used [^{11}C]raclopride and a stimulant challenge (oral methylphenidate) to measure dopamine release in methamphetamine abusers and showed that it was blunted compared to controls, as reported previously in cocaine abusers. This study also followed the methamphetamine abusers for 9 months at an outpatient drug rehabilitation program with an intensive behavioral treatment and showed that response to treatment was associated with greater dopamine release. In addition, the methamphetamine abusers who responded to

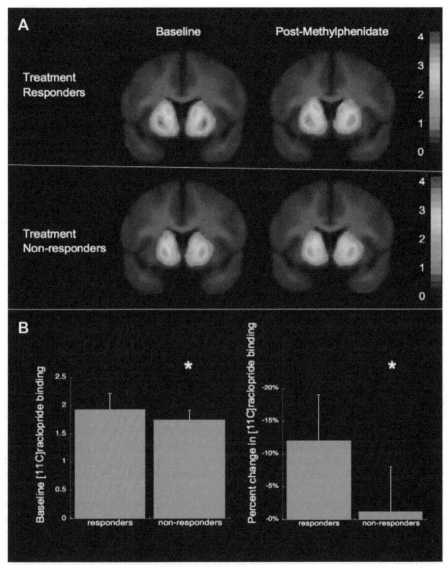

Fig. 2. A recent study in treatment seeking cocaine abusers showed that both [^{11}C]raclopride D$_2$ receptor binding (BP$_{ND}$) and presynaptic dopamine release (ΔBP$_{ND}$) were higher in subjects who responded to treatment versus those who did not. PET scans (*A*) from the treatment responders (*top*) and nonresponders (*bottom*) are shown, at baseline (*left*) and after (*right*) 60 mg PO methylphenidate administration to obtain ΔBP$_{ND}$. The color bar shows the values for BP$_{ND}$. (*B*) Bar graphs illustrating the differences between the treatment responders and nonresponders in the limbic striatum for (*left*) BP$_{ND}$ (premethylphenidate D$_{2/3}$ receptor binding) and (*right*) ΔBP$_{ND}$, the percent decrease in methylphenidate-induced [^{11}C]raclopride binding. (*Reprinted from* Martinez D, Carpenter KM, Liu F, et al. Imaging dopamine transmission in cocaine dependence: link between neurochemistry and response to treatment. Am J Psychiatry 2011;168(6):634–41; with permission.)

treatment did not differ from the controls in both PET outcome measures. These findings are consistent with our study in cocaine abusers, and suggest that impaired dopamine transmission predicts a failure to respond to intensive behavioral treatment in stimulant abusers.

Alcohol and Heroin

In addition to stimulant abuse, imaging studies using this technique have shown that presynaptic dopamine release is blunted in alcohol and heroin dependence.[43,44,70] Thus, the decrease in presynaptic dopamine release measured with PET is not selective for cocaine dependence alone, and, like reduced baseline D_2 receptor binding, it appears to occur across addictions. However, the study by our group in heroin-dependent subjects also used a measure of drug-seeking behavior, and correlated the choice to self-administer heroin with the PET outcome measures.[70] In this study there was no correlation between either outcome measure or the choice to self-administer drug, suggesting that dysregulation in dopamine transmission may be similar across different addictions, but that the correlation between neurochemistry and drug-seeking behavior appears to vary with the particular drug of abuse.

Imaging Dopamine Transmission in Addiction: Clinical Correlates

Taken together, these studies provide some insight into the alterations in dopamine transmission that occur in addiction. The findings in the preceding text show that the administration of a number of drugs of abuse to control subjects produced a measurable increase in presynaptic dopamine that can be measured with PET imaging. In addition, this increase in endogenous dopamine is consistent with animal studies showing that most drugs of abuse increase striatal dopamine, which plays a crucial role in their reinforcing effects. However, in addicted individuals, the administration of stimulants that are known to induce presynaptic dopamine release has been shown to have little effect on the presynaptic dopamine neurons. A number of these studies show that addicted individuals have not only blunted dopamine release but also a reduction in the positive subjective effects of stimulant administration. These findings suggest that addiction is associated with a decrease in dopamine transmission, and show that addiction extends far beyond simply the "high" that drugs induce.

Notably, both studies that have investigated the correlation between dopamine transmission and treatment response show that the stimulant-dependent subjects who failed to respond to treatment were those who had the greatest reduction in presynaptic dopamine release. Importantly, both studies also found that there was no difference in dopamine transmission in the stimulant-dependent subjects who responded to treatment and the control group. These findings suggest that low striatal dopamine transmission may occur in a subset of dependent individuals who are the most refractory to treatment.

Addiction: Compulsive Behavior Perpetuated by Low Dopamine Transmission

The role of dopamine in the striatum is among the most studied phenomena of the brain. For almost a half-century, it has been shown that striatal dopamine is a crucial component of reward and reward-based learning.[71] The NAc, contained within the ventral striatum in humans, serves as a hub of the brain's reward pathways, and plays a central role in selecting adaptive, motivated behavior.[72] In animal studies, deficits in dopamine signaling in the NAc have been shown to impair operant conditioning, response inhibition, and behavioral flexibility.[73] Lesions of the NAc result in a profound deficit in the animals' ability to choose appropriately between two reinforcers: they impulsively and consistently choose a lesser reward over a delayed reinforcer of greater value.[74] These findings suggest that dopamine signaling is critical for making the shift between competing reinforcers. Thus, in the setting of low dopamine transmission a behavior that is ingrained is carried out, even in the presence of an alternative reward of greater value. In other words, low dopamine transmission in addiction appears to be consistent with a habit, rather than playing a role in mediating a "high."

Treatment of Addiction Through Increasing Dopamine?

This information can then be used in treatment development. Previous clinical trials have investigated the effect of medications that increase striatal dopamine transmission as treatment for cocaine dependence, and some report success, whereas others do not (for review see Ref.[75]). One reason for this inconsistency may be that medications that are known to increase dopamine transmission in some addicted subjects may have no effect in more refractory patients. Future treatments that increase striatal dopamine transmission, particularly in refractory patients, need to be explored. This could possibly include medications that improve dopamine transmission by increasing presynaptic stores in the striatum.[76] Another approach may be to increase dopamine transmission by targeting other receptor systems, such as the κ, glutamate, or acetylcholine receptors (for review see Ref.[77,78]). In addition, it may be necessary to combine pharmacotherapies that increase striatal dopamine with behavioral treatments that work to change behavior while dopamine is at work.

Additional Neurocircuitry

Based on this body of literature, the majority of functional imaging studies have focused on investigating the dopamine receptors and dopamine transmission in the basal ganglia. There is mounting evidence that additional circuits are engaged in the development of addiction, including[79]:

1. Mesolimbic dopamine system
2. Ventral striatum
3. Ventral striatum/dorsal striatum/thalamus circuits
4. Dorsolateral frontal cortex/inferior frontal cortex/hippocampus circuits
5. Extended amygdala.

In addition, although dopamine transmission in the nucleus accumbens does play a key role in mediating the positive reinforcement of drugs of abuse,[6] other receptor system are also clearly affected in the development of addiction.[80] At present, radiotracers are available to image the dopamine receptors and transporters, serotonin receptors/transporters, γ-aminobutyric acid (GABA) and glutamate receptors, opioid receptors, and others.

IMAGING STUDIES OF PSYCHOSTIMULANT ABUSE: BEYOND D$_2$ RECEPTORS
Dopamine Transporters in Stimulant Abuse

In addition to the dopamine D$_2$ receptors and presynaptic dopamine release, imaging studies have also investigated other receptors and transporters. One of the most consistent findings seen in imaging studies of methamphetamine dependence is a decrease in dopamine transporter (DAT) binding in the striatum. As shown in **Table 1**, seven published imaging studies in humans have shown a decrease in the DAT in methamphetamine abusers compared to controls.[81–87] In addition, the percent

Table 1
Published studies in human methamphetamine abusers listed in order of least to greatest percent decrease in DAT reported

Study	Number of Volunteers	Abstinence Average (Range)	% Decrease DAT
Johanson et al[85]	MA: 16 HC: 18	3.4 y (3 m–18 y)	Caudate, 16; putamen, 12
McCann et al[86]	MA: 6 HC: 10	3.3 y (4 m–5 y)	Putamen, 25; caudate, 23
McCann et al[87]	MA: 22 HC: 17	2.4 y (8 m– >10 y)	Caudate, 23; putamen, 17
Iyo et al[84]	MA: 11 HC: 9	9 m[a] (0 m–18 m)	Ventral striatum, 26; caudate/putamen, 20
Volkow et al[83]	MA: 15 HC: 18	6 m (0.5 m–36 m)	Caudate, 28; putamen, 21
Sekine et al[81]	MA: 11 HC: 9	5.6 m (7d–1.5 y)	Ventral striatum, 20; caudate/putamen, 20
Chou et al[82]	MA: 7 HC: 7	Days (not specified)	Whole striatum, 30

The average abstinence is the average time of abstinence before the PET scan reported in the study. Abstinence is provided as average and range.
Abbreviations: d, days; HC, healthy control; m, months; MA, methamphetamine abuser; y, years.
[a] Estimated average; actual data not provided.

decrease in the dopamine transporter appears to correlate with the duration of abstinence before scanning (less abstinence, greater loss of DAT). These studies are consistent with imaging studies in nonhuman primates, which also show that methamphetamine exposure results in a significant decrease in the DAT, which can take months to years to recover.[88–93] The mechanism behind this reduction in transporter density appears to involve a number of mechanisms, including oxidative stress, activation of transcription factors, DNA damage, excitotoxicity, and various apoptotic pathways that result in frank injury to the dopamine neurons (for review see Ref.[94]).

Cocaine

Interestingly, PET studies of the DAT in cocaine dependence show that, unlike methamphetamine, cocaine has a much less dramatic effect. In a study of cocaine abusers abstinent for 96 hours, Malison and colleagues[95] showed a 20% increase in the DAT compared to matched controls. However, imaging studies performed at either 5 ± 8 days or 42 ± 7 days of abstinence show no difference in BP between healthy controls and cocaine abusers.[42,96] This suggests that the DAT is elevated in very early abstinence, but does not appear to differ from controls after this time point. Even though cocaine abusers and methamphetamine abusers both show blunted dopamine release, the mechanism mediating this difference likely varies between the two drugs of abuse. Thus, whereas the loss of dopamine transmission in methamphetamine abuse results from injury to the dopamine neurons, blunted dopamine transmission in cocaine abusers most likely results from other factors, such as dysregulation of the neurotransmitters that regulate dopamine transmission.

Serotonin and Opiate Receptors

Although the majority of imaging studies in addiction have focused on the dopamine receptors and dopamine transmission in the basal ganglia, there is mounting evidence that additional circuits and other neurotransmitters also play a crucial role in the development of addiction.[80] In cocaine dependence, imaging studies have also investigated alterations in the serotonin transporter and μ opioid receptor. Cocaine directly affects the serotonin system, and altering serotonin transmission in human subjects affects craving and the subjective effects of cocaine.[97–99] However, only one imaging study has been performed in humans to measure the serotonin transporter, and this study showed that the transporter was increased in the brain stem in cocaine abusers who had been abstinent for 4 to 8 days.[100] Three imaging studies have measured the μ receptor using [^{11}C]carfentanil in cocaine dependence. These studies show that cocaine dependence is associated with an increase in μ receptor BP in the anterior cingulate, frontal and temporal cortex, caudate, and thalamus compared to controls, and remains elevated even after months of abstinence.[101,102] This group also showed that regional brain μ receptor binding in cocaine-dependent subjects was a significant predictor of time to relapse to cocaine use.[103]

ALCOHOL DEPENDENCE

Ethanol affects numerous neuronal receptor and channels.[104] As described briefly in the preceding text, ethanol clearly has an effect on dopamine signaling, although the exact mechanism remains uncertain.[104] Imaging studies have used the radiotracer [^{11}C]raclopride to investigate whether acute ethanol administration to healthy humans produces striatal dopamine release that can be measured with PET. Two studies have shown that acute alcohol administration results in [^{11}C]raclopride displacement[61,62] while others have not.[105,106] Importantly, a recent study showed that [^{11}C]raclopride displacement induced by ethanol varied by gender: men had a much larger effect compared to women, and percent dopamine release correlated with the positive subjective effects in men, but not in women.[62]

Alcoholism Interferes with Dopamine Signaling

However, like stimulant dependence, studies in alcohol-dependent subjects show that striatal dopamine signaling is impaired once dependence sets in. Several PET and SPECT studies have measured striatal D_2 receptor BP in alcohol dependence,[41,43,44,107–111] and seven of these show that D_2 receptor BP is decreased compared to that in matched controls (two show nonsignificant decreases). As described in the preceding text, studies imaging stimulant-induced dopamine release have shown this to be blunted in alcohol-dependent subjects compared to controls.[43,44] Studies using alcohol as a challenge to release dopamine have been performed only in healthy controls but not in alcohol-dependent subjects. Other parameters of dopamine transmission in alcohol dependence have been studied with imaging, overall supporting the hypothesis that striatal dopamine signaling is impaired in alcohol dependence (for review see Ref.[112]).

Other Neurotransmitter Systems Affected in Alcoholism: Serotonin

The other receptor systems that have been imaged in alcohol dependence include the serotonin, opiate, and GABA receptor systems. Imaging studies of the serotonin system have focused on the serotonin transporter, given the important role of the serotonin system in vulnerability to alcohol-induced aggression.[113] Overall, the results of these studies are mixed in that some studies have reported a decrease in the serotonin transporter and other studies have not.[114–118] One of the studies also investigated the serotonin 1A receptor,[118] but showed no difference between the alcohol-dependent and control subjects, while another study imaged the serotonin 1B receptors and found an increase in binding in the ventral striatum of alcohol-dependent subjects compared with controls.[119] Given the importance of the serotonin system in alcohol dependence, the fact that the findings from these are not consistent is surprising, particularly given that the imaging studies of dopamine are very consistent. One possibility is that the alterations in dopamine signaling reported in alcohol dependence are not specific to alcoholism (see earlier), but belie a vulnerability to addiction. In addition, it appears from the imaging studies of the serotonin system in alcoholism that differences in gender, genotype, and aggression may explain why there is less uniformity in these results.[112,113] Thus, further imaging studies of the serotonin system in alcohol dependence should be performed to understand better how these factors affect serotonin transmission and play a role in the development of alcoholism.

Opiate Receptors

The other neurotransmitter systems that play a crucial role in alcohol dependence are the opiate receptors and GABA. Several studies have measured the μ receptor in alcohol dependence using the μ receptor selective radiotracer [^{11}C]carfentanil. An early study in eight alcohol-dependent men after 4 days of abstinence reported a decrease in μ receptor BP in the prefrontal cortex compared to controls, with no differences in other cortical regions.[120] However, a subsequent study of 25 alcohol-dependent subjects scanned after weeks of abstinence showed that alcohol dependence was associated with an increase in μ receptor BP in the ventral striatum compared to the control subjects, with no difference in other brain regions studied.[121] These findings are in agreement with another imaging study in 20 alcohol-dependent subjects showing significantly higher μ receptor BP compared to controls in several brain regions including the ventral striatum.[122] In addition, there was an inverse relationship between [^{11}C]carfentanil BP_{ND} and craving.[122]

GABA

With respect to the GABA system, imaging studies have focused on measuring the $GABA_A$ receptor, given the direct role it plays in ethanol intoxication and withdrawal. Seven PET and SPECT studies have been conducted to look at this receptor in alcohol dependence. Three showed that alcohol dependence is associated with a decrease in the $GABA_A$ receptor binding in the frontal cortex, anterior cingulate, cerebellum, and parietal and temporal cortices.[123–125] In contrast, two studies reported no difference in $GABA_A$ receptor binding between alcohol-dependent subjects and healthy controls,[126,127] and two studies showed an increase in $GABA_A$ receptor binding in alcohol-dependent subjects compared to controls.[128,129] An important issue with respect to these discrepancies is not only the number of subjects included (some studies had a very small cohort) but also time of abstinence to the time of scanning. The study of Staley and colleagues[129] imaged early and later in abstinence and showed that radiotracer binding at the $GABA_A$ receptor varies with duration of abstinence and likely shifts across the different stages of alcohol dependence (for review see Ref.[130]).

CANNABIS DEPENDENCE
THC Induces Dopamine Release

Four imaging studies have examined the effect of Δ^9-THC on dopamine release in vivo, including an anecdotal case report.[63,131–133] Unlike studies using a stimulant to produce dopamine release in the brain, the studies using THC as a challenge to release dopamine show very different results. In one study, THC inhalation was found to reduce [^{11}C]raclopride binding in the ventral striatum and the precommissural dorsal putamen compared to placebo, consistent with an increase in dopamine levels in these regions in a small pilot study.[63] However, a study using the synthetic cannabinoid dronabinol as a challenge reported no significant difference in THC-induced [^{11}C]raclopride binding (but an increase in psychosis-like symptoms).[132] In addition, Barkus and colleagues compared intravenous THC to placebo in 11 healthy men using SPECT with [^{123}I]IBZM, and found no significant change in the caudate or putamen.[133] Overall, these studies suggest that there may be a small effect of acute THC on dopamine release in the human striatum, but that this effect is difficult to measure. Given that the increase in striatal dopamine may be slightly larger with a stimulant challenge compared to acute THC inhalation,[134,135] it is possible that the effect of chronic THC use on dopamine is present, but not large enough to be measurable with these imaging methods.

D_2 Receptors Are Not Affected in Cannabis Dependence

As described, the abuse of most drugs of abuse (cocaine, methamphetamine, alcohol, heroin, and nicotine) has been shown to be associated with a reduction in D_2 receptor binding. Thus, one would expect the same finding in cannabis abuse. However, imaging studies investigating the dopaminergic system in chronic cannabis users have not seen any difference in [^{11}C]raclopride BP_{ND} in chronic cannabis-dependent subjects compared to controls.[134,136,137] Sevy and colleagues [136] reported that although cannabis-dependent subjects had lower normalized glucose metabolism in the right orbitofrontal cortex and bilateral putamen with [^{18}F]FDG, there was no difference in striatal D_2 receptor availability compared to controls. One other study retrospectively evaluated a data set of [^{11}C]raclopride scans of volunteers who had also reported cannabis use and compared D_2 binding to data from a control sample without any reported use. No difference in D_2 binding was found, or any correlation with lifetime frequency of use and D_2 binding potential.[138]

Is Dopamine Transmission Affected by Chronic Cannabis Use?

Similarly, imaging studies in addiction to cocaine, methamphetamine, heroin, and alcohol dependence are associated with a reduction in presynaptic dopamine release. Only one imaging study to date has evaluated changes in dopamine release in addition to D_2 receptor density in chronic, recently abstinent, cannabis users with the amphetamine challenge paradigm and [^{11}C]raclopride, and found no difference to healthy controls.[134] Subjects in our sample, however, reported only mild to moderate cannabis use, while meeting *Diagnostic and Statistical Manual of Mental Disorders*, 4th ed. (DSM-IV-TR) criteria for dependence. It is conceivable that more severe cannabis use may lead to measurable changes in the dopaminergic system. Interestingly, dopamine release in the associative striatum correlated positively with age at onset of the drug use, providing further evidence that the adolescent brain may be more vulnerable to chronic effects of the drug.

Endogenous Cannabinoid Receptors

The endocannabinoid system, however, may be more directly affected, and imaging studies have recently become possible with the development of the inverse agonist radiotracer [^{18}F]FMPEP-d$_2$ [(3R,5R)-5-(3-[18F]Fluoromethoxy-d2)phenyl)-3-((R)-1-phenyl-ethylamino)-1-(4-trifluoromethyl-phenyl)-pyrrolidin-2-one]. A recent study by Hirvonen and colleagues[138] demonstrated a reversible and regionally selective downregulation of brain cannabinoid CB1 receptors in chronic, heavy cannabis users. Downregulation of CB1 receptor correlated with the years of cannabis smoking, was limited to cortical regions, and returned to normal levels after 1 month of monitored abstinence from the drug. Downregulation of endocannabinoid receptors may contribute to tolerance to cannabis, while the dopaminergic system plays a secondary role, but further studies are needed to understand the interplay better.

SUMMARY

Neuroimaging studies have been crucial in understanding changes in the various neurotransmitter systems implicated in addiction in the living human brain. Predominantly reduced striatal dopamine transmission appears to play an important role in psychostimulant, alcohol and heroin addiction, while addiction to cannabis may be mediated primarily by the endocannabinoid system. However, the study of other neurotransmitter systems likely involved in addiction, for example glutamate, has been limited by the number and quality of available radiotracers, and data on changes in these systems in the most common addictions are emerging only now. Further studies are needed to understand fully how the interplay of various neurotransmitter systems contributes to addiction and to ultimately help to develop more effective treatment approaches.

REFERENCES

1. Koob GF. Hedonic homeostatic dysregulation as a driver of drug-seeking behavior. Drug Discov Today Dis Models 2008;5(4):207–15.
2. Carlezon WA Jr, Wise RA. Rewarding actions of phencyclidine and related drugs in nucleus accumbens shell and frontal cortex. J Neurosci 1996;16(9):3112–22.
3. Devane WA, Axelrod J. Enzymatic synthesis of anandamide, an endogenous ligand for the cannabinoid receptor, by brain membranes. Proc Natl Acad Sci U S A 1994;91(14):6698–701.
4. Vogel Z, Barg J, Levy R, et al. Anandamide, a brain endogenous compound, interacts specifically with cannabinoid receptors and inhibits adenylate cyclase. J Neurochem 1993;61(1):352–5.
5. Wise RA, Rompre PP. Brain dopamine and reward. Annu Rev Psychol 1989;40:191–225.
6. Koob GF, Le Moal M. Drug addiction, dysregulation of reward, and allostasis. Neuropsychopharmacology 2001;24(2):97–129.
7. Robinson TE, Berridge KC. Addiction. Annu Rev Psychol 2003;54:25–53.
8. Koob GF. Neural mechanisms of drug reinforcement. Ann N Y Acad Sci 1992;654:171–91.
9. Wise RA. The role of reward pathways in the development of drug dependence. Pharmacol Ther 1987;35(1–2):227–63.
10. Wise RA. Roles for nigrostriatal—not just mesocorticolimbic—dopamine in reward and addiction. Trends Neurosci 2009;32(10):517–24.
11. Schultz W. Multiple dopamine functions at different time courses. Annu Rev Neurosci 2007;30:259–88.

12. Grace AA. The tonic/phasic model of dopamine system regulation and its implications for understanding alcohol and psychostimulant craving. Addiction 2000; 95(Suppl 2):S119–28.

13. Carson RE. Parameters estimation in positron emission tomography, in positron emission tomography: principles and applications for the brain and the heart. In: Phelps ME, Mazziotta JC, Schelbert HR, editors. New York: Raven Press; 1986. p. 347–90.

14. Slifstein M, Laruelle M. Models and methods for derivation of in vivo neuroreceptor parameters with PET and SPECT reversible radiotracers. Nucl Med Biol 2001;28(5): 595–608.

15. Innis RB, Cunningham VJ, Delforge J, et al. Consensus nomenclature for in vivo imaging of reversibly binding radioligands. J Cereb Blood Flow Metab 2007;27(9): 1533–9.

16. Breier A, Su TP, Saunders R, et al. Schizophrenia is associated with elevated amphetamine-induced synaptic dopamine concentrations: evidence from a novel positron emission tomography method. Proc Natl Acad Sci U S A 1997; 94(6):2569–74.

17. Dewey SL, Smith GS, Logan J, et al. Striatal binding of the PET ligand ^{11}C-raclopride is altered by drugs that modify synaptic dopamine levels. Synapse 1993;13(4): 350–6.

18. Innis RB, Malison RT, al-Tikriti M, et al. Amphetamine-stimulated dopamine release competes in vivo for [^{123}I]IBZM binding to the D2 receptor in nonhuman primates. Synapse 1992;10(3):177–84.

19. Laruelle M, Iyer RN, al-Tikriti M, et al. Microdialysis and SPECT measurements of amphetamine-induced dopamine release in nonhuman primates. Synapse 1997; 25(1):1–14.

20. Laruelle M, Abi-Dargham A, van Dyck CH, et al. SPECT imaging of striatal dopamine release after amphetamine challenge. J Nucl Med 1995;36:1182–90.

21. Volkow ND, Wang G, Fowler RS, et al. Therapeutic doses of oral methylphenidate significantly increase extracellular dopamine in the human brain. J Neurosci 2001; 21(2):RC121.

22. Martinez D, Greene K, Broft A, et al. Lower level of endogenous dopamine in patients with cocaine dependence: findings from PET imaging of D(2)/D(3) receptors following acute dopamine depletion. Am J Psychiatry 2009;166(10):1170–7.

23. Cropley VL, Innis RB, Nathan PJ, et al. Small effect of dopamine release and no effect of dopamine depletion on [^{18}F]fallypride binding in healthy humans. Synapse 2008; 62(6):399–408.

24. Riccardi P, Baldwin R, Salomon R, et al. Estimation of baseline dopamine D2 receptor occupancy in striatum and extrastriatal regions in humans with positron emission tomography with [^{18}F] fallypride. Biol Psychiatry 2008;63(2):241–4.

25. Verhoeff NP, Hussey D, Lee M, et al. Dopamine depletion results in increased neostriatal D(2), but not D(1), receptor binding in humans. Mol Psychiatry 2002;7(3): 233, 322–8.

26. Laruelle M, D'Souza CD, Baldwin RM, et al. Imaging D2 receptor occupancy by endogenous dopamine in humans. Neuropsychopharmacology 1997;17:162–74.

27. Laruelle M, Al-Tikrity M, Abi-Dargham A, et al. D-amphetamine-induced reduction of dopamine D2 availability in primates: comparison between [^{123}I]IBF and [^{123}I]IBZM. Soc Neurosci Abstr 1994;20:644.

28. Laruelle M. Imaging synaptic neurotransmission with in vivo binding competition techniques: a critical review. J Cereb Blood Flow Metab 2000;20(3):423–51.

29. Volkow ND, Fowler JS, Wolf AP, et al. Effects of chronic cocaine abuse on postsynaptic dopamine receptors. Am J Psychiatry 1990;147(6):719–24.

30. Volkow ND, Fowler JS, Wang GJ, et al. Decreased dopamine D2 receptor availability is associated with reduced frontal metabolism in cocaine abusers. Synapse 1993; 14(2):169–77.

31. Volkow ND, Wang GJ, Fowler JS, et al. Decreased striatal dopaminergic responsiveness in detoxified cocaine-dependent subjects. Nature 1997;386:830–3.

32. Martinez D, Broft A, Foltin RW, et al. Cocaine dependence and d2 receptor availability in the functional subdivisions of the striatum: relationship with cocaine-seeking behavior. Neuropsychopharmacology 2004;29(6):1190–202.

33. Martinez D, Carpenter KM, Liu F, et al. Imaging dopamine transmission in cocaine dependence: link between neurochemistry and response to treatment. Am J Psychiatry 2011;168(6):634–41.

34. Nader MA, Morgan D, Gage HD, et al. PET imaging of dopamine D2 receptors during chronic cocaine self-administration in monkeys. Nat Neurosci 2006;9(8):1050–6.

35. Martinez D, Slifstein M, Narendran R, et al. Dopamine D1 receptors in cocaine dependence measured with PET and the choice to self-administer cocaine. Neuropsychopharmacology 2009;34(7):1774–82.

36. Volkow ND, Change L, Wang GJ, et al. Low level of brain dopamine D2 receptors in methamphetamine abusers: association with metabolism in the orbitofrontal cortex. Am J Psychiatry 2001;158(12):2015–21.

37. Lee B, London ED, Poldrack RA, et al. Striatal dopamine d2/d3 receptor availability is reduced in methamphetamine dependence and is linked to impulsivity. J Neurosci 2009;29(47):14734–40.

38. Wang GJ, Smith L, Volkow ND, et al. Decreased dopamine activity predicts relapse in methamphetamine abusers. Mol Psychiatry 2011. DOI: 10.1038/mp.2011.86. [Epub ahead of print].

39. Dalley JW, Fryer TD, Brichard L, et al. Nucleus accumbens D2/3 receptors predict trait impulsivity and cocaine reinforcement. Science 2007;315(5816):1267–70.

40. Wang GJ, Volkow ND, Fowler JS, et al. Dopamine D2 receptor availability in opiate-dependent subjects before and after naloxone-precipitated withdrawal. Neuropsychopharmacology 1997;16(2):174–82.

41. Hietala J, West C, Swälahti E, et al. Striatal D2 dopamine receptor binding characteristics in vivo in patients with alcohol dependence. Psychopharmacology [Berl] 1994;116(3):285–90.

42. Volkow ND, Wang GJ, Fowler JS, et al. Decreases in dopamine receptors but not in dopamine transporters in alcoholics. Alcohol Clin Exp Res 1996;20(9):1594–8.

43. Martinez D, Gil R, Slifstein M, et al. Alcohol dependence is associated with blunted dopamine transmission in the ventral striatum. Biol Psychiatry 2005;58(10):779–86.

44. Volkow ND, Wang GJ, Telang F, et al. Profound decreases in dopamine release in striatum in detoxified alcoholics: possible orbitofrontal involvement. J Neurosci 2007;27(46):12700–6.

45. Fehr C, Yakushev I, Hohmann N, et al. Association of low striatal dopamine d2 receptor availability with nicotine dependence similar to that seen with other drugs of abuse. Am J Psychiatry 2008;165(4):507–14.

46. Wang GJ, Volkow ND, Logan J, et al. Brain dopamine and obesity. Lancet 2001; 357(9253):354–7.

47. Volkow ND, Wang GJ, Fowler JS, et al. Overlapping neuronal circuits in addiction and obesity: evidence of systems pathology. Philos Trans R Soc Lond B Biol Sci 2008;363(1507):3191–200.

48. Volkow ND, Fowler JS, Wang GJ. Role of dopamine in drug reinforcement and addiction in humans: results from imaging studies. Behav Pharmacol 2002;13(5–6): 355–66.
49. Melis M, Spiga S, Diana M. The dopamine hypothesis of drug addiction: hypodopaminergic state. Int Rev Neurobiol 2005;63:101–54.
50. Wagner FA, Anthony JC. From first drug use to drug dependence; developmental periods of risk for dependence upon marijuana, cocaine, and alcohol. Neuropsychopharmacology 2002;26(4):479–88.
51. Volkow N, Li TK. The neuroscience of addiction. Nat Neurosci 2005;8(11):1429–30.
52. Morgan D, Grant KA, Gage HD, et al. Social dominance in monkeys: dopamine D2 receptors and cocaine self-administration. Nat Neurosci 2002;5(2):169–74.
53. Martinez D, Orlowska D, Narendran R, et al. Dopamine type 2/3 receptor availability in the striatum and social status in human volunteers. Biol Psychiatry 2010;67(3): 275–8.
54. Volkow ND, Wang GJ, Begleiter H, et al. High levels of dopamine D2 receptors in unaffected members of alcoholic families: possible protective factors. Arch Gen Psychiatry 2006;63(9):999–1008.
55. Volkow ND, Wang GJ, Fowler JS, et al. Prediction of reinforcing responses to psychostimulants in humans by brain dopamine D2 receptor levels. Am J Psychiatry 1999;156(9):1440–3.
56. Volkow ND, Wang GJ, Fowler JS, et al. Brain DA D2 receptors predict reinforcing effects of stimulants in humans: replication study. Synapse 2002;46(2):79–82.
57. Volkow ND, Wang GJ, Fowler JS, et al. Relationship between psychostimulant-induced "high" and dopamine transporter occupancy. Proc Natl Acad Sci U S A 1996;93(19):10388–92.
58. Volkow ND, Wang GJ, Fowler JS, et al. Reinforcing effects of psychostimulants in humans are associated with increases in brain dopamine and occupancy of D(2) receptors. J Pharmacol Exp Ther 1999;291(1):409–15.
59. Drevets WC, Gautier C, Price JC, et al. Amphetamine-induced dopamine release in human ventral striatum correlates with euphoria. Biol Psychiatry 2001;49(2):81–96.
60. Brody AL, Mandekern MA, Olmstead RE, et al. Ventral striatal dopamine release in response to smoking a regular vs a denicotinized cigarette. Neuropsychopharmacology 2009;34(2):282–9.
61. Boileau I, Assaad JM, Pihl RO, et al. Alcohol promotes dopamine release in the human nucleus accumbens. Synapse 2003;49(4):226–31.
62. Urban NB, Kegeles LS, Slifstein M, et al. Sex differences in striatal dopamine release in young adults after oral alcohol challenge: a positron emission tomography imaging study with [^{11}C]raclopride. Biol Psychiatry 2010;68(8):689–96.
63. Bossong MG, van Berckel BN, Boellaard R, et al. Delta 9-tetrahydrocannabinol induces dopamine release in the human striatum. Neuropsychopharmacology 2009; 34(3):759–66.
64. Di Chiara G, Imperato A. Drugs abused by humans preferentially increase synaptic dopamine concentrations in the mesolimbic system of freely moving rats. Proc Natl Acad Sci U S A 1988;85(14):5274–8.
65. Malison RT, Mechanic KY, Klummp H, et al. Reduced amphetamine-stimulated dopamine release in cocaine addicts as measured by [^{123}I]IBZM SPECT. J Nucl Med 1999;40(5 Suppl):110P.
66. Wu JC, Bell K, Najafi A, et al. Decreasing striatal 6-FDOPA uptake with increasing duration of cocaine withdrawal. Neuropsychopharmacology 1997;17(6):402–9.

67. Martinez D, Narendran R, Fottin RW, et al. Amphetamine-induced dopamine release: markedly blunted in cocaine dependence and predictive of the choice to self-administer cocaine. Am J Psychiatry 2007;164(4):622–9.

68. Higgins ST, Budney AJ, Bickel WK, et al. Incentives improve outcome in outpatient behavioral treatment of cocaine dependence. Arch Gen Psychiatry 1994;51(7):568–76.

69. Higgins ST, Sigmon SC, Wong CJ, et al. Community reinforcement therapy for cocaine-dependent outpatients. Arch Gen Psychiatry 2003;60(10):1043–52.

70. Martinez D, Saccone PA, Liu F, et al. Deficits in dopamine D(2) receptors and presynaptic dopamine in heroin dependence: commonalities and differences with other types of addiction. Biol Psychiatry 2012;71(3):192–8.

71. Wise RA. Addictive drugs and brain stimulation reward. Annu Rev Neurosci 1996; 19:319–40.

72. Sesack SR, Grace AA. Cortico-basal ganglia reward network: microcircuitry. Neuropsychopharmacology 2010;35(1):27–47.

73. Goto Y, Grace AA. Limbic and cortical information processing in the nucleus accumbens. Trends Neurosci 2008;31(11):552–8.

74. Cardinal RN, Pennicott DR, Sugathapala CL, et al. Impulsive choice induced in rats by lesions of the nucleus accumbens core. Science 2001;292(5526):2499–501.

75. Grabowski J, Shearer J, Merrill J, et al. Agonist-like, replacement pharmacotherapy for stimulant abuse and dependence. Addict Behav 2004;29(7):1439–64.

76. Schmitz JM, Mooney ME, Moeller FG, et al. Levodopa pharmacotherapy for cocaine dependence: choosing the optimal behavioral therapy platform. Drug Alcohol Depend 2008;94(1–3):142–50.

77. Shippenberg TS, Zapata A, Chefer VI. Dynorphin and the pathophysiology of drug addiction. Pharmacol Ther 2007;116(2):306–21.

78. Lester DB, Rogers TD, Blaha CD. Acetylcholine-dopamine interactions in the pathophysiology and treatment of CNS disorders. CNS Neurosci Ther 2010;16(3):137–62.

79. Koob GF, Volkow ND. Neurocircuitry of addiction. Neuropsychopharmacology 2010;35(1):217–38.

80. Nestler EJ. Is there a common molecular pathway for addiction? Nat Neurosci 2005;8(11):1445–9.

81. Sekine Y, Iyo M, Ouchi Y, et al. Methamphetamine-related psychiatric symptoms and reduced brain dopamine transporters studied with PET. Am J Psychiatry 2001;158(8):1206–14.

82. Chou YH, Huang WS, Su TP, et al. Dopamine transporters and cognitive function in methamphetamine abuser after a short abstinence: a SPECT study. Eur Neuropsychopharmacol 2007;17(1):46–52.

83. Volkow ND, Chang L, Wang GJ, et al. Association of dopamine transporter reduction with psychomotor impairment in methamphetamine abusers. Am J Psychiatry 2001;158(3):377–82.

84. Iyo M, Sekine Y, Mori N. Neuromechanism of developing methamphetamine psychosis: a neuroimaging study. Ann N Y Acad Sci 2004;1025:288–95.

85. Johanson CE, Frey KA, Lundahl LH, et al. Cognitive function and nigrostriatal markers in abstinent methamphetamine abusers. Psychopharmacology [Berl] 2006; 185(3):327–38.

86. McCann U, Wong DF, Yokoi F, et al. Reduced striatal dopamine transporter density in abstinent methamphetamine and methcathinone users: evidence from positron emission tomography studies with [^{11}C]WIN-35,428. J Neurosci 1998; 18(20):8417–22.

87. McCann UD, Kuwabara H, Kumar A, et al. Persistent cognitive and dopamine transporter deficits in abstinent methamphetamine users. Synapse 2008;62(2):91–100.

88. Melega WP, Lacan G, Desalles AA, et al. Long-term methamphetamine-induced decreases of [(11)C]WIN 35,428 binding in striatum are reduced by GDNF: PET studies in the vervet monkey. Synapse 2000;35(4):243–9.

89. Hashimoto K, Tsukada H, Nishiyama S, et al. Protective effects of N-acetyl-L-cysteine on the reduction of dopamine transporters in the striatum of monkeys treated with methamphetamine. Neuropsychopharmacology 2004;29(11):2018–23.

90. Hashimoto K, Tsukada H, Nishiyama S, et al. Protective effects of minocycline on the reduction of dopamine transporters in the striatum after administration of methamphetamine: a positron emission tomography study in conscious monkeys. Biol Psychiatry 2007;61(5):577–81.

91. Villemagne V, Yuan J, Wong DF, et al. Brain dopamine neurotoxicity in baboons treated with doses of methamphetamine comparable to those recreationally abused by humans: evidence from [^{11}C]WIN-35,428 positron emission tomography studies and direct in vitro determinations. J Neurosci 1998;18(1):419–27.

92. Harvey DC, Lacan G, Tanious SP, et al. Recovery from methamphetamine induced long-term nigrostriatal dopaminergic deficits without substantia nigra cell loss. Brain Res 2000;871(2):259–70.

93. Volkow ND, Chang L, Wang GJ, et al. Loss of dopamine transporters in methamphetamine abusers recovers with protracted abstinence. J Neurosci 2001;21(23):9414–8.

94. Cadet JL, Krasnova IN. Molecular bases of methamphetamine-induced neurodegeneration. Int Rev Neurobiol 2009;88:101–19.

95. Malison RT, Best SE, van Dyck CH, et al. Elevated striatal dopamine transporters during acute cocaine abstinence as measured by [^{123}I] beta-CIT SPECT. Am J Psychiatry 1998;155(6):832–4.

96. Wang GJ, Volkow ND, Fowler JS, et al. Cocaine abusers do not show loss of dopamine transporters with age. Life Sci 1997;61(11):1059–65.

97. Aronson SC, Black JE, McDougle CJ, et al. Serotonergic mechanisms of cocaine effects in humans. Psychopharmacology [Berl] 1995;119(2):179–85.

98. Satel SL, Krystal JH, Delgado PL, et al. Tryptophan depletion and attenuation of cue-induced craving for cocaine. Am J Psychiatry 1995;152(5):778–83.

99. Walsh SL, Preston KL, Sullivan JT, et al. Fluoxetine alters the effects of intravenous cocaine in humans. J Clin Psychopharmacol 1994;14(6):396–407.

100. Jacobsen LK, Staley JK, Malison RT, et al. Elevated central serotonin transporter binding availability in acutely abstinent cocaine-dependent patients. Am J Psychiatry 2000;157(7):1134–40.

101. Zubieta JK, Gorelick DA, Stauffer R, et al. Increased mu opioid receptor binding detected by PET in cocaine-dependent men is associated with cocaine craving. Nat Med 1996;2(11):1225–9.

102. Gorelick DA, Kim YK, Bencherif B, et al. Imaging brain mu-opioid receptors in abstinent cocaine users: time course and relation to cocaine craving. Biol Psychiatry 2005;57(12):1573–82.

103. Gorelick DA, Kim YK, Bencherif B, et al. Brain mu-opioid receptor binding: relationship to relapse to cocaine use after monitored abstinence. Psychopharmacology [Berl] 2008;200(4):475–86.

104. Sulzer D. How addictive drugs disrupt presynaptic dopamine neurotransmission. Neuron 2011;69(4):628–49.

105. Yoder KK, Constantinescu CC, Kareken DA, et al. Heterogeneous effects of alcohol on dopamine release in the striatum: a PET study. Alcohol Clin Exp Res 2007;31(6): 965–73.

106. Salonen I, Hietala J, Laihinen A, et al. A PET study on the acute effect of ethanol on striatal D2 dopamine receptors with [^{11}C]raclopride in healthy males. Hum Psychopharmacol Clin Exp 1997;12(2):145–52.

107. Volkow ND, Wang G-J, Fowler JS, et al. Decreases in dopamine receptors but not in dopamine transporters in alcoholics. J Nucl Med 1996;37:33P.

108. Volkow ND, Wang GJ, Maynard L, et al. Effects of alcohol detoxification on dopamine D2 receptors in alcoholics: a preliminary study. Psychiatry Res 2002; 116(3):163–72.

109. Heinz A, Siessmeier T, Wrase J, et al. Correlation between dopamine D(2) receptors in the ventral striatum and central processing of alcohol cues and craving. Am J Psychiatry 2004;161(10):1783–9.

110. Rominger A, Cumming P, Xiong G, et al. [(18) F]fallypride PET measurement of striatal and extrastriatal dopamine D(2/3) receptor availability in recently abstinent alcoholics. Addict Biol 2012;17(2):490–503.

111. Heinz A, Siessmeier T, Wrase J, et al. Correlation of alcohol craving with striatal dopamine synthesis capacity and D2/3 receptor availability: a combined [^{18}F]DOPA and [^{18}F]DMFP PET study in detoxified alcoholic patients. Am J Psychiatry 2005; 162(8):1515–20.

112. Martinez D, Kim JH, Krystal J, et al. Imaging the neurochemistry of alcohol and substance abuse. Neuroimag Clin N Am 2007;17(4):539–55, x.

113. Heinz AJ, Beck A, Meyer-Lindenberg A, et al. Cognitive and neurobiological mechanisms of alcohol-related aggression. Nat Rev Neurosci 2011;12(7):400–13.

114. Heinz A, Jones DW, Bissette G, et al. Relationship between cortisol and serotonin metabolites and transporters in alcoholism. Pharmacopsychiatry 2002;35(4):127–34.

115. Heinz A, Jones DW, Mazzanti C, et al. A relationship between serotonin transporter genotype and in vivo protein expression and alcohol neurotoxicity. Biol Psychiatry 2000;47(7):643–9.

116. Szabo Z, Owonikoko T, Peyrot M, et al. Positron emission tomography imaging of the serotonin transporter in subjects with a history of alcoholism. Biol Psychiatry 2004;55(7):766–71.

117. Brown AK, George DT, Fujita M, et al. PET [^{11}C]DASB imaging of serotonin transporters in patients with alcoholism. Alcohol Clin Exp Res 2007;31(1):28–32.

118. Martinez D, Slifstein M, Gil R, et al. Positron emission tomography imaging of the serotonin transporter and 5-HT(1A) receptor in alcohol dependence. Biol Psychiatry 2009;65(2):175–80.

119. Hu J, Henry S, Gallezot JD, et al. Serotonin 1B receptor imaging in alcohol dependence. Biol Psychiatry 2010;67(9):800–3.

120. Bencherif B, Wand GS, McCaul ME, et al. Mu-opioid receptor binding measured by [^{11}C]carfentanil positron emission tomography is related to craving and mood in alcohol dependence. Biol Psychiatry 2004;55(3):255–62.

121. Heinz A, Reimold M, Wrase J, et al. Correlation of stable elevations in striatal mu-opioid receptor availability in detoxified alcoholic patients with alcohol craving: a positron emission tomography study using carbon 11-labeled carfentanil. Arch Gen Psychiatry 2005;62(1):57–64.

122. Weerts EM, Wand GS, Kuwabara H, et al. Positron emission tomography imaging of mu- and delta-opioid receptor binding in alcohol-dependent and healthy control subjects. Alcohol Clin Exp Res 2011;35(12):2162–73.

123. Abi-Dargham A, Krystal JH, Anjilvel S, et al. Alterations of benzodiazepine receptors in type II alcoholic subjects measured with SPECT and [I-123]iomazenil. Am J Psychiatry 1998;155(11):1550–5.

124. Lingford-Hughes AR, Acton PD, Gacinovic S, et al. Reduced levels of GABA-benzodiazepine receptor in alcohol dependency in the absence of grey matter atrophy. Br J Psychiatry 1998;173:116–22.

125. Gilman S, Koeppe RA, Adams K, et al. Positron emission tomographic studies of cerebral benzodiazepine-receptor binding in chronic alchoholics. Ann Neurol 1996; 40:163–71.

126. Litton JE, Neiman J, Pauli S, et al. PET analysis of [^{11}C]flumazenil binding to benzodiazepine receptors in chronic alcohol-dependent men and healthy controls. Psychiatry Res 1993;50(1):1–13.

127. Lingford-Hughes AR, Acton PD, Gacinovic S, et al. Levels of gamma-aminobutyric acid-benzodiazepine receptors in abstinent, alcohol-dependent women: preliminary findings from an ^{123}I-iomazenil single photon emission tomography study. Alcohol Clin Exp Res 2000;24(9):1449–55.

128. Jalan R, Turjanski N, Taylor-Robinson SD, et al. Increased availability of central benzodiazepine receptors in patients with chronic hepatic encephalopathy and alcohol related cirrhosis. Gut 2000;46(4):546–52.

129. Staley JK, Gottschalk C, Petrakis IL, et al. Cortical gamma-aminobutyric acid type A-benzodiazepine receptors in recovery from alcohol dependence: relationship to features of alcohol dependence and cigarette smoking. Arch Gen Psychiatry 2005; 62(8):877–88.

130. Krystal JH, Staley J, Mason G, et al. Gamma-aminobutyric acid type A receptors and alcoholism: intoxication, dependence, vulnerability, and treatment. Arch Gen Psychiatry 2006;63(9):957–68.

131. Voruganti LN, Slomka P, Zabel P, et al. Cannabis induced dopamine release: an in-vivo SPECT study. Psychiatry Res 2001;107(3):173–7.

132. Stokes PR, Mehta MA, Curran HV, et al. Can recreational doses of THC produce significant dopamine release in the human striatum? NeuroImage 2009;48(1): 186–90.

133. Barkus E, Morrison PD, Vuletic D, et al. Does intravenous Δ^9-tetrahydrocannabinol increase dopamine release? A SPET study. J Psychopharmacol 2011;25(11): 1462–8.

134. Urban N, Sliftstein M, Thompson JL, et al. Dopamine release in chronic cannabis users: a [^{11}C]raclopride positron emission tomography study. Biol Psychiatry 2012. [Epub ahead of print].

135. Abi-Dargham A, Kegels LS, Martinez D, et al. Dopamine mediation of positive reinforcing effects of amphetamine in stimulant naive healthy volunteers: results from a large cohort. Eur Neuropsychopharmacol 2003;13(6):459–68.

136. Sevy S, Smith GS, Ma Y, et al. Cerebral glucose metabolism and D2/D3 receptor availability in young adults with cannabis dependence measured with positron emission tomography. Psychopharmacology [Berl] 2008;197(4):549–56.

137. Stokes PR, Egerton A, Watson B, et al. History of cannabis use is not associated with alterations in striatal dopamine D2/D3 receptor availability. J Psychopharmacol 2012;26(1):144–9.

138. Hirvonen J, Goodwin RS, Li CT, et al. Reversible and regionally selective downregulation of brain cannabinoid CB(1) receptors in chronic daily cannabis smokers. Mol Psychiatry 2011. DOI: 10.1038/mp.2011.82. [Epub ahead of print].

Index

Note: Page numbers of article titles are in **boldface** type.

A

Addiction medicine, patient-centered medical home model in, 474
  psychiatrists specializing in and addiction psychiatrists
    as personal physician, 474–475
    on patient-centered medical home team, 475
    roles for, 474
Addiction medicine training, **461–480**
  current deficits in, 464, 466
    clinical skills, 466–467
    lack of emphasis on addiction medicine training in nonpsychiatric residencies,
      468
    perceptions and stigma of addiction, 467
  current state of, addiction problems outpacing caregivers, 462–463
    American Board of Addiction Medicine addiction programs and characteristics,
      464, 466
  deficits in, 464, 466
    clinical skills, 466–467
    lack of emphasis in nonpsychiatric residencies, 468
    perceptions and stigma of, 467
  fellowships in, 463–464, 466
  improving in medical school, case-based learning, 469
    integration in medical specialties, 469
    mandatory psychiatric rotations, 468–469
  improving in residency, 469–470
    addiction medicine training scale, 470
    chief resident immersion training, 472
    expanding scope of, 471
    integration in primary care residencies, 471–472
    integration over four years of residency, 470–471
    reflection techniqes in, 470
  in medical school, current, 463
    improving, 468–469
  in residency programs, characteristics of, 463–464
    current state of, 463–464
    improving, 468–472
    vs. in primary care specialties, 463
  physician contributions to, 465
  screening, brief intervention, and referral for treatment protocol, for primary care
    physicians, 472–473
    for trauma patients, 473
    outcomes with, 473

Psychiatr Clin N Am 35 (2012) 543–555
http://dx.doi.org/10.1016/S0193-953X(12)00039-1
0193-953X/12/$ – see front matter © 2012 Elsevier Inc. All rights reserved.

Moving?

Make sure your subscription moves with you!

To notify us of your new address, find your **Clinics Account Number** (located on your mailing label above your name), and contact customer service at:

Email: journalscustomerservice-usa@elsevier.com

800-654-2452 (subscribers in the U.S. & Canada)
314-447-8871 (subscribers outside of the U.S. & Canada)

Fax number: 314-447-8029

Elsevier Health Sciences Division
Subscription Customer Service
3251 Riverport Lane
Maryland Heights, MO 63043

*To ensure uninterrupted delivery of your subscription, please notify us at least 4 weeks in advance of move.

Printed and bound by CPI Group (UK) Ltd, Croydon, CR0 4YY

03/10/2024

01040357-0002